Praise for *Tiny and Full*™ and Jorge Cruise

"Lose weight without cutting out your favorite food groups."
–Redbook

"This challenge helped me get past years-long plateau—I
haven't been this skinny since high school."
–Allure

"Women are losing up to 11 pounds a week on Jorge
Cruise's weight-loss plan. And it's so easy!"
–First For Women

"An entire pizza is only 300 calories, wow!"
–Wall Street Journal

"Jorge Cruise takes a three-pronged approach to weight loss and overall health."
–Harper's BAAZAR

"A more sustainable approach to plant-based eating, talk about results."
–Life & Style

"Jorge knows how to make low-calorie vegetable focused recipes delicious."
–OK! Magazine

"Super healthy breakfasts that are also super delicious, we swear."
–Teen Vogue

"Avoid Packing On The Pounds with Jorge Cruise."
–Us Weekly

"Celebrity Trainer Jorge Cruise gives the easiest tips to keep that fab figure."
–E! News

"Start your day by energizing with 200 calorie meals and feel
like you've cheated by dinner with Jorge's pizza."
–Mario Lopez, Host of Extra!

"I really love the concept behind this. It's about eating plant-based
meals, losing weight and most importantly, never being hungry."
–Daily Burn

"A prime weapon in the battle to lose weight."
—Fox News

"Jorge Cruise helps you get model-slim without starving."
—*Examiner*

"Jorge gets it right. His recipes make eating smart easy. I recommend them highly."
—Andrew Weil, M.D., author of *Why Our Health Matters*

"Eat sweets and still lose weight!"
—Meredith Viera

"Jorge Cruise guarantees we're going to be looking beautiful in that bathing suit."
—CNN

"Jorge, again, is on to something; belly fat is surely an indicator of poor health."
—Suzanne Somers, actress and bestselling author of *Breakthrough: Eight Steps to Wellness*

"I'm eternally grateful to Jorge for creating a simple lifestyle plan."
—Christiane Northup, M.D., #1 *New York Times* bestselling
author of *The Wisdom of Menopause*

"Jorge knows what he's talking about. Follow his book—lose the weight."
—Chris Robinson, fitness expert and author of *The Core Connection*

"Jorge Cruise will keep you looking and feeling your best."
—David Kirsch, author of *The Ultimate New York Body Plan*

"Jorge continues to inspire and make losing weight fun and part of your life forever."
—Mariel Hemingway, author of *Healthy Living from the Inside Out*

"Sets you up to win!"
—Anthony Robbins, bestselling author

"Eat well without dieting or going to the gym with Jorge's
strategies for breakfast, lunch and dinner."
—Mehmet Oz, M.D., Host of the *Dr. Oz Show*

"When it comes to your health, forward thinking will allow you to
avoid obesity and disease and achieve longevity. Jorge's program springs
from progressive science that can truly change your body."
—Ray Kurzweil, world-renowned scientist and author of *The Singularity Is Near: When
Humans Transcend Biology* and *Fantastic Voyage: Live Long Enough to Live Forever*

tiny and full ™

Other Books by Jorge Cruise

The Three Choices™

Stubborn Fat Gone!™

Happy Hormones, Slim Belly™

The 100™

Inches Off!™ Your Tummy

The Aging Cure™

The Belly Fat Cure™

The Belly Fat Cure™ Diet

The Belly Fat Cure™ Sugar & Carb Counter

The Belly Fat Cure™ Fast Track

The Belly Fat Cure™ Quick Meals

Body at Home™

The 12-Second Sequence™

The 3-Hour Diet™

The 3-Hour Diet™ Cookbook

The 3-Hour Diet™ for Teens

The 3-Hour Diet™ On the Go

8 Minutes in the Morning®

8 Minutes in the Morning® for Extra-Easy Weight Loss

8 Minutes in the Morning® to a Flat Belly

8 Minutes in the Morning® to Lean Hips and Thin Thighs

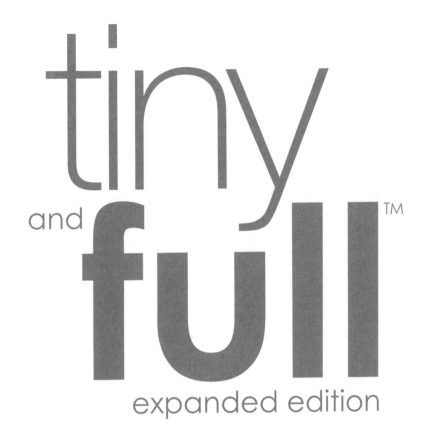

tiny and full™

expanded edition

Eat More, Weigh Less, and Turn Off Hunger All Day

Jorge Cruise

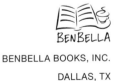

BENBELLA BOOKS, INC.

DALLAS, TX

The reference material in this book was compiled using a number of sources, and all information was accurate at the time of printing. Internet addresses given in this book were accurate at the time the book went to press.

BlueBerry Banana O's, 2016 © and ® /™ of General Mills, used with permission

Trademarks:

The Three Choices™	Tiny and Full™	Jorge Cruise™
8 Minutes in the Morning™	3-Hour Diet™	Belly Fat Cure™
The 100™	Stubborn Fat Gone!™	Think Fit™
Move Fit™	Eat Fit™	Hi-Lo Yoga™
Thyroid Boost™	Belly Burn™	Fitness Begins in the Kitchen™

BenBella Books, Inc.
10440 N. Central Expressway
Suite #800
Dallas, TX 75231
www.benbellabooks.com
Send feedback to feedback@benbellabooks.com

Printed in the United States of America
10 9 8 7 6 5 4 3 2 1

Trade paperback ISBN: 978-1-944648-50-3
e-ISBN: 978-1-944648-51-0

Distributed by Perseus Distribution
www.perseusdistribution.com

To place orders through Perseus Distribution:
Tel: (800) 343-4499
Fax: (800) 351-5073

E-mail: orderentry@perseusbooks.com

Special discounts for bulk sales (minimum of 25 copies) are available.
Please contact Aida Herrera at aida@benbellabooks.com.

To my husband, Sam,

for making coming home

always the best part of my day.

Contents

Foreword

Jorge has always had, and continues to have, a unique ability to take complicated information and make it simple and accessible. In particular, I consider him genuinely gifted when it comes to seeing an easy way into an important healthy behavior change that most people find intimidating. That is certainly the case with Tiny and Full™, which addresses the many good reasons for eating more plant-based diets that many of us talk about all the time. But then, in that inimitable Jorge Cruise style, the book serves up a brilliantly simple insight that never dawned on the rest of us: being plant-based until lunch!

Suddenly, what might have seemed an imposing burden of change is bite-size, and manageable. Suddenly, you can get there from here—and then, perhaps, keep going.

As a physician focused on disease prevention and health promotion, Jorge knows that "tiny," the use of which he explains, is his choice but not mine. While he is quite right about waist circumference as a potent indicator of metabolic health, and the waist to hip ratio in women an indicator of reproductive health that has had implications for attractiveness and sex appeal throughout history and across all cultures, you certainly don't need to be "tiny" to be healthy, and my focus is health and vitality. If we take the liberty of interpreting "tiny" to mean a healthy waist circumference, then we are aligned. It's not about size; it's about vitality.

I particularly appreciate how Jorge combines insights about motivation, behavior change science, and the benefits of plant-based eating to offer the empowering simplicity of this plan. Frankly, I like how it conforms to my personal experience as well. I am a very disciplined person, fully committed to practicing what I preach. Even so, I find it much easier to practice that discipline, and get my workouts in, in the morning. At the end of a long and challenging day, I like to kick back and relax like everyone else.

The focus of my career, including the newly launched True Health Initiative, is all about leveraging the incredible, and all-too-often neglected, power of lifestyle as medicine. The centerpiece of a health promoting lifestyle is a diet of wholesome foods, mostly plants, in sensible combinations. The clever and innovative guidance in that direction served in Tiny and Full™ is moderate and manageable, encouraging and inviting. My hope is that you accept the invitation to join Jorge, and step in the direction of the true, vibrant beauty that only health and vitality confer.

David L. Katz, MD, MPH, FACPM, FACP
is the founding director (1998) of Yale University's Yale-Griffin Prevention Research Center, and current President of the American College of Lifestyle Medicine.

He earned his BA degree from Dartmouth College (1984); his MD from the Albert Einstein College of Medicine (1988); and his MPH from the Yale University School of Public Health (1993). He completed sequential residency training in Internal Medicine, and Preventive Medicine/Public Health. He is a two-time diplomate of the American Board of Internal Medicine, and a board-certified specialist in Preventive Medicine/Public Health. He has received two Honorary Doctorates.

Dr. Katz has published roughly 200 scientific articles and textbook chapters, and 15 books to date, including multiple editions of leading textbooks in both Preventive Medicine and nutrition. He has made important contributions in the areas of lifestyle interventions for health promotion; nutrient profiling; behavior modification; holistic care; and evidence-based medicine. A widely supported nominee for the position of U.S. Surgeon General, Dr. Katz has been recognized by Greatist.com as one of the 100 most

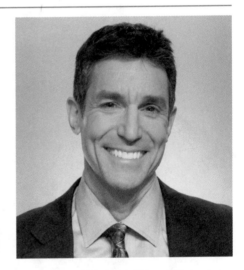

influential people in health and fitness in the world for the past 3 years (2013-). He is recognized globally for expertise in nutrition, weight management, and the prevention of chronic disease, and has a social media following of well over half a million. He has delivered addresses in numerous countries on four continents, and has been acclaimed by colleagues as the "poet laureate" of health promotion. In 2015, Dr. Katz established the True Health Initiative to help convert what we know about lifestyle as medicine into what we do about it, in the service of adding years to lives and life to years around the globe.

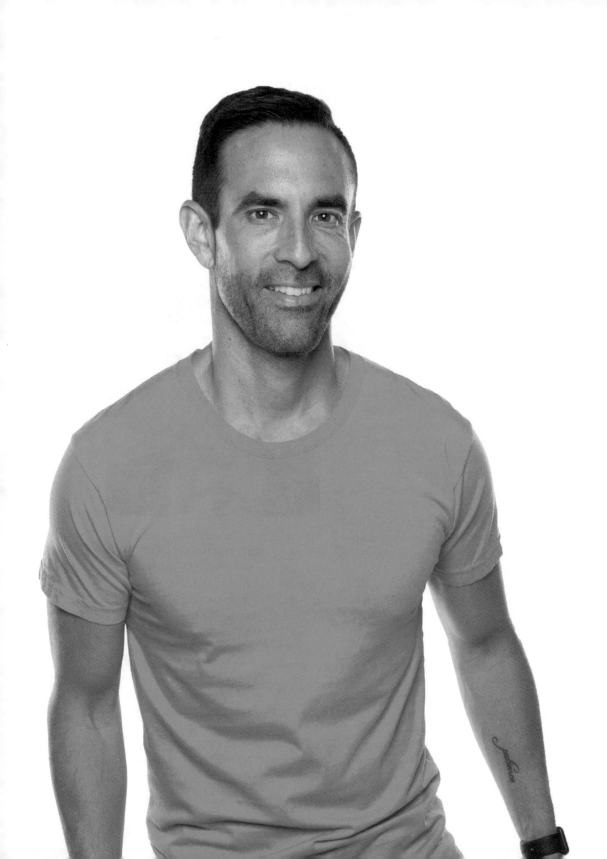

Welcome

Dear Friends,

I am so happy that you are here and that I have the opportunity to be your health coach and trainer. In this book, I will teach you how to eat off the pounds (because . . . yes, it's possible!), turn off hunger, and get you the results you deserve.

Before you begin, it's important that you know that Tiny and Full is not a diet. Diets are restrictive and based on negative reinforcement techniques that don't work. No more starvation tactics, jazzercising, or spending hours on a treadmill, because on this plan fitness begins in the kitchen.

There will be no cutting back or removing food on this plan, in fact you will be eating MORE instead of less. With Tiny and Full you will discover what scientists and researchers call "tiny-calorie foods" which are foods that are big in size so that you stay FULL, but low in calories so that you stay TINY.

This simplified approach of eating more while cutting calories will allow you to turn off hunger and have a nutrition plan that becomes a lifestyle, not a diet.

And in this special edition of Tiny and Full you now will have the power of the Thyroid Boost to help restore and unbreak your metabolism. If you have low energy, constipation, or a weight gain plateau, it's time to unbreak your metabolism. It's time to take a look at the background of your body, specifically the master gland of metabolism, the thyroid. With my Thyroid Boost meal planners and recipes you will protect and restore the thyroid as well as rev up your metabolism, increase energy, eliminate belly fat, and shed the pounds once and for all.

I look forward in guiding you every step of the way for the next 12 weeks, over which you will lose 2 to 4 pounds every single week. You will soon be eating your way to confidence, vitality, and optimal health!

I am so glad you're here and I can't wait for you to get the results you deserve. Happy reading!

Your coach,

Jorge Cruise

Part One

The Eat It Off Revolution

1 Ready for Tiny

> "Your waistline is your lifeline."
> —JACK LALANNE

Getting "Ready for Tiny" means many things. First and foremost, you must understand that *Tiny* is a frame of mind. It's a shift from thinking that you have to settle for *some* weight loss and a *little* less flab, to owning that you not only have the power to be perfectly Tiny, you deserve nothing less. Yes, you have the right to be Tiny!

What exactly is Tiny?

Tiny isn't about vanity or some narcissistic need to stand in front of the mirror obsessing about being the fairest of them all. It's the understanding that you have the absolute inherent power and right to be as red-carpet gorgeous, fit, and healthy as any Kardashian-Jenner. Tiny doesn't have an age limit, and it isn't just about looks—being Tiny *is* about being healthy. Tiny is about getting you the results that empower you to live your healthiest life ever. In fact, far from being fanatical, Tiny is actually *the* number one indicator of health and fitness—having a Tiny Waist *is* epic health, inside and out. *Your outside beauty indicates your inside health.*

Did you get that? Both things, inner beauty and outer beauty, are inherently related. Looking and feeling good on the outside—fitting effortlessly in your skinny jeans, being a showstopper in your little black dress, rocking that swimsuit—is a reflection of your inner health. That's what having a Tiny Waist gives you: outer beauty and inner health. The great reality is that having a Tiny Waist is a reliable gauge of underlying whole-body wellness, vitality, and health. With this knowledge, you can and *should* embrace being beautiful, without fear of being labeled egotistical or superficial. A small waist gives you beauty, energy, and confidence; attracts other people to you; *and* lowers your risk for all diseases. We'll get into this in great detail on the next pages, but for now, know that having a healthy waist circumference—having a Tiny Waist—frees you to be the best *you* ever. When you harness this powerful mind-set—the mind-set of Tiny—you are Ready for Tiny.

Now…

Are *you* Ready for Tiny?

First, we must address three points:

1. How a Tiny Waist equals health

2. How to get a Tiny Waist

3. How to beat THE problem: hunger!

After we've covered these points, you'll be ready to commit to your health for the next 12 weeks—to promise yourself that you will get a Tiny Waist, which will free you to be the best *you* ever. You'll be free to wear that swimsuit with joy and free to never diet again.

Let's start by taking a deeper look at how slimming your middle will give you an overall body and mind health makeover.

A Tiny Waist Equals Health

If you want to be healthy, you've got to have a tiny waist circumference. Now I'm not saying you need to go out and grab one of the waist-trainers you see on Instagram. But, I am saying that measuring your waist is a great indicator of health and disease. In 2009, I had the great privilege of sitting down with Dr. Mehmet Oz for an interview. I'll never forget that day. Despite an incredibly busy schedule of filming his own show, Dr. Oz had invited me and my team to film a short video for my readers while he was on a layover in New York. That day I learned some vital distinctions about waist circumference that I'd never before considered. I came away from our talk with a thrilling new insight—that wanting, no, *needing* a slender waist truly isn't about vanity but is instead an essential requirement for true health and fitness. Your waist circumference, Dr. Oz told me, simple as it seems, is a key marker of health, vitality, disease, happiness, lower risk of heart disease, stroke, and many cancers. It's also the main attraction, or detraction, when choosing partners—and not for the trivial reasons you might suspect.

According to the research of Devendra Singh, an evolutionary psychologist at the University of Texas who published the pioneering findings on the significance of attractiveness and waist size, first impressions are belly-based. Singh's research on waist-to-hip ratio spans 1993 through 2010, until just before he passed away. He was the first to reveal the link between having a Tiny Waist and attractiveness and health. One such study found that attractiveness is gauged by waist circumference—with thin being in, and fat being out. Singh's paper reviewed three separate studies which all concluded that men define the attractiveness of women based on their low waist-to-hip ratio (more on waist-to-hip ratio on page 7):

- The first study had men rate the attractiveness of pageant contestants over the past 30 to 60 years. The raters consistently decided that the tinier the waist, the more attractive the women.

- The second study found that college-age men find females with small waists more attractive, healthier, and of greater value as reproductive partners than women with thicker waists.

- And in the final study, men aged 25 to 85 were found to prefer women with smaller waists and rated them as being more attractive and having a higher fertility rate.

What does this mean? Six-pack-sizzle and the hotness factor aside, these men are not making superficial choices. Singh concluded that these preferences for slim waists are actually linked to health. These men were really being attracted to health. It's easy to think that the unrealistic photoshopped pictures of beauty that we often see promoted in media images are what sway men to choose slim-waisted women, but, in reality, women with Tiny Waists *are* healthier. In a jointly published study from a prominent university in Spain and the University of Wisconsin, researchers found that higher amounts of belly fat in women are linked to increased risks for ovarian disease and infertility. Even more shocking, according to a study published in the *Journal of the American Medical Association*, increased waist size is consistently linked to increased risks of cardiovascular disorders, adult-onset diabetes, elevated plasma lipids, hypertension, cancer (endometrial, ovarian, and breast), gallbladder disease, and premature mortality in women. So this fondness for Tiny-Waisted women is really a natural tendency to select a healthier partner.

And men aren't the only ones "sizing up" their potential mates—women find slim-waisted men more attractive as well. In a study published in the *Journal of Personality and Social Psychology*, two experiments were conducted to examine how females choose mates:

- In the first group, college-age women rated normal weight male figures with lean and thick waists. The women consistently rated males with leaner abs as being more attractive, healthy, and as containing positive qualities than the men with thicker waists.

- Women ages 18 to 69 rated men with a variety of waist sizes. All women, regardless of their age, education, or income, rated men with the healthiest waists more favorably than those with thicker middles.

And the links to waist size and health in men are just as evident as they are in women. Studies done by researchers in Texas, Australia, and Sweden connected high levels of belly fat in men directly to low levels of available testosterone. These investigators speculate that levels of abdominal fat on a man convert testosterone to estrogen, which lowers sperm count and causes lack of muscle. Experts who study mate choice and attractiveness speculate that the trend for choosing mates based on Tiny Waists comes from our evolutionary history. This preference for Tiny Waists, researchers believe, is in fact a deeply ingrained evolutionary adaptation that dates back more than 160,000 years.

According to researchers who study ancient humans, it seems that our ancestors instinctively knew to avoid mates with large bellies because they were an indicator of poor health. These ancient humans didn't have the constant stream of 24/7 media telling them how to choose a mate. They had to go by instinct to tell them which man or woman would make the best partner in terms of provider, protector, and reproductive partner. So, the idea of "sizing someone up" may have had its start back among prehistoric humans. Besides doing a general once-over for a healthy body size and shape, it turns out that belly size is an easy to spot and reliable indicator of a high-quality or poor-quality mate. As for Paleolithic women, the researchers speculate that they had a biological instinct not to choose a big-bellied caveman because he wouldn't be a strong protector, efficient provider, or good reproductive partner. On the flip side, if a Paleolithic man saw a woman with a large belly, researchers think his instinct would alert him that she was either pregnant (and therefore unavailable) or might have a hormonal imbalance such as ovarian disease, which could decrease her ability to reproduce.

The bottom line is that whether you are male or female, a high waist circumference is a marker of serious health issues, and "a hot body is an instinctual sign of health," as Dr. Oz so beautifully states in his book, *YOU: Being Beautiful, The Owner's Manual to Inner and Outer Beauty*.

So, stop feeling guilty about wanting a Tiny Waist. It's hardwired. Accept that having outer beauty is a reflection of inner health. This is your new mind-set. You aren't shallow, vapid, or vain—you want a Tiny Waist because you want optimal health. Looking smoking hot is just something you'll have to live with.

What is a Tiny Waist?

Your waist-to-hip ratio is the measurement that best shows how Tiny—or not—your waist is. Figuring it out only requires a fabric tape measure, you, and some very simple math. If you've ever seen one of my Tiny Talks on Facebook Live, you'll know that I am a huge advocate of measuring your waist weekly. All you have to do is take a tape measure, and while sucking your belly in, measure your waist at the level of your belly button. Next, measure your hips at the largest point around your bottom. Finally, divide your waist size by your hip size. An ideal ratio is 0.7 for women and 1.0 for men. Canadian researchers said that this test is an ideal and inexpensive way to predict something as serious as heart disease.

If your waist circumference is higher than these results, don't fret. This book is designed to help you eat off the pounds over the course of the next 12 weeks. *Tiny and Full*™ will give you long-lasting, sustainable results. You'll get the body you want, and it will stay the body you dreamed of forever.

How to Get a Tiny Waist

You have to cut calories. Period.

There.

I said it.

I didn't come to this conclusion easily, folks. I've been a calorie-bashing, fruit-banishing, nut-noshing, spinach-with-chicken-salad-eating enthusiast for years now. I have published books, posted blogs, and tweeted regularly and passionately about only "counting the calories that count," or worse, "not counting calories at all." But, calories are the key to weight loss, and I've finally seen the light.

Whatever the diet, this is the new reality—you must create a calorie deficit if you want to shed pounds, lose belly fat, and get a Tiny Waist. Now I know that this isn't really "new," but for some time now, the most popular diets, from Atkins to South

Beach, The Paleo Solution to The Primal Blueprint, and yes, The Belly Fat Cure to The 100 (those two are mine), all promise weight loss without tracking or counting calories, or at least not all calories. To be fair, many of these plans (and my diets always) do provide menus that are low-calorie, so they do result in weight loss (as long as the reader follows the menu to the letter). The faulty premise of most of these diets is the claim that you'll naturally eat less because you'll be eating more filling and slowly digestible foods, and also that you won't be eating foods (refined sugars and flours that spike insulin) that cause fat accumulation. Unfortunately, these claims don't hold. The first idea—that you'll naturally eat less—doesn't hold because most of us don't stop eating just because we feel full. Many physical, emotional, and psychological reasons regulate how much food we consume and when we stop eating. Brian Wansink, professor of consumer behavior at Cornell and author of *Mindless Eating,* has conducted several clever studies that show repeatedly that the more food you put in front of you, the more you eat. It doesn't matter what it is—we humans always eat more than we should. We are simply lousy at randomly limiting ourselves to an appropriate amount of calories. Secondly, while avoiding refined sugars and flours is still a good rule of thumb, if you *don't* cut overall calories, you *won't* see weight loss. There is no one food component that causes fat accumulation, as some fat enthusiasts argue. Finally, diets that focus on cutting out an entire food group—all fruits and grains, for example—are too severe and are unsustainable even when they do cut calories. The result is that most people eventually go off these plans and binge on the forbidden foods.

The idea of fat accumulation as being the result of insulin-spiking foods (all carbs and sugars) is one that I once wholeheartedly endorsed, but in the light of more recent and accurate studies, I now reject this theory. I was one of many who loved the message of Gary Taubes, an engaging and gifted journalist, who has written many books and articles that claim carbohydrates are solely responsible for obesity and fat accumulation. Taubes argues that it's impossible to lose weight while eating carbohydrates, but that you can achieve weight loss by eating as many calories as you desire as long as you cut out all carbs and sugars. This all boils down to the way that insulin, says Taubes, spiked by carbohydrate-rich foods, causes fat to be accumulated. The research does not bear out, however. More recent and careful studies provide evidence which shows that more calories, regardless of type, means more weight, and vice versa.

In 2015, a new National Institutes of Health study published in *Cell Metabolism* examined the effects of low-carb and low-fat, calorie-controlled diets on 19 obese men and women. The participants stayed in a metabolic unit for two weeks so the researchers could control, regulate, and record all food intake and activity. Each group cut their daily calorie intake by 30 percent. Half of the group cut carbs (low carb), and the other half cut fat (high carb). After the two weeks, the subjects took a break for a few weeks, and then they came back and repeated the study, with the two groups switching diets. Interestingly, the average participant lost about a pound of fat over two weeks, and about four pounds of weight, but the high-carb group lost *more* body fat (the high-carb group lost 463 grams of fat on average, compared to 245 grams in the low-carb dieters). Further, the researchers predicted that had the diets continued over the following six months, the people in the high-carb group would have ended the study losing six more pounds than the low-carb group. This directly debunks the popular low-carb theory purported by Taubes which claims that low-carb diets are more effective for fat loss because they lower levels of insulin and therefore liberate fat from fat tissue. This dispels the theory that only low-carb diets can help people shed fat. The bottom line is, once again, overall calories matter most for weight loss. (For more on my philosophical transformation, see page 7.)

For the record, I still believe that refined sugars and flours and overly processed foods cause serious health issues, but they aren't the reason for weight gain or loss—that's all about calories. You can just as easily lose weight eating 1,200 calories of Twinkies as you would eating the same amount of lean protein, vegetables, fruit, and whole grains (for proof, see the "Cutting Calories Any Way You Please" box on page 11). Other health problems arise when you dedicate your diet to junk food, but we'll get into that later. The bottom line is that when it comes to weight loss—just weight loss—it's simple math. Eat fewer calories than you burn, and you will lose weight.

Marion Nestle, professor of human nutrition at New York University, inspired much of the Tiny and Full™ philosophy that I now believe to be the best method for losing weight. In her book, *Why Calories Count*, she uses studies to show that cutting calories is the only reliable method for reducing weight. This is not a new idea. The whole idea of what a calorie is—a measurement of the energy, heat, or work in a food, or the energy or work that is expended in physical activity—was discovered and solidified in the 1800s. Scientists have long understood that to maintain weight, you must have a balance between the number of calories you consume and the number you expend. To lose weight, you must consume less food than you expend, or you must expend more calories in exercise than you consume in food. What you eat doesn't really matter in this equation. Consider these studies:

- In a study published in the *Journal of the American Dietetic Association*, nutrition researchers from Texas Woman's University found that regardless of the components of a diet, as long as the participants stuck to the calorie restrictions, they lost weight. The study separated women into three groups of at least 11 per group and had them eat 1,200-calorie diets of 25, 45, or 75 percent of carbohydrates with variations on fats and protein.

- In a 2001 review, researchers from the US Department of Agriculture and the University of California compared the high-protein, low-carb Atkins diet; the low-fat, high-carb Ornish plan; and the low-fat, moderate-carbohydrate Weight Watcher program. The study found that all three resulted in equal weight loss as long as the calories didn't exceed 1,400 to 1,500 calories per day. The researchers concluded that the major determinant of weight loss was calorie balance. All people succeed at losing weight when they eat fewer calories than they burn, regardless of protein, fat, and carbohydrate levels. In addition, the subjects all reported similar effects on hunger and satisfaction despite the diet followed.

- In a study published in 2009, researchers compared four diets: low fat, average protein; low fat, high protein; high fat, average protein; and high fat, high protein. Nearly 80 percent of the 200 people followed the dietary restrictions, all of which required the men and women to cut 750 calories off their daily intake. At the end of six months, the participants, regardless of diet group, had lost an average of nine pounds. All groups reported equal levels of hunger and diet satisfaction, and all had similar improvements in insulin and cholesterol. Because the weight loss was low, and the calorie cutting was high, the investigators revisited the results and concluded that most participants had only reduced their calories by 250 per day. (The participants self-recorded their calories.)

This isn't rocket-science, we've known for a while that cutting calories is how to get a Tiny Waist. But the truth is, cutting calories isn't the *only* way to get a Tiny Waist. There are actually three new scientifically proven ways to reduce waist circumference that I've discovered:

1. Phytochemicals: Foods such as blackberries, eggplant, and even dark chocolate contain certain phytochemicals that actually ignite your body's belly burning cells. I know what you are thinking, how can dark chocolate burn off my belly fat? Well, it's because of the phytochemicals found within that dark chocolate that you CAN burn your belly fat off. A phytochemical is a chemical compound that occurs naturally in plants. Some are responsible for color and other organoleptic properties, such as the deep purple of blueberries and the smell of garlic. We'll explore which phytochemicals burn belly fat, what foods contain them, and how to successfully incorporate these foods into your diet in Chapter 3.

2. Thyroid boost: If you've had a lack of energy, constipation, or a sudden weight gain that just won't come off, you may be having symptoms of an

When it comes to weight loss, it really doesn't matter how you slice away the excess calories—reduce your intake, and you'll drop the pounds. There are no promises of great health here, and I don't recommend any of the following diets, but when it comes to moving the needle on the scale down, cutting calories is the key. The following outrageous examples illustrate just how crazy diets can be:

- **Twinkies:** To show that all calories—even the emptiest—count, an overweight Kansas State University nutrition professor put himself on a self-professed Twinkie Diet where he ate one of the Hostess treats every three hours, and interspersed the Twinkies with snacks of Doritos chips, sugary cereals, and Oreos. He limited himself to roughly less than 1800 calories a day of the overly processed, highly refined, sugar-and-fat-filled diet and lost 27 pounds over the course of 10 weeks. The professor to date hasn't released any health issues resulting from his diet.

- **Baby food:** Yes, this Hollywood fad of substituting baby food for two, or possibly three, meals a day does result in weight loss. Celebrity trainer Tracy Anderson started this gimmick for cutting calories and controlling portions, and although it does cause weight loss (as long as you are cutting your calories), most people who tried it reported that the weight quickly returned when they started eating adult food again. This diet is an Internet phenomenon and isn't published anywhere, but it makes sense when you use baby food, which is around 20 to 100 calories per jar, to replace a meal that would typically be 300 to 500 calories.

underactive thyroid. If you are experiencing any one of these symptoms I recommend consulting with your doctor. But I would encourage you to be proactive with your testing. Some doctors misdiagnose the thyroid treatment due to a lack of testing, so it's important to take multiple in-depth tests to help support your thyroid to the fullest. However, there are natural nutrition remedies that can help boost your thyroid with the right minerals and nutrients to repair the thyroid. Now, how does this help you get a Tiny Waist? Well, the thyroid is master gland of metabolism. The thyroid's main job is to metabolize our food, in other words break down our food and release energy into our body to keep us awake and alert. If your thyroid is underactive it can't metabolize food, resulting in a broken metabolism. If you feel that you may have an underactive thyroid, I hope you consult with your doctor and continue reading as I further explain how to repair your thyroid in Chapter 3.

3. False belly fat: Do you have a history of eating processed foods? Is your belly fat hard instead of jiggly? Do you experience frequent constipation? If you've answered yes to any of these questions, you may be experiencing what I call false belly fat. What is false belly fat? Well false belly fat isn't actually fat, it's built-up waste in your colon from the consumption of nutritionless foods. Eating the wrong kind of food makes you prone to this false fat as well as raising risk for visceral fat. Eating foods that high in fiber and water help promote regularity that eliminates this false fat. We'll explore more on the foods that eliminate false belly fat and the importance of healthy digestion in Chapter 3.

I'll explain all about bringing health into Tiny and Full™ and how to get a Tiny Waist in the next chapter, but for now, I'm focusing on just the aspect of losing weight—nothing else. It's an important concept to understand. One thing we have plenty of in our society is constant access to plenty of highly nutritious foods. What we lack is moderation, and in regard to weight loss, moderation is the central concern.

THE Problem: Hunger!

The central problem when it comes to cutting calories—what you need to do to get Tiny—is hunger! Your body does not like to be denied food. If you are deprived of calories, you'll want food and you'll want it right *now*. You'll be so bombarded with hunger signals incessantly telling you to eat that you'll become increasingly irritated, aggressive, and even angry. This concept is so common and pervasive that the term "hangry," an amalgam of "hungry" and "angry," has been added to the *Oxford Dictionaries* to describe this phenomenon of being bad-tempered, agitated, or irritable as a result of being hungry. You might even get hangry regularly, or love someone who does. Interestingly, a natural brain chemical, the neuropeptide Y that is released when you are hungry, is the same chemical your brain secretes when you feel angry or aggressive. This reaction is thought to be part of your evolutionary being that developed to protect you from going without food for too long. We didn't always have the plentiful open access to food that we have today. Back in the days of the hunter-gatherer, humans had to be prepared for times when food was scarce. Being aggressive and greedy about food was key to survival, which is

On My Revelation

I have not recommended fruit for years due to its Sugar Calories, but I've discovered new research that has opened my eyes to how we look at food in relation to weight loss. As I continue to do research, I can't help but find indisputable evidence that there is another approach to weight loss that is more effective than just focusing on Sugar Calories. And today I am happily enjoying bowls full of watermelon and am leaner than I've ever been before.

Sugar Calories is the term I used in my books The 100 and Happy Hormones, Slim Belly, to define any carbohydrate calorie. It's an accurate term in that all carbohydrates are "read" as sugar by your body—hence Sugar Calories. The mistake I made was to say that all Sugar Calories are equal. They aren't. There are good sugars and bad sugars. The second misstep I took was following the advice of writers such as Gary Taubes, who argued persuasively that it was carbohydrate calories that caused weight gain. The truth is that too many calories cause weight gain, whatever food components they come from.

Knowledge exists in a flowing and changing state, and this includes nutrition and weight-loss research. Remember, once upon a time, we thought the world was flat. Several explorers were brave enough to venture out farther and discover the truth. In a similar vein, I have never believed in resting on my laurels. When I discover that I can share a better message for weight loss and health, I am always willing to update my philosophy to reflect the latest and most accurate science available. So, after much research, thought, and even internal struggle over accepting this science, I now have no lingering doubts that the most effective approach to weight loss is to consider all calories. That's it. All calories count.

Do I still think it's important to avoid refined sugars and flours? Absolutely. It's a great first step and vital to your health. However, just avoiding these empty calories won't cause weight loss in the way I once believed it would. I have discovered that "counting only Sugar Calories," along with the research relating to insulin and its effects on fat accumulation, is not as critical a factor to weight loss as watching your overall calories. In fact, it's actually quite insignificant.

So, I bring this information to you with the sincere hope that you will continue to trust me to bring you the latest dietary science and the most effective ways to lose weight and improve your health.

Here's to a big bowl of watermelon, grapes, and strawberries! You'll soon learn all about celebrating the one natural source of sweetness that will help you get the Tiny Waist you've always dreamed of having—and you'll find that fruit is an essential part of feeling Full while being Tiny!

why we don't act with grace when we are hangry. So while it isn't always pretty, hanger makes sense. Think about it. If our caveman forefather had been chill about the freshly killed wildebeest he worked so hard to hunt and had graciously invited the folks from the neighboring cave clan to join himself and his family, he and his might have starved. Being greedy and ravenous isn't our most civilized behavior, but when you are in a state of hanger, it's understandable.

Your body is a magnificent machine that is always working to maintain balance. Hunger is simply a signal to your body that it's out of balance. The feeling is unpleasant for a good reason. What you feel when you are deprived of food is your brain beckoning your body to eat. When you diet by cutting calories from your daily allotment, you naturally feel hungrier. Let's say you have a smaller breakfast than usual, and then you plan on having your lunch at the midday hour just like you normally do—only this time you are functioning on less than your average amount of calories (and remember, you'll be eating a smaller lunch portion as well). Your body takes notice of such things. As time passes since your last meal, the nutrients in your bloodstream (your blood glucose) begin to drop. If the drop is far enough, your brain will see it as an emergency situation. Initially, you feel the pangs of hunger, and you might get a headache, snarl at someone, or grow weak and fatigued. You might begin to have trouble concentrating. Your thoughts will increasingly turn to food, and you'll begin to obsess about when you can eat. Eventually, you'll be able to think of nothing else. The result in almost every circumstance is that you will eat. Now, if you are really pumped up about losing some weight and cutting calories, you might be able to stick to your plan for a few days, but being hungry day in and day out gets old pretty fast.

One survey from the UK found that women start about three different diets per year, and quit on or around day 19. Yep. According to the researchers, by day 5, two-thirds had already cheated on their weight-loss plan. In another poll conducted by British researchers, 1,000 women reported that they quit their diets by week 5. As early as week 2, 25 percent had quit, and 50 percent dropped out by week 4. Not one woman reached her goal.

The other problem that comes with cutting calories is that your body's calorie-burning engine (your metabolism) slows down in proportion to the calories you cut and also to the weight you lose. If you want to continue to lose weight, you have to eat fewer and fewer calories as the number on the scale goes down; otherwise, you won't continue to lose weight. As time goes on, this gets tiresome, and, eventually, most of us bag the diet and overeat. Or, we diet for a certain amount of time, thinking that when we reach our goal, we'll get to splurge and eat again. And when you splurge, the weight comes back with a vengeance. Remember, your body thinks you've been starving it, so it greedily replaces whatever you've lost—and fast. This situation is why yo-yo dieting is as common as rain in Seattle. Consider the following studies that illustrate the common struggles with calorie cutting and hunger:

- In a Minnesota study, researchers put 19 men on a severe calorie-restricted diet, largely composed of potatoes. At the end of the six-month study, the men had become lethargic, depressed, irritable, cold, and lost all libido while they were eating a diet that severely limited their calories. They were constantly obsessed with thoughts of food. Their muscles grew weak, endurance declined dramatically, and they lost muscle mass.

- In a study that examined the heart health of 18 voluntary calorie-restricting, antiaging enthusiasts, researchers at Washington University in St. Louis found that while they were about 20 percent leaner and had lower blood pressure, cholesterol, and markers of inflammation than a comparison group of "normal" eaters, the calorie restrictors were open about other difficulties. These members of the Calorie Restriction Society, who believe that the choice to reduce calorie intake will extend their life spans, report constant experiences of hunger and cold. Women report menstrual irregularities, testosterone levels will decrease in men, and many say that they obsess about food and alienate family members and friends with their lifestyle choices.

- Of dieters who lose weight, 80 to 95 percent of them gain it back within a year or two, according to a 2010 National Health and Nutrition Examination Survey. Researchers speculate that cutting calories too severely, or following a rigid diet that cuts out certain food groups entirely, make most diets unsustainable and leave dieters too hungry. It's better to focus on avoiding highly processed foods and to eat moderately.

- In a Columbia University study, researchers underfed men and women to make them lose 10 to 20 percent of their weight. Not surprisingly, hunger increased while metabolism plummeted. After the studies ended, the subjects quickly regained the weight.

I have worked with many A-list stars who have horror stories of rigid self-starving plans they've put themselves on to lose weight. The dieting is miserable, and the weight loss is always temporary. It reminds me of the movie *The Devil Wears Prada*. While the movie is fictional, it's based on a true-life story of the fashion industry and how it glorifies the ultra-twiggy ideal for women. One of the all-too-real exchanges is between the editorial assistants Emily (played by Emily Blunt) and Andy Sachs (played by Anne Hathaway):

Emily: Andrea, My God! You look so chic.

Andy Sachs: Oh, thanks. You look so thin.

Emily: Really? It's for Paris. I'm on this new diet. Well, I don't eat anything, and when I feel like I'm about to faint, I eat a cube of cheese. I'm just one stomach flu away from my goal weight.

And another between the fashion director Nigel (played by Stanley Tucci) and Andy Sachs:

Andy Sachs: So none of the girls here eat anything?

Nigel: Not since two became the new four and zero became the new two.

Andy Sachs: Well, I'm a six . . .

Nigel: Which is the new fourteen.

These examples are unfortunately all too real for many women who want to achieve the ideal thinness factor. But it doesn't have to be this way. You don't have to starve or deprive yourself to have a Tiny Waist. You can be Tiny and Full™—and feel great having it all!

So how can you lose weight by cutting calories without suffering from feelings of deprivation and hunger? How can you counter the basic biological desire to eat that occurs when you restrict calories to lose weight? This is the weight-loss paradox—to get and maintain a Tiny Waist requires eating tiny amounts of food, which leads to being hangry and then, often, to binging and regaining weight. Being hungry or hangry obviously isn't the answer.

The good news is that I have a solution that works! There is no reason to suffer. No longer will you have to cut portions and deprive yourself, because I'm going to teach you how to eat more while cutting calories. I know it seems impossible, but it's true, you can actually feel Full and have a Tiny Waist! Feeling Full is not being stuffed like a Thanksgiving turkey. It's important to understand the difference. People who have dieted for decades have often lost touch with the internal signals the body gives to alert them to levels of satiation. Feeling Full, not uncomfortably stuffed, is the feeling of being satisfied, content, and *not* hungry. When you are a healthy "Full," you aren't thinking about food. You know that you have nourished yourself appropriately and don't need to eat again for a few hours. You could eat more, but if you did, you would cross from being Full to being uncomfortably bloated and distended. Being Full is being energized, comfortable, relaxed, and happy. Are you Ready for Full? Then, turn the page.

2 Ready for Full

17

Are you ready to banish hunger and deprivation forever? You may believe that the only way to lose weight, the only way to get a Tiny Waist, is to starve yourself and to suffer the pangs of hunger and deprivation—but that isn't true. If you have a long history of dieting, it might seem impossible, but you are about to learn that you can have both—a Tiny Waist and a Full belly. In the previous chapter, I explained the necessity of creating a calorie deficit (eating fewer calories than you burn) for weight loss, but that doesn't mean that you have to feel like you are starving. In fact, you can feel Full at all times. There is a better way, and that's what you'll learn in these next pages. Getting Ready for Full means absorbing the knowledge outlined in this chapter. After you've read these pages, you'll never have to feel starved or deprived again. You'll never again find yourself *off* a diet binging because you're ravenous, and you'll never again go *on* a depriving diet struggling for a slim waist because Tiny and Full™ isn't a diet that you go *on* or *off*. It's a lifestyle plan that you'll love so much, you'll never have to think about dieting again.

What is Full?

Being Full is both a way of eating and a frame of mind. When it comes to eating, the concept of Full is about being satisfied, not stuffed. This will be our main focus. I'm going to teach you how to take practical steps to eat so you are always satisfied. Never again will you feel ravenous or restricted.

The other perspective of Full, just like with Tiny in the previous chapter, is having a mind-set of Full. Being "Full of mind" means being filled with vitality, energy, wisdom, knowledge, confidence, happiness, and peace. When someone says, "I have a full life," isn't that what they mean? Having a Full mind-set can also be applied to your attitude in regards to food and eating. Knowing that you deserve to eat healthy foods that nourish you and propel you to become Tiny is having a Full attitude about your style of eating. Being Full, in this sense, means that you don't have to worry about eating or have to think of food as something to fear, restrict, or forbid. When I say you are going to eat Full, I am saying that you are going to eat a balanced diet packed with nutrients, vitamins, minerals, and antioxidants, but this is not a food plan that is devoid of empty or harmful calories (I'll explain more in the next section).

To bring this concept together, I want you to understand that having a Full life means being *Full*-filled in all areas of your life, as well as being free and confident to accomplish everything on your life's bucket list. Plus, Full goes hand in hand with Tiny. If you remember from the previous chapter, when you are Tiny, you are beautiful inside and out—because being beautiful on the outside is an exterior reflection of your interior health. Being Full, in your attitude and in your style of eating, is how you will get to be Tiny. When your life is *Full*, you will be Tiny—and when you are *Tiny*, your life will be Full. Put both together, and you will be filled with epic health, serenity, happiness, and confidence.

Now, let's move on to the nutritional aspect of how to eat to always feel Full, but not overstuffed or starving.

Ready?

Three things:

1. Calorie density: To get you FULL-ly prepared to be Full, first we need to discuss the concept of calorie density, so you'll understand how to choose foods to be Tiny, while never feeling hungry or deprived again.

2. Optimal eating: We'll explore how veganism maximizes low-calorie density and boosts your health so you can always be Full. These strategies for Full Eating to get a Tiny Waist will help you to never feel deprived or hungry.

3. The problem: Eating vegan all day, every day, deprives you of vital nutrients and is not sustainable. We'll explore the shortcomings of veganism.

By the end of this chapter, you'll have both components of what it takes to be Tiny and Full™. You will effortlessly create a new lifestyle you can follow with ease! You will be free, once and for all, from yo-yo dieting, gimmicks, and fad diets, and you'll have the clarity and focus you need to reach the freedom, health, and beauty you've always desired.

Not All Foods Will Fill You Equally

In the previous chapter, Ready for Tiny, I shared how I've come to a new under-standing, based on overwhelming research, that to be truly and forever Tiny, you must watch your overall calorie intake. This presents a problem—hunger. Your body is incredibly sensitive to the calories it is accustomed to getting on a daily basis. When you cut calories, it makes you feel hungry, which can set up a dangerous reaction of overeating. You might be able to stick to a reduced-calorie plan for a few weeks, but when you feel empty from the lack of calories you are used to having, it becomes increasingly difficult to stick to your goal to get that Tiny Waist. Obsessive thoughts about food, irritability, and hunger eventually win.

Fortunately, there is a simple and clear solution—being Full! I'm not being flippant here because there is a trustworthy method that you can use to plan your meals and to eat foods that will keep you satisfied, while cutting calories so you can get Tiny. The secret to being steadily Full while lowering your calorie intake begins with understanding that not all foods are created equal. While a calorie is always a calorie, some foods are more *calorie dense* than others. What does that mean? A calorie-dense food has lots of calories, or energy, packed into a relatively small package. Let's take a closer look at this essential concept.

What is calorie density?

Barbara Rolls, nutrition professor and researcher at Penn State and author of *The Ultimate Volumetrics Diet,* coined the term "calorie density" to describe how foods vary in the number of calories they pack into each bite. Calorie density refers to the number of calories (or the amount of energy) contained in a gram of food. Foods with a lower calorie density provide fewer calories per gram than foods with a higher calorie density. Basically, for the same amount of calories, you can eat a larger portion of a food that is low in calorie density than a food that is high in calorie density. For example, let's say you'd like to eat a snack of about 150 calories. If you choose a small bag of Doritos from your office vending machine (a high-calorie-density food), you can have 11 chips to reach this quota. However, if you decide to have a bowl of strawberries (a low-calorie-density food), you can have 37 strawberries for the same 150 calories. Not only do the portion sizes look dramatically different—barely a handful of chips versus an overflowing bowl of juicy fruit—the first snack offers you nothing but salt, sugar, and empty calories that won't fill you up at all, while strawberries are low in fat and full of all natural flavors and colors, fiber, minerals, antioxidants, and vitamins (for more examples of calorie density and how it affects portion size, see the following picture of the varying sizes of 100-calorie snacks).

Eating these lower-calorie-density foods isn't a trick—you are actually filling your stomach with more food (by volume or weight), but you eat far fewer calories. That is calorie density in action. And it works! Researchers from the University of Alabama at Birmingham, Harvard, Spain, and many others, along with the Penn State researchers led by Rolls, have conducted a wealth of studies which show that lowering the calorie density of foods helps you to feel Full while eating fewer calories. Again and again, this research shows that you can lose weight while keeping your belly consistently and steadily Full. Consider these examples:

- Stay Full, eat less, be Tiny: Researchers from the Centers for Disease Control and Prevention conducted a survey of more than 7,000 adults and found that when compared to high-calorie-density foods, those who ate diets full of larger amounts of low-calorie-density foods ate fewer calories overall, even though they ate more food by weight. Remember, low-calorie-density foods fill up your plate, and your belly, without filling you with the calories that cause weight gain. This study, published in *The American Journal of Clinical Nutrition*, found that people with diets highest in fruits and vegetables (the lowest-calorie-density foods) ate the least calories and had the lowest rates of obesity.

- Size matters: In a study published in *Physiology & Behavior*, researchers from Pennsylvania State University and the Bell Institute of Health and Nutrition found that size matters more than calorie count. For three days, the researchers had 36 women consume varying formulas of a milk-based liquid food—496 calories in 10 ounces (a little over a cup), 987 calories in 20 ounces (nearly three cups), or 496 calories in 20 ounces (also nearly three

Which would you choose?

Here's what 100 calories of different snacks looks like. You can eat any of these and still eat the same amount of calories, but which ones do you think would fill you up the most?

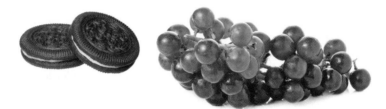

2 Oreo cookies (100 calories) or 62 grapes (100 calories)

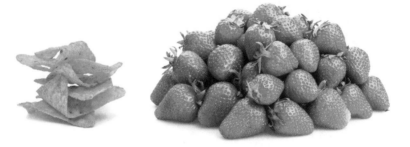

8 Dorito chips (100 calories) or 25 medium strawberries (100 calories)

cups). The three milk drinks varied based on volume (size; some were larger than others), and calorie density (the amount of calories per gram of drink; some had more calories than others). All drinks tasted similar and had the same nutrient composition. The women all rated the drinks as tasting similar and being equally enjoyable, but how satisfying—*how Full*—each drink made the woman feel was directly related to how large the drink was. The largest drink for the least calories was just as satisfying as the largest drink with the most calories. Again—you can be Full on less.

- Cut calories effortlessly: In another study, jointly published by Pennsylvania State University, the University of Alabama at Birmingham, Pennington Biomedical Research Center, Kaiser Permanente, Duke University, and Johns Hopkins Medical Center, researchers found that successful weight loss occurred when calorie density was reduced. When more than 650 overweight and obese men and women were divided into three groups, those who ate the lowest-calorie-density foods consumed the least calories, compared to groups that had higher-calorie-density foods. It gets even more impressive when you consider that compared to the highest-calorie-density diet group, the lowest-calorie-density diet group lost the most weight (5.3 pounds in the high-density group versus 13 pounds in the low-density group). The low-calorie-density group also decreased their calorie intake per day more (500 for the low-calorie-density group, while the high-calorie-density group only cut 100 calories per day). Plus, the low-calorie-density group increased the weight of the food they ate per day by 300 grams, while the high-calorie-density group didn't change the weight significantly at all. Again, this means that the people eating the low-calorie-density foods visually saw more food on their plates and felt more food in their bellies, while eating an average of 500 calories less a day than the high-calorie-density group did.

- Let them eat soup!: In a trial with 200 overweight men and women, researchers at Penn State, led by Rolls, tested the effect of incorporating either a low-calorie-density food or a high-calorie-density food into a reduced-calorie diet. The study found that reducing calorie density by adding a low-calorie-density soup into the diets of men and women was the main predictor of weight loss during the first two months of the study. Did you get that? The researchers *added* a food—the low-calorie-density soup, which was basically vegetables in broth—and that alone helped the subjects who had soup to lose weight. In addition, this strategy increased the amount of weight lost and the success at maintaining the loss.

- **Eat more veggies and fruits:** In another Penn State study, Rolls and colleagues tested the effect of lowering calorie density on a group of 97 obese women. The first group was directed to increase the amount of water-rich foods, such as vegetables and fruits, and to lower fat. The second group was told to restrict portions and to reduce fat. A year later, the group told to eat more fruits and vegetables had a greater reduction in calorie density and lost more weight than the group told to simply restrict portions. I love this positive strategy. Instead of telling the participants to cut foods, the researchers told them to eat *more* fruits and vegetables—and the group that was told to eat more lost the weight!

Our goal is to mimic the research you've just read about to eat the most nutrient-rich, but calorie-light foods to maintain a constant feeling of fullness while creating a calorie deficit that results in steady and sustainable weight and fat loss.

How will we do this?

Let's get to it.

Bulking up the portions

What makes the biggest difference in portion sizes are water and air. The quality of being filling also comes from fiber in foods, but that won't necessarily change the portion size. The examples given so far have been foods that have more water (and vitamins, fiber, minerals, and antioxidants), but you can also achieve this same effect, of larger portions, by whipping in, or whipping up, various meals, which you'll learn about in later chapters (think yummy smoothies and shakes). Weight-loss researchers say this is an important concept because what you see affects how Full you feel. The previous research examples all provide proof that this is true. The research by Rolls and her colleagues emphasizes that we all hold inherent beliefs about how much food we need to see on our plates or in our bowls to feel satisfied. When you see a full plate of food, your brain registers that you will be receiving enough nourishment, and you feel more satisfied. Once again, this shows that it's what you *see* on your plate that matters, not how many calories are *in* the food on your plate. This is good news because it means you can eat a low-calorie, highly nutritious meal and be sufficiently Full. The result is weight loss without ever feeling hungry or deprived.

Understanding the calorie density of various foods

All foods are made up of a blend of various macronutrients—fat, carbohydrates, protein, water, fiber, and sometimes alcohol. Combined, these components determine the calories in a given food and the calorie density (see the following image). It's helpful to look at each macronutrient separately to see where calorie density of a food is highest:

- Fat has 9 calories per gram, making it the most calorie dense of all macronutrients.

- Alcohol has 7 calories per gram and rates almost as high as fat. Alcohol is a special commodity as well because it isn't metabolized like other foods. Based on this, it should be consumed sparingly.

- Both protein and carbohydrates (including all sugars) come in at 4 calories per gram.

- Fiber, while also a carbohydrate, is only partially digestible, and so it comes in at 2 calories per gram.

- Water is the one and only true "free" nutrient because it has 0 calories, and 0 calorie density. It adds weight and volume without any calories—so the "wetter" the better. The more water in a food means the more food you'll see on your plate, in your bowl, or filling your cup.

How to calculate calorie density

You can calculate the calorie density of any food. Simply turn to the nutrition label of any package of food in your kitchen (or look up nonpackaged items on calorieking.com), and look for the serving size and the calories per serving. Let's consider a 5-ounce single serving of plain, nonfat Greek yogurt. The serving size in grams is 130, and the calorie per serving is 90. To calculate the calorie density, divide the calories per serving by the grams per serving. Here, 90 divided by 130 is .69, meaning that the calorie density of this yogurt is .69.

Calories per serving ÷ Grams per serving = Calorie density per serving

or

90 ÷ 130 = .69

You can get a reasonable idea of how calorie dense a food is by using this calculation on any food and then using the following chart as a guide.

Quick Tip: If the number of grams per serving of a food is larger than the calories per serving, the food is a low-calorie-density food, and you can safely include it in your diet.

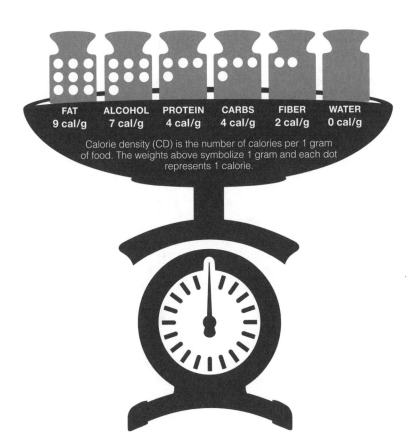

Calorie density (CD) is the number of calories per 1 gram of food. The weights above symbolize 1 gram and each dot represents 1 calorie.

However, you won't have to worry about calculating the calorie density of the foods you'll be eating. I've done all the work for you in the Tiny and Full™ Foods list in Chapter 7 as well as this quick-reference guide of foods that fall in the four Tiny and Full™ categories:

The Tiny and Full™ Levels

Level 1 (80%)

Plant-Based Food

Soups
- Chunky vegetable soup
- Black bean soup
- Lentil soup

Vegetables
- Cucumber
- Spinach
- Zucchini
- Broccoli
- Green beans
- Bell pepper

Fruits
- Watermelon
- Strawberries
- Grapefruit
- Blackberries
- Orange
- Pineapple
- Raspberries
- Blueberries
- Lemon
- Lime

Non-Dairy
- Silk® Unsweetened Vanilla Almondmilk 30 calories
- Tiny and Full® Chocolate Protein Shake (TinyandFull.com)
- Tiny and Full® Vanilla Protein Shake (TinyandFull.com)

Condiments
- Cinnamon
- Mustard
- Balsamic vinegar
- Himalayan salt
- Black pepper
- Garlic

Beverages
- Water
- Coffee
- Green tea
- San Pellegrino Water
- LaCroix Sparkling Water

Animal-Based Food

Soups
- Chicken broth
- Beef broth

Level 2 (20%)

Plant-Based Food

Soups
- Tomato soup
- Split pea

Vegetables
- Sweet potato
- Green peas
- Kidney beans
- Lima beans
- Corn

Fruits
- Mango
- Grapes
- Banana

Cereals, Grains
- Cheerios®
- Brown rice
- Oatmeal
- Quinoa

Snack
- Popcorn, air popped
- Tiny and Full® Fiber Bar Dark Chocolate Coconut (TinyandFull.com)
- Tiny and Full® Fiber Bar Chocolate Mint (TinyandFull.com)
- FiberOne® Chewy Bar

Animal-Based Food

Meat, Poultry, Fish
- Chicken breast, roasted, no skin
- Tuna, light, canned in water
- Tilapia
- Turkey breast, roasted, no skin
- Ham, extra lean

Soups
- Clam chowder, prepared with almondmilk
- Chunky bean with ham soup

Dairy
- Yoplait® Yogurt GREEK Whips!

Condiments
- Sour cream, fat-free
- Ranch dressing, fat-free

Level 3 (Dip)

Plant-Based Food

Vegetables
  Hummus
  Potatoes

Fruits
  Avocado

Breads
  Tortilla, corn
  Pita, gluten free
  Bread, gluten free

Desserts
  Chocolate, dark

Animal-Based Food

Dairy
  Cream cheese, light
  Feta cheese
  Mozzarella cheese, light
  Swiss cheese, reduced fat
  Parmesan cheese

Meat, Poultry, Fish, Eggs
  Egg, hard-boiled
  Sirloin steak, lean, broiled
  Salmon, farmed, baked
  Pork chop, center loin, broiled
  Ground beef, lean, broiled

Desserts
  Frozen yogurt

Condiments
  Mayonnaise, light

Level 4 (Avoid)

Plant-Based Food

Breads, Crackers
  Rice crackers
  Mary's Gone Crackers®

Desserts, Snack Foods, Candy
  Brownies
  Donuts
  Cake
  Trail mix
  Potato chips, baked
  Potato chips, regular
  Tortilla chips, regular
  Granola bar, hard

Nuts
  Peanut butter, reduced-fat
  Almonds, dry-roasted
  Peanuts, roasted
  Peanut butter, regular
  Pecans, dry-roasted
  Almond butter

Condiments
  Berry jam
  Olive oil
  Coconut oil

Animal-Based Food

Dairy
  Butter

Meat
  Pork spareribs
  Bacon

Hunger Signals:
When to Start Eating and When to Stop

One key part of being Tiny and Full™ is to understand your hunger and fullness signals. If you've been following one diet plan or another over the past several years, you've likely lost the ability to listen to the small quiet voice inside that tells you when to start eating and when to stop eating. When you are starving, that inner voice isn't so quiet—it screams; ditto for when you are stuffed. The problem is that if you wait until your body is shrieking for food or wailing because you are bloated beyond comfort, it's too late. The damage is done, and you're either going to be inhaling food like a thousand-dollar Dyson, or you're going to be in agony, popping Tums all night and beating yourself up for going overboard. That's why you have to learn to listen for the subtler signals. Start making use of the following scale right away to help you get back in touch with your hunger and full signals.

Throughout the day, check in and see how you are feeling on a hunger or fullness level. Rate your hunger on the scale of 1 to 10. You want to aim to eat when you are at a 3–4 and to stop when you are around 5–6.

1—Ravenous, weak, dizzy, jittery, headache; hangry. Can't concentrate. Stomach acid is churning. You don't care what you eat, but you must eat—now!

2—Stomach growling, cranky, feel a headache coming on, can't stop thinking about food.

3—Stomach is starting to growl, stomach feels empty, eating would be enjoyable now.

4—Could eat something, may feel the first pangs or gurgles of hunger; you notice your first thoughts of food.

5—Full, satisfied, neither hungry or full; your stomach doesn't feel bloated at all.

6—Perfectly and pleasantly full, relaxed, and comfortable.

7—Starting to feel a little uncomfortable. Food stops tasting as good. Stomach feels a bit stretched. You start to feel sleepy.

8—Need to unbutton your pants; you know you've gone too far, and you feel regret.

9—Your stomach hurts, feeling heavy and uncomfortable; clothes feel tight.

10—You are so overstuffed it hurts. You are in a food coma. You feel sick. You are Thanksgiving-dinner-full.

Optimizing Low-Calorie-Density Eating

So now you know all about the science of calorie density, and it makes sense. Still, it can be challenging to stick to this strategy all day every day. Of course, I've found the perfect solution—don't I always? What's the best way to low-calorie-density eating and staying Full, losing weight, and getting that Tiny Waist? My investigation of the facts led me again and again to see that a diet focused on plant-based eating is the way to go.

You will also want to know how to prepare foods to give you the fullest portions and nutrients while having the lowest calories. The simplest ways to achieve this are to use high-calorie-density foods as condiments and low-calorie-density foods as the foundation of all meals and snacks. Envision breakfasts of brightly colored fruit salads—strawberries, watermelon, blueberries, mangoes, melons—topped with a smattering of sliced almonds, sunflower seeds, or pepitas. Or you might have a large frothy fruit shake made with pea protein, whipped up with ice to fill a large glass. Lunches can be stir-fried zucchini, carrots, snow peas, and celery with small portions of lean chicken and fish on top. A large chef or spinach salad or a veggie-based casserole is on tap for dinner. These are all simple ways to add bulk without the calories.

It's all about being plant-based

Did you notice that many of these strategies use fruits and vegetables? That's because eating a plant-based diet is the one best option for superior health and for eating a low-calorie-density diet. It isn't as daunting as it sounds, and a diet rich in plants is fundamentally healthier. Let's take a closer look at what it means to eat plant-based.

The benefits of eating plant-based

More and more people are turning to a plant-based diet for the health benefits. Plant-based eaters report increased energy, better mood and mind-set, weight loss, and younger-looking skin. The scientific research on people who eat the most fruits and vegetables and the least animal protein show that those on plant-based diets have the lowest levels of chronic disease and longer life spans. The plant sources of these diets tend to be packed with nutrients but not calories. These diets are naturally higher in fiber, folic acid, Vitamins C and E, potassium, magnesium, and phytochemicals, and they are lower in saturated fats (see "The Natural Nutrient Benefits of Eating Plant-Based" box on page 30). It's easy to see that eating plant-

The Natural Nutrient Benefits of Eating Plant-Based

In addition to being naturally lower in calorie density, the following nutrients are inherently more present in plant-based diets:

- **Fiber:** Dietary fiber includes all parts of plant foods that your body can't digest or absorb. Fiber passes pretty much intact through your digestive tract. Why is this good? Fiber helps your body lower blood cholesterol and blood sugar levels, helps you have regular and painless bowel movements, and has been shown to lower the risk of cancers, heart disease, type 2 diabetes, and obesity. Fiber-rich foods include navy beans, pinto beans, kidney beans, lentils, black beans, prunes, pears, mangoes, almonds, pistachios, and pumpkin. I recommend 30 grams of fiber a day for all my clients.

- **Folic acid:** Folic acid is a B vitamin that helps your body make healthy new cells. Both men and women need folic acid, but it's particularly important to women before and during pregnancy because it helps prevent major birth defects. Folic acid keeps your blood healthy and protects you from anemia; it's also been shown to increase heart health and protect against cell changes that can cause cancer. Foods rich in folic acid include lentils, beans, peas, dark green vegetables, okra, asparagus, and citrus fruits.

- **Vitamin C:** This is one of the most powerful and effective nutrients. Vitamin C is necessary for the growth, development, and repair of all body tissues. Scientific studies of vitamin C show that it reduces stress, reduces the duration and intensity of the common cold, protects against stroke risk, guards eyesight, reduces overall inflammation, decreases cancer risk, protects your heart, and even slows the aging process of your skin. Vitamin C boosts the body's ability to absorb iron, enhances the immune system, increases wound healing, and helps in the maintenance of bones, teeth, and cartilage. This vitamin is also considered an antioxidant for its role as protector against free radicals and toxins such as cigarette smoke. Most fruits offer an excellent source of vitamin C, as do some vegetables, including tomatoes; red, yellow, and orange bell peppers; dark leafy greens; broccoli; and more.

- **Vitamin E:** In the past few years, the information about the benefits of taking vitamin E as a supplement has become unclear. However, vitamin E in foods such as almonds, hazelnuts, seeds, Swiss chard, spinach, and kale is safe and shown to be key for strong immunity, strong vision, and healthy skin.

- **Potassium:** This mineral is part of every cell in your body, and it helps your cells to function properly. It helps your nerves and muscles to communicate, assists in the regulation and maintenance of healthy blood pressure, and plays a vital role in helping your heart to beat properly. Some examples of potassium-rich foods are: dark leafy greens, potatoes, squash, avocados, mushrooms, and bananas. If you find yourself overly tired, irritable, or grumpy, it could be a sign that your potassium is too low. Other signs of low potassium include cramping, feelings of overall weakness, and nausea.

- **Magnesium:** I've written about magnesium before. It's an essential nutrient for many reasons, but one reason that caught my attention recently was a study in *The Journal of Intensive Care Medicine*, which reported that being deficient in magnesium doubles your risk of dying compared to those who have sufficient magnesium. Besides this attention-grabbing research, magnesium has long been known to reduce stress and enhance relaxation. Magnesium also reduces the risk of insomnia, reduces cramps, boosts mood, keeps kidneys healthy, and has been associated with reducing chronic diseases such as heart disease, diabetes, osteoporosis, and certain cancers. Magnesium-rich foods include almonds, dark leafy greens, peas, nuts, and whole grains.

- **Phytochemicals:** These biologically active compounds in plants are made up of several beneficial properties, including the reduction of waist circumference and antioxidants. Scientists are still learning the benefits of these naturally occurring compounds, but they believe them to be largely responsible for the protective health benefits in plant-based foods. Phytonutrients are found in fruits, vegetables, whole grains, legumes, herbs, spices, nuts, and seeds.

based is a great strategy for eating low-calorie-density foods because, as I've already mentioned, the lowest-calorie-dense foods are plant foods—fruits and vegetables. These are also the foods that are the most jam-packed with nutrients, vitamins, minerals, fiber, and antioxidants. Not convinced? Check out just a sampling of the research on the benefits of going plant-based:

- **Boosts immunity and prevents disease:** In a study published in the *Journal of the National Cancer Institute,* researchers from the Harvard School of Public Health found that of more than 100,000 men and women, those who ate the most fruits and vegetables had lower rates of heart disease, cancer, and death of any type than those who ate the least fruits and vegetables.

- **Protects your heart:** A UK review study of dietary habits that analyzed 12 studies, including more than 278,000 men and women for 11 years, found that those who ate the highest levels of fruits and vegetables had the lowest rates of heart disease. The researchers, from St. George's University of London, determined that individuals who had fewer than three servings per day of fruit and vegetables had a 17 percent greater risk of heart disease or heart attacks than those who ate five or more servings of plant foods per day.

- **Lowers stroke risk:** In another review study by the same UK research group as above, investigators analyzed stroke risk among people and correlated it with fruit and vegetable consumption. Of the eight studies and more than 250,000 men and women that spanned the course of 13 years, the researchers found that individuals who ate fewer than three servings of fruit and vegetables per day had the highest risk of stroke compared to those who ate five or more servings of fruits and veggies per day. The protective effects of fruits and vegetables were so strong that they led the researchers to strongly advise eating a minimum of five servings per day.

- **Keeps blood pressure low:** In a *Journal of American Medical Association* review of 32 scientific studies, researchers from Japan, Pennsylvania, and Washington, DC, found that eating a vegetarian diet influenced healthy blood pressure. The researchers analyzed more than 21,000 men and women and found that those who ate a vegetarian diet reduced their average systolic blood pressure by nearly 7 mm/Hg and nearly 5 mm/Hg diastolic blood pressure. Those who ate animal protein didn't lower their blood pressure. Another study that analyzed the effects of plant foods on blood pressure, published in *The New England Journal of Medicine*, found that when 459 men and women ate either a diet low in fruits and vegetables or rich in fruits and vegetables for three weeks, those in the high plant food group lowered their blood pressure by 11.4 and 5.5 mm/Hg points. The low vegetable and fruit group didn't lower their blood pressure at all.

- Reduces bad cholesterol: In a Brazilian study, researchers from the Catholic University at São Paulo found that those following a plant-based diet had LDL cholesterol that was 44 percent lower than those who ate a traditional diet. The researchers collected blood samples from 76 men and women who were separated into groups according to diet styles.

- Reduces diabetes risk: In a study published in *Diabetes Care*, researchers followed more than 71,000 women, ages 38 to 63, for 18 years. During the follow-up phase of the study, the Tulane University researchers found that those who reported a diet high in fruit and leafy green vegetables had a lower rate of diabetes than those who didn't eat many plant foods. In addition, those women who reported high fruit juice consumption had an increased risk of diabetes. Fruit juice is really just an isolated and concentrated form of the fruit, but without the nutritional benefits.

- Protects your eyes: From a study of more than 39,000 women, Harvard researchers found that munching on fruits and vegetables preserves eye function. After the initial assessment, the researchers did a follow-up 10 years later and found that the women who had the highest intake of fruits and vegetables had a 10 to 15 percent lower risk of having cataracts than those who ate the lowest amounts of plant foods.

- Lowers cancer risk: Eating deep yellow and dark green fruits and vegetables and eating onions and garlic are all associated with a lower risk of colorectal cancer, according to a University at Buffalo, School of Public Health study reported in the *American Journal of Clinical Nutrition*. Using findings of more than 3,000 men and women who were screened for colorectal cancers and comparing them to more than 29,000 control subjects, the researchers detected a reduced risk for these types of cancers among those who had the lowest risk of cancers. In addition to this research, many experts who study plant-based diets and cancer risks say that the high consumption of whole fruits, vegetables, and legumes provides a powerful and regular dosing of phytochemicals that protect against many cancers. As mentioned earlier, phytochemicals are the active compounds found in plant-based foods. Because plant-based diets consume considerably more of the foods that have been shown in scientific research to be protective against many types of cancers—including legumes, total fruit and vegetables, tomatoes, allium vegetables, fiber, and vitamin C—it's reasonable to

What It Really Means to Be Plant-Based

When I say "plant-based," I mean in the truest, most natural form of a whole food (minimally processed), plant-based diet. One can technically live on Coke, potato chips, and processed tofu dogs, but that is not the "plant-based" diet I support. I encourage the healthiest, most natural form of plant-based possible, which means eating whole, minimally processed foods.

conclude that those following a plant-based diet are more highly protected from many types of cancers.

- Reduces the risk of weight gain: People who follow diets that are rich in vegetables and fruits are less likely to gain weight over the same time period than those who have diets scarce in plant foods. In a study published in the *American Journal of Clinical Nutrition,* researchers analyzed the data of more than 89,000 men and women from five countries. Those who ate the most fruits and vegetables had the lowest changes in weight. In another study from the journal *Nutrition* that followed the dietary patterns of more than 10,000 men and women for 10 years, researchers from the Department of Preventive Medicine and Public Health at the University of Navarra, Spain, found that those who consumed the most fruits and vegetables had the least weight gain, compared to those who didn't consume as many fruits and vegetables.

To sum it up—to eat plant-based is to be healthy, slim, energized, happy, and confident. Unfortunately, there's a snag or two when it comes to being a full-time plant-eater.

The Flaw

While a plant-based diet is good for you and good for the world, there's a problem— or three. A plant-based diet does have superior health benefits because of diets with higher amounts of fiber, folic acid, vitamins C and E, potassium, magnesium; many phytochemicals; and lower intake of saturated fats—but this style of eating also comes with potential health risks. Eating this way all day every day means missing out on key nutrients if you're not careful, being exposed to some health risks, and dealing with the rigidity and limiting quality of a full-time plant-based lifestyle makes it unsustainable for the majority of people who attempt to follow the regimen. Celebrities from former President Bill Clinton to Beyoncé have tried the life-style and found it lacking.

Clinton explained to my good friend and celebrity chef Rachael Ray that he had to come to terms with the fact that he wasn't getting the quality protein and nutrients while eating a 100 percent plant-based diet. Clinton's doctor, Mark Hyman, expressed concern to the president, telling him, "It's hard to be plant-based and eat enough good, quality protein, and not have too much starch." On the other side of celebrity-hood, diva-musician Beyoncé and her husband Jay Z recently launched a line of plant-based meal plans. Beyoncé has said that she feels more energy and an enhanced glow to her skin from eating the plant-based way but admitted that she doesn't follow the strategy full time.

Missing nutrients

Several key nutrients are often lacking in a plant-based diet, including vitamins, minerals, and essential fatty acids. The nutritional adequacy of plant-based diets for weight management was recently discussed in great detail in a paper published in *The American Journal of Clinical Nutrition*. The review discusses information from the National Health and Nutrition Examination Survey (NHANES), a program of studies designed to assess the health and nutritional status of adults and children throughout the United States. The author concludes that while plant-diets do help in maintaining healthier weights, they are at greater risk for deficiencies in vitamin B_{12}, zinc, and protein as compared to those who eat animal protein. It's important to take a closer look at these nutrient risks and the health issues associated with them.

Vitamin B_{12}

Men and women need 2.4 mcg of this vitamin daily. Vitamin B_{12} is essential for having healthy blood cells and maintaining a healthy nervous system. A deficiency in this vitamin can cause abnormal neurologic and psychiatric symptoms that can include psychosis, nerve damage, disorientation, dementia, mood and motor disturbances, lack of energy, and difficulty concentrating. In a University of Wisconsin study, researchers tested the blood of 83 men and women who were attending the American Vegetarian Society Conference to determine vitamin B_{12} levels. The results of the study, published in the *Annals of Nutrition & Metabolism,* found that 92 percent of those only eating plants were deficient in the vitamin, compared to lacto-vegetarians (47 percent were deficient), and semi-vegetarians (just 20 percent were deficient). B_{12} is found only in animal proteins, including eggs, dairy, poultry, beef, fish, and dairy products. Although some plant foods, including mushrooms, tempeh, miso, and sea vegetables, are reported to have some vitamin B_{12}, they are not reliable. These foods contain an inactive form of the vitamin, and not only can it not be absorbed, it interferes with the absorption of active B_{12}; so many plant-based eaters need to take a B_{12} supplement to maintain levels. If you are interested in supplementing with vitamin B12, I encourage you to check out my Tiny and Full™ B_{12} Boost packed with 5,000 mcg of B_{12} and made from 100 percent natural sources available at tinyandfull.com.

Vitamin D

Vitamin D is known to be highly beneficial in protecting bone health and reducing heart disease, type 2 diabetes, high blood pressure, and cancer risk. The scientific evidence suggests that plant-based populations often have low vitamin D levels, which is associated with an increased risk of some cancers. In an Oxford University study, researchers found that of more than 65,000 men and women, those who were plant-based had the lowest levels of vitamin D, compared to all other eating styles. Compared to the meat eaters, the plant eaters' average vitamin D level was 75 percent lower. In another study, Finnish investigators followed the vitamin D status and bone health of 28 women for one year. The women were separated into three groups: plant-eaters, plant-eaters who consume dairy, and meat eaters. Blood and urine samples were collected over the course of 12 months, and the plant-eaters were found to have consistently lower levels of vitamin D and lower bone density than either the vegetarians or omnivores. The bone density in the plant-eaters was 12 percent lower than in the omnivores.

Iron

The daily iron quota for adult women, ages 18 to 50, is 18 mg. For men, and for women after menopause (mid-50s for most), the daily requirement is 8 mg per day. Surprisingly, those following a 100 percent plant-based diet do not show an increased risk for iron deficiency anemia, but they do tend to have lower iron stores. While you can get sufficient iron from dark leafy greens and beans in a vegan diet, it takes focus and work. Low iron increases your risk for anemia, a condition that can cause constant fatigue.

Zinc

Meat, seafood, and animal products are high in zinc. Interestingly, many plant-based foods tend to lower the absorption of zinc. Zinc is essential for metabolism, immunity, and healing.

Calcium

Adults age 18 to 50 need 1,000 mg of calcium daily. Those over age 51 need 1,200 mg daily. Most of you know that calcium is important for bones and overall health. The most common source of dietary calcium comes from dairy products, and without these, plant-eaters are at risk of having lower calcium levels, which can put their bone health in danger.

Omega-3s

One hundred percent plant-based diets do not include fish or eggs, which are the main sources of these healthy heart- and memory-protecting fats. There are plant-based fatty acids that can be converted to omega-3s, but not with any great efficiency. When tested, plant-eaters tend to have lower blood concentrations of omega-3s. In a study published in the *American Journal of Clinical Nutrition,* researchers from the University of Oxford found that of 196 men, those who were 100 percent plant-based had the lowest levels of omega-3 fatty acids when compared to meat eaters.

Protein

Animal protein contains all the essential amino acids our bodies need. Amino acids are key for muscle mass and bone health. Many plant-eaters don't meet their protein requirements, which puts them at an increased risk of anemia and lowers their access to many of the nutrients already described.

You are almost completely Ready for Tiny and Ready for Full. You know now that you deserve to be Tiny, and you deserve to be Full. You've established the necessary mind-set to have and be the success you've always dreamed about. You know that having a Tiny Waist means both inner and outer beauty, that being Full means never feeling hungry or deprived, and that optimizing a plant-based lifestyle is the key to being both Tiny and Full™.

We have just one last glitch to sort through—the dilemma. The dilemma comes from the fact that although following a sole plant-based lifestyle is beneficial in so many obvious ways, it's ultimately difficult to sustain and can be lacking essential nutrients. While you do increase fiber, vitamins, minerals, and antioxidants, and lower risks of many chronic diseases by eating plant-based, not to mention the effortless path to slim living—it's hard to follow. So, what's the answer? Is there a way to get the best of both worlds? That's what I'm about to reveal to you. You know I wouldn't leave you hanging. You are just a page turn away from learning everything you need to know about how to incorporate everything positive about the plant-based lifestyle, while leaving all the negatives behind in the dust. In the next chapter we'll put all the pieces together, and you'll start taking the actions to get you going on becoming Tiny and Full™ forever. Turn the page to find out why being Tiny and Full™ will transform your life!

"Every morning is a fresh start. Embrace it."

—JORGE CRUISE

3 Ready to Eat

39

So here we are. We've discussed getting Tiny and being Full for epic health; you've learned how to make the most of the calories you are going to eat by optimizing low-calorie-density foods; and you know all about the pros and cons of eating plant-based. Now we've arrived at the time to put all the pieces together so that you can get started on the path to living a Tiny and Full™ life forever. Here's the plan:

1. Ready? First, we're going to discuss how setting the stage for success first thing in the morning will keep you strong all day long.

2. Set? Second, I'll teach you how you'll continue to eat healthy throughout the day to feel consistently Full, energized, and inspired—all while losing weight.

3. Go! Third, we'll get started. I'll walk you through how Tiny and Full™ will be working in your life on a daily basis.

Let's get started now.

Start Your Day Plant-Based

When you start off your day by eating the most powerful, healing, and cleansing foods, you'll set the stage for success all day long. In Chapter 2, you learned how a plant-based diet is one of the healthiest and most healing diets available—for your body, and for the entire planet—all by relying on plant-based foods and reducing your intake of animal protein. Unfortunately, you also learned that a plant-based diet misses some vital nutrients that come from eating a more balanced diet and that the majority of people find that eating plant-based all day long is too rigid, limits options too drastically, and ultimately is not sustainable long-term. Still, I want you to eat plant-based. But that doesn't mean that you have to eat plant-based all day long for the rest of your life. You can actually get all the benefits of a plant-based lifestyle on a part-time basis. I'm going to teach you a realistic, satisfying, and fulfilling way of eating plant-based that will allow you to get a Tiny Waist in 12 weeks and to continue eating for epic health and happiness for the rest of your life. You'll pump up your levels of all nutrients, you'll lower your calorie intake while always feeling Full, you'll slash your risk of chronic diseases, and you'll boost your levels of energy and immunity.

The plant-based solution

By following plant-based eating principles each and every morning, you'll start your day off ahead of the game by nourishing your body with excellent sources of plant-based foods that are also naturally low in calorie density. You can eat satisfying and full plates, bowls, and cups of food that will lower your overall calories without you ever feeling hungry or deprived. Being plant-based in the morning is like giving yourself a daily detox. You'll cleanse your body each morning and then continue to eat a healthy balanced diet throughout the rest of the day. You really can optimize your health and happiness and be Tiny and Full™ by front-loading your morning with fruits and veggies. You will also reap these other benefits:

- Enjoy younger-looking skin, stronger nails, and more luxurious hair.

- Reduce the intensity of PMS symptoms.

- Decrease body odor.

- Boost your immunity.

- Lose weight.

- Lower your blood pressure.

- Protect your eyesight.

- Reduce your risk of heart disease, high cholesterol, diabetes, cancer, osteoporosis, obesity, and stroke.

- Increase your energy.

- Feel happier and more relaxed.

- Help the planet by reducing greenhouse gases.

By eating plant-based in the morning and eating low-calorie-density foods all day long, you'll maximize your nutrient intake, feel Full all day, and reduce calories to get a Tiny Waist in 12 weeks!

Morning is magical

You could eat plant-based any time of the day, but there are a number of reasons, backed by research, that starting your day with a successful action such as eating vegan sets the stage for you to be successful all day long. Why? Morning is when your willpower is strongest.

Roy Baumeister, director of social psychology at Florida State University and author of *Willpower: Rediscovering the Greatest Human Strength,* has published numerous studies which show that determination and drive are almost always strongest in the morning hours when you are fresh. That's because willpower is like a muscle. It's strongest when it's been given adequate rest and restoration. Also like a muscle, as willpower is used, as you go through the day, it becomes fatigued. What drains willpower is resisting trigger foods, making healthy decisions, dealing with difficult people, driving in traffic, being awake—basically just dealing with the normal demands of everyday life such as your work, partner, kids, your house, daily chores, and so on. That's why people tend to make healthier decisions in the morning, but by evening time, they are too tired to stick to healthy goals. Research shows that when your willpower is drained, you are more susceptible to overeating because the impulse control center in your brain becomes more vulnerable.

You can protect your willpower by starting your day plant-based. According to Baumeister's research, the key is practicing healthy actions on a daily basis such as starting off with the healthiest, most energizing, and nourishing meal possible for breakfast. This strategy works both because you start off your day consciously by choosing foods that are good for you and because you set the tone for eating healthy and low-calorie-density foods all day long. You'll eat less while feeling Full. You'll have front-loaded your motivation muscle, and you'll strengthen your willpower to stave off temptations later in the day. It's an automated way to stay Full while eating the least amount of calories.

The other component of morning magic is that the physiological and biological chemical reactions of digesting breakfast help you stay Full throughout the day and lower your susceptibility to overeating later in the day. In one study, UK brain researchers from the Imperial College London used MRI scans to study the effects of skipping breakfast. The researchers found that the MRI scans of the people who ate breakfast didn't elicit dramatic brain changes when shown pictures of pizza, cake, or chocolate. However, when the researchers viewed the MRIs of people who skipped their morning meal, they saw brains that lit up like a fireworks show on the 4th of July. The areas of the brain that were stimulated in the breakfast-skippers were the areas that control impulse, appetite, and cravings. This section explains the powers of phytochemicals, the Thyroid Boost, and False Belly Fat and how these three eating techniques can help get rid of your stubborn fat once and for all.

The Power of Plants

Earlier in Chapter 1, I shared with you that the only way to get a tiny waist was by cutting calories. Fortunately, science has proven me wrong and there are three new scientifically proven plant-based ways to reduce your waist circumference. This section explains the powers of phytochemicals, the Thyroid Boost, and False Belly Fat and how these three eating techniques can help get rid of your stubborn fat once and for all.

Phytochemicals

It's hard to believe that certain foods can actually help burn belly fat, but it's true! Foods high in certain phytochemicals can reduce your belly fat. How? Well, a plant-based meal triggers a series of hormonal changes that dampen hunger and fire up metabolism. "Plant foods supply phytochemicals that prevent the body from secreting abnormal levels of fat-storage hormones," explains Joel Fuhrman, M.D., an Ivy League–trained nutrition expert. Even better: Front-loading the diet with veggies and whole grains primes the body to burn calories eaten later in the day instead of storing them as fat, Dr. Fuhrman says. "You're flooding the body with phytochemicals that don't let fat cells grow." So what are these phytochemicals? Well, as you know, a phytochemical is a compound found in plants.

There are three types of phytochemicals linked to burning belly fat: Catechin (cat-a-kin), Anthocyanin (an-tho-sy-a-nin), and Thylakoid (thi-la-koy-d). A Catechin is a phytochemical found in plant-based sources that reduces waist circumference, lowers body mass index, and aids in weight loss. The ingestion of plants with high levels of catechins can prevent and improve many lifestyle-related diseases, specifically obesity. The next belly burning phytochemical is Anthocyanin. Anthocyanin is found in many dark pigmented fruits and vegetables such as blackberries and eggplant. Anthocyanin directly tells muscle and fat cells to increase their use of fat for energy, resulting in weight loss. The last phytochemical, Thylakoid helps us maintain a healthy weight by releasing cholecystokinin into our body. Cholecystokinin is a hormone produced by the gastrointestinal tract that encourages a feeling of fullness and decreased desire for food. In addition, Thylakoid also aids in weight loss and improves obesity-related risk-factors. You can find this phytochemical in mostly dark green vegetables like kale and spinach.

If you are someone who would like to starting burning your belly fat with these phytochemicals, you are in luck! I've included these belly burning foods in your 12-week meal planners and shopping lists and I've even identified which of the 80 recipes contain belly burning ingredients with recipe icons so you can start burning with ease. Below I've included a list of the top foods for each belly burning phytochemical.

Catechin:

- blackberries
- raspberries
- cherries
- apples
- pears
- beans
- fava beans
- red table wine
- black grapes
- brewed black tea
- brewed green tea
- cocoa
- dark chocolate
- milk chocolate
- barley

Anthocyanin:

- acai
- black currant
- aronia
- eggplant
- blood orange
- blackberry
- black raspberry
- raspberry

- blueberries
- cherries
- plums
- red currant
- purple corn
- concord grapes
- purple cauliflower
- cranberries
- red cabbage
- beetroot
- plums
- kale

Thylakoid:

- spinach
- cabbage
- lettuce
- kale
- collard
- broccoli
- mustard greens
- seaweed
- dandelion greens

Thyroid boost

In Chapter 1, I asked if you were experiencing any of the following symptoms of an underactive thyroid: lack of energy, constipation, and weight gain. If you are experiencing any of these symptoms I suggest you consult with your doctor to help repair your thyroid medically. But, first I would like to share with you some nutritional remedies that may help repair your broken thyroid. As you know, the thyroid is the master gland of metabolism, controlling the process of metabolizing our food. With a weak thyroid, the food we eat won't be metabolized correctly. Luckily there are certain tweaks to your diet that can actually help boost your thyroid.

The first thyroid boosting remedy is going gluten-free. I know going gluten-free sounds difficult, but it's not as hard as you think. I've even created a Thyroid Boost meal planner for you that is 100 percent gluten-free. Why gluten? Well, most low-thyroid issues fall on the autoimmune spectrum. This means that we have to identify what triggers our immune system to attack the thyroid. When gluten is consumed, it passes through your gut lining and enters your bloodstream, where your immune system identifies it and attacks it with antibodies. The problem is that your immune system oftens mistakes gluten for your thyroid and ends up attacking your thyroid instead. This case of mistaken identity is why going gluten-free will help prevent your body from attacking your thyroid, not to mention increase your energy and aid in weight loss.

The second thyroid boosting remedy is fueling your body with foods rich in iodine and selenium. Iodine deficiency is the most common cause of hypothyroidism worldwide, so it's important to have a diet rich in iodine. The reason why is because iodine is essential for making the thyroid hormone. Without iodine, you may develop hypothyroidism or further damage your thyroid. I recommend incorporating iodine-rich foods into your diet; the American Thyroid Association recommends 150 micrograms (mcg) **per day** for adult men and women, 220 mcg for pregnant women, and 290 mcg for lactating/breastfeeding women. Foods rich in iodine are: seaweed, cod fish, yogurt, turkey breast, navy beans, tuna, strawberries, and baked potato. The other plant-based thyroid boosting nutrient is selenium. Selenium supports the thyroid hormone synthesis and metabolism, helps protect the thyroid gland from damage, and is essential for the conversion of T3 and T4 hormones. The American Thyroid Association recommends 400 micrograms per day for adult men and women. I've included iodine and selenium rich foods in your Thyroid Boost meal planner as well as in the recipe icons labeled Thyroid Boost.

False belly fat

When you have belly fat (not the kind you can pinch), you have what is known as visceral belly fat. Visceral belly fat sits deep inside the abdominal region, wraps itself around vital organs like your kidneys and liver, and pushes out your belly. Even "skinny" people can have this protruding belly—and it's just as dangerous to them. Research has confirmed that belly fat is, without question, the most dangerous fat of all to have on our bodies. Here's more on how belly fat is connected to the three biggest killers:

Heart disease

Belly fat is dangerous because it releases inflammatory molecules called interleukin-6 (IL-6) into portal vein blood. Higher levels of these molecules are connected to higher levels of C-reactive protein, which is in turn connected to chronic inflammation.

Inflammation is associated with arterial stiffness and heart disease. Inflammation causes your arteries to "swell in" and cause problems in circulation. To make matters worse, if you've only been feeding your body a diet of sugar and refined carbs, those same arteries will begin to fill up with LDL, or "bad" cholesterol. Your body responds by sending in white blood cells to help attack the inflammation—but this attack actually releases toxic infection-fighters that eventually land on your arteries, creating holes. These holes fill up with platelets and essentially scab over, adding even more and more buildup. The combination of these events leads to heart disease/heart attack.

Diabetes

Visceral fat is also believed to lead to disease through your "portal vein." When blood travels from your abdominal organs to the liver it uses the portal vein. Scientists believe that when you have too much visceral fat stored in your omentum, it begins to dump fatty acids and hormones directly into the liver, which causes it to produce too much glucose. Your body then starts producing more insulin to try and manage the glucose. This cycle causes your body to become insulin resistant, which leads to type 2 diabetes.

Cancer

Since visceral fat is mostly metabolized by the liver into fatty acids and then released into the blood, it results in an excess of insulin. Insulin can contribute to the growth of cancerous cells. Abdominal fat cells also help convert adrenal hormones into a type of estrogen, which has been linked to increased risk of breast cancer. Overall, belly fat disrupts your body's hormone balance, which can lead to cancer.

When you lose belly fat, you will begin to lower your risk for the top three killers. And there's more: getting rid of your belly fat will greatly reduce your risk of sexual dysfunction, including lowered libido and erectile dysfunction. You'll also notice increased energy—research has connected belly fat to higher levels of fatigue, so losing it will help wipe out that constant tired feeling. And of course, you will experience an incredible increase in self-confidence!

What is false belly fat?

When you lose up weight on this, or any, program, not all of it will be from fat (or muscle or water)—a lot of it will be waste that has built up inside your body. Especially if you are someone who would describe their belly fat as hardened instead of jiggly. I call this waste built up in your body "false" belly fat, but my nine-year-old likes to call it what it really is: poop. Fecal matter has gotten stuck in your intestines because your diet may have been full of overly processed foods that are gluing your insides together! (Gross, right?)

Ideally, you should be having up to three healthy bowel movements a day. If your gut flora is at a proper level, you shouldn't have a problem with your body cleansing itself naturally. However, most of my clients when they start working with me are going one to two times *a week*! If you're not going to the bathroom enough, you might have one of those firm, hard bellies that sticks out. That's from built-up waste in your intestines. You've got to get rid of that false belly fat!

Below is the Bristol Stool Chart that describes what healthy and unhealthy bowel movements look like. Your goal is to get to Type 4. This is a normal, healthy bowel. Type 3 is acceptable as well, however Type 4 is ideal.

BRISTOL STOOL CHART

	Type 1	Separate hard lumps	Very constipated
	Type 2	Lumpy and sausage like	Slightly constipated
	Type 3	A sausage shape with cracks in the surface	Normal
	Type 4	Like a smooth, soft sausage or snake	Normal
	Type 5	Soft blobs with clear-cut edges	Lacking fibre
	Type 6	Mushy consistency with ragged edges	Inflammation
	Type 7	Liquid consistency with no solid pieces	Inflammation

Now the only way to achieve optimal bowel movements is by eating plant-based, fiber-rich foods. These type of foods help promote movement of material through your digestive system and increase the size and quality of your stool. I recommend you get 30 grams of fiber a day. That is why I encourage you to eat plant-based foods, especially in the morning. These foods are powerful and your body can benefit from the power of plants. If you think you may need extra support for your false belly fat I recommend using a probiotic daily. A celebrity client of mine took our Tiny and Full probiotic and trained with me over the course of 12 weeks and lost 50 pounds of belly fat due to her use of a probiotic and consumption of plant-based and fiber-rich foods. A probiotic supplement provides 10 billion active cultures. These cultures help restore your gut flora and keep your intestinal tract moving, helping your body rid itself of trapped waste and unwanted false belly fat.

In Chapter 4, you'll find the Tiny and Full™ meal planners that provide you with a daily plant-based breakfast plan complete with plenty of juicy fruits and savory vegetables, along with protein. It's important to include protein, especially if you are like me and have a hard time making it until lunch. Protein will help keep you Full and satisfied for the hours between meals. I've found a plant-based protein powder that I love because it provides 10g of satisfying protein you need while still allowing you to eat plant-based in the morning (see the "Plant-Based Protein Powder," box on page 48 for more information). Now that we've determined your breakfast routine, it's time to talk about the rest of the day.

All-Day Healthy Eating

Now that you know how to start your day off right, we can talk about how you'll keep eating healthy throughout the day to be Tiny and Full™. In the next section, you'll be given meal planners that will make eating the Tiny and Full™ way a no-brainer. And in the section after that I've even included icons on each recipe that indicates which ones: help burn belly fat with phytochemicals; boost your thyroid with iodine- or selenium-rich foods; turn off hunger with high-volume, low-calorie ingredients; and which ones are low in sugar for those of you who are diabetic, need to watch your insulin levels, or need to monitor sugar intake. But it's important for you to understand the logic behind this new way of plant-based eating. This will be especially helpful for those unavoidable occasions when you might be stuck without this book or a prepacked meal. I want you to always be prepared to keep your calorie density low and to never feel hungry or deprived.

Remember the Tiny and Full™ Levels Chart on page 26? I suggest that you make a copy of that page and carry it in your pocket or purse. You can also take a picture with your smartphone or visit TinyandFull.com to get a digital copy. You can make sure to eat low-calorie-density foods all day by choosing the foods listed in Level 1 as your base and as often as possible, then use those foods in Levels 2 to 4 as sparingly by adding from Level 2 first (which includes lean protein), and using Level 3 as a condiment. Your Level 1 foods are your go-to foods for feeling satisfied on fewer calories. Here you'll find lots of vegetables and fruits, which are full of nutrients but with a very low calorie density. Try to minimize or avoid Level 4 as much as possible. Use Level 4 oils, such as olive oil, in moderation.

Next, read on for my favorite all-day healthy eating tips.

Plant-Based Protein Powder

Plant-based diets typically lack protein, and protein is an important part of breakfast because it helps keep you Full for longer than just fruits and vegetables. Research on breakfast shows that protein helps people to feel less hungry later in the day (people who eat just carbs for breakfast or skip breakfast tend to eat more calories throughout the day and more calories overall). While fruits and vegetables are highly nutritious, they are also quickly digested and can leave you craving more sustenance. Thankfully, I've discovered a fantastic solution to getting protein while sticking with plant-based eating in the morning—pea protein powder. It's a relatively new addition to the protein powder family and is showing a lot of promise in the nutrition research community. Why go for your pea protein? Let's count the ways:

- **It's planet-friendly:** As discussed in the previous chapter, reducing your intake of animal protein is a great way to be more planet-friendly.

- **It's delicious:** Protein pea powder is delicious and comes in all the typical flavors—vanilla, chocolate, and unflavored. You can create delectable, creamy, frothy, fully satisfying, and fully plant-based shakes.

- **It's gluten free:** If you are among the estimated 10 percent of people who struggle with gluten or grain intolerance, or if you've been diagnosed with celiac disease, pea protein powder is a great option for you. It's 100 percent gluten free.

- **It helps you stay Full:** Pea protein powder is made from isolating the protein in peas, so it's high in protein. At about 10–20 grams per scoop of powder, pea protein powder will keep you feeling Full and satisfied all morning long. In a study published in *Nutrition Journal*, researchers found that pea protein was just as satisfying as protein powder made with casein (made from milk protein) and more filling than protein powders made with whey and egg.

- **It blends beautifully:** Many protein powders have a chalky, clumpy, or grainy texture or tendency. Not pea protein powder. It dissolves easily in water and blends into a creamy smooth shake. Even without a blender, pea protein powder blends easily in a shaker bottle.

- **It's hypoallergenic:** Many people have allergens to protein powders that contain whey, egg, soy, and casein (a milk protein). These ingredients can cause gas, bloating, and digestive discomfort. According to the Food Allergy Research & Education Organization, eight foods account for 90 percent of all allergic reactions: milk, eggs, peanuts, tree nuts, soy, wheat, fish, and shellfish. Peas are not among these. Pea protein powder is free of all allergens, making it the perfect choice.

There are many great pea protein powders on the market. I suggest one that is low in sugar and free of artificial additives. You can find my pea protein powder—made from incredible non-GMO, North American yellow peas and available in vanilla, chocolate, and plain flavors—at TinyandFull.com.

49

Ready to Eat

Make meat a condiment

Use meat and animal products as condiments. The Western way of eating makes meat the star of the show, which means too many calories and often too many heart-clogging fats. Instead of ordering or grilling up a huge slab of steak, choose a lean cut, and slice it into small pieces. Build bigger meals by incorporating your side dishes and your protein together. Instead of having a small serving of vegetables on the side of your plate, stir fry up a generous portion of vegetables, such as zucchini, red bell peppers, spinach, carrots, and snow peas; or mix up a large colorful salad of greens, peppers, tomatoes, carrots, shredded cabbage, and cucumbers, and top with chosen bits of protein. Your belly will be Full, but you'll stay way under your calorie quota.

Soup equals satisfaction

When liquids are combined with solid food, your body treats it as a whole meal, says Barbara Rolls, author of *The Ultimate Volumetrics Diet*. This seems to trigger your brain to feel satisfied. Your eyes see a large portion, your senses of taste and smell are fed, and you feel Full. When Rolls serves soup in her lab, she sees her subjects shave 20 percent of the calories off the meal that follows. There is an enormous body of research on soup and weight loss that began back in the 1980s. These studies consistently find that when people eat soup, they cut calories—up to four times as much as people who don't include this liquid food in their diets. For reasons not fully understood, drinking water separately doesn't provide the same satiating effects as eating it mixed in with food to make a soup.

Go big

When you are making your lunches and dinners, think large in terms of size, but low in terms of calories. Make a plentiful plate or container of salad, a big bowl of soup, or a generous dish of stir-fried vegetables. By using a foundation of vegetables and water (in soups), you'll create satisfying meals that will stay well within your calorie range.

Prep your fruits and veggies

Make sure to keep a container of clean veggies such as sliced cucumbers, baby carrots, sugar snap peas, celery sticks, and grape tomatoes for quick low-calorie-density snacking. Ditto on the fruits—I love to keep a bowl of strawberries, cubed melon, and grapes always in my fridge for quick snacking.

Rate your hunger

Remember to use the 1 to 10 hunger rating scale on page 28 from Chapter 2. Starting today, pay attention to how you feel. Start listening to the signals your body gives you about feeling hungry. How do you feel right now? Is your stomach growling or aching? Do you feel pleasantly Full? Before eating your next meal or snack, ask yourself, "Am I hungry right now?" After putting this query to yourself, use the scale to rate your hunger, with 1 being starving, and 10 being so stuffed you can't move. Don't stop there. As you eat your meal, pause and check in again, asking, "Am I still hungry?" When your rating reaches a 4 or 5, it's time to stop. If you aren't sure, put down your utensils, wait for five minutes or so, and then ask yourself again if you're hungry. Stay conscious throughout your entire meal. It may help to keep your eating area quiet and without distractions from a television or computer. It might even help to eat a meal or two in solitude. Over time, you will naturally begin to recognize your healthy hunger and full signals.

How to Get Started

Before you turn to the next section and start following the meal plans, it's important to do some prep work and then to continue to track your progress in several different ways. Below you'll find directions on how to set a baseline for yourself, your weight, and your waist and hips, as well as how to track your progress daily and weekly to keep your motivation optimally revved.

But first, let me summarize the steps to getting started:

- Take a weekly selfie.

- Weigh yourself daily.

- Choose your calorie goal.

- Take a weekly measurement of your waist and hips.

- Write down your accountability partners.

- Join me socially.

- Sign the Success Contract.

Take a weekly selfie

During the next 12 weeks, you'll be taking pictures once a week to track your progress. You'll also track your weight, but it's important to follow the progress you see in your photos. There are many changes you'll be able to detect in your photos that a scale won't show you. This is especially important when you want to lose a moderate or small amount of weight. Without visible evidence of your body's changes, you won't be able to notice the subtle improvements that can be seen in a picture. Here's how to take your selfie:

- Set a reminder on your phone and/or computer calendar so you'll have an automated alarm that triggers you to take your picture.

- Always shoot your picture at the same time of the day, on the same day of the week. I recommend recording your photo first thing in the morning, before you have breakfast.

- Wear the same clothes for each picture. I recommend something form fitting, or, even better, wear a bikini, bathing suit, or a bra and underwear.

- Take your photo in the same location, same background, and same lighting.

- Make sure your photo captures your entire body.

- Take two pictures each week. Take one picture with you facing front and another shot that captures your profile (a side view).

- Stand in the same posture, with your feet together, and your hands slightly away from your sides.

- Don't pose. Don't suck in your belly, or try to hide your thighs. Stand in a relaxed manner.

Weigh yourself daily

It used to be that you were only supposed to weigh yourself once a week, but no more. Today's nutritionists will tell you, and I agree, that you can keep your motivation at its highest by stepping on the scale once each morning. According to a recent study published in the *Journal of the Academy of Nutrition and Dietetics*, weighing yourself every day boosts motivation and leads to greater weight loss. For the study, researchers asked 91 men and women, ages 18 to 60, to either weigh themselves daily or to weigh themselves once a week. At the end of six months, the daily weighers lost 13 to 14 pounds, while the weekly weighers lost about

7 pounds. These daily scale-steppers also reduced the calories they consumed each day, increased exercise, and reduced television-viewing time more than those who weighed themselves less often. Still not convinced? In another study, University of Minnesota researchers tracked the weighing habits of 1,800 men and women who were trying to lose weight. The researchers found that those who did a daily weigh-in lost an average of 12 pounds over two years, while those who weighed weekly lost only 6 pounds. Not only did the daily weight watchers lose twice as much weight, they were less likely to regain the weight lost.

How to track your weight

First, choose a goal weight that is healthy and realistic. Take a moment to think about the history of your weight gains and losses over the past years. What was your lowest weight ever? Where does your weight seem to settle when you are taking action to be your healthiest ever? If you feel daunted by the amount of weight you have to lose, focus on reducing your weight by 10 percent to start. If you weigh 180, you'll focus on losing 18 pounds. Then, when you reach 162, you'll lose 16 pounds, and so on. In this way, your weight loss will feel more attainable, and you'll stay more motivated. Plus, setting up mini-achievements will give you more opportunities to reward yourself—another great way to stay motivated!

Baseline weight

Tomorrow morning, as soon as you wake up, step on the scale, and write your baseline weight in the space below:

Baseline Weight _____ .

Daily weight

Each morning from now until day 84, repeat your scale-stepping action first thing in the morning, and write your weight in the provided tracker on page 60. Don't fret if you see some fluctuations. Your weight can go up a pound or two based on retained liquid, sodium, or due to your menstrual period, but as long as you follow the Tiny and Full™ menus and meal planners, you'll steadily lose one to two pounds a week.

Choose your calorie goal

Based on your weight, choose your calorie level. In the next section of the book, you'll begin your menus and meal planners. You select your calorie level based on your current weight. You may need to adjust your calorie level as you lose weight. Please refer to the following chart.

Current Weight	Women: Calories Per Day	Men: Calories Per Day
Below 150 lbs	1,200	1,400
150–199	1,400	1,600
200–249	1,600	1,800
250–299	2,000	2,000
Over 300 lbs	For every 50 lbs. over 300, add 100 additional calories per day	For every 50 lbs. over 300, add 100 additional calories per day

Take a weekly measurement of your waist and hips

In Chapter 1, we discussed the importance of measuring your weight and keeping track of your waist-to-hip ratio. As a quick review, your waist-to-hip ratio is the measurement that shows the size of your waist in relation to your hips. A healthy waist-to-hip ratio for women is 0.7, and for men, it's 1.0. To take this measurement, take a fabric tape measure, and while sucking in your belly, measure your waist at the level of your belly button. Next, measure your hips at the largest point around your bottom. Finally, divide your waist size by your hip size. For example, if you have hips that are 46 inches and a waist that is 40 inches, then your waist-to-hip ratio is 0.86. Write all three measurements in the appropriate spaces in the tracker that starts on page 60. Seeing the inches melt off your body is a great way to stay motivated. Plus, a healthy waist circumference—35 inches for women, 40 inches for men—has been linked to better health as well. The Nurses' Health Study, one of the largest and longest studies to date that measures abdominal obesity, found that after 16 years, women who have the largest waist circumferences had nearly double the risk of dying from heart disease, an increased risk of dying from cancer, and an increased risk of dying from any cause, compared to women with the lowest waist circumferences.

Write down your accountability partners

I want you to bring all the pieces together by creating your own team of support, by signing the following Success Contract, and by committing to checking in with me on the social media sites I'm including below. To ensure your success, make a commitment to yourself, track your weight and waist, take those selfies, and enlist a group of friends (me included!) and family to support your efforts.

Your group of cheerleaders can include family members, coworkers, and good friends—anyone you feel comfortable communicating with openly and honestly. People in your inner support team must be caring and nonjudgmental, and they must be willing to listen to you and support you. Start by thinking of three people you'd like to invite into your inner support team. List their names (just their names for now) in the blanks on the left below:

Name and Contact Info: _____   Text Contact: _____

Name and Contact Info: _____   Phone Contact: _____

Name and Contact Info: _____   Accountability Contact: _____

Now I want you to appoint each person a contact category and write it in the blank space above, along with his or her contact information.

Here are the types of contact categories to choose from:

- Text contact: Designate one of the three people you listed as your texting contact, and fill in her cell phone number in the contact information area. Anytime you feel that you need to reach out for encouragement, shoot a text to this person, and tell her how you're feeling. Feel free to designate more than one person to this category. Invite friends and family who have weight to lose to join you on this journey.

- Phone contact: In the second space, list a friend or family member as a phone buddy, and fill in his home, work, and cell phone numbers. This buddy will help you when you need immediate support.

- Accountability contact: The last person on your inner support team is your accountability contact. This person will help you stay accountable for your weight-loss goal by talking to you for up to 15 minutes every night during your first week, preferably at the end of each day.

Join me socially

Please join the Tiny and Full™ community to share with me and with others following the Tiny and Full™ path to epic health and happiness. You'll find motivational tools and community support, and you'll also be able to cheer others on in their weight-loss journeys. Join me at these social media sites to post your photos and share your journey of success:

- Facebook.com/TinyandFull

- Instagram.com/TinyandFull

- Twitter.com/TinyandFull

- TinyandFull.com

- #TinyandFull

Sign the Success Contract

Please read the short commitment contract on page 58. I encourage you to rewrite this in your own hand. Feel free to personalize this Success Contract, adding any details that will help remind you of your internal motivation for wanting to change your life for the better. Use this written oath as a reminder to yourself that you are making YOU a priority. I know you want to look and feel healthy, but you've got to lay the mental foundation first. Think about the journey you are about to embark on. Do you want this? There are going to be good days, and, I won't lie, you will have some days where you'll struggle. Life will keep coming with all its ups and downs, no matter what you decide to do for yourself. You will be better armed with this book and all the powerful Tiny and Full™ tools in your back pocket, but ultimately *you* are the key. You must believe in yourself, believe that you can do this, and believe that you deserve a better life, better health, and more happiness. I already know that you deserve all of this—but you have to do your part by signing the following contract. This document that you'll write and sign is nonnegotiable, binding, and permanent. After you sign this commitment contract, there's no going back. You are promising to live your best life ever, to feed yourself only the best foods, and to treat your body with the utmost respect.

Selfie, Weight, Waist Tracker

Track the weekly and daily dates of your progress photos, your weight, and your shrinking waist and hips all in one place. Jot the date for your selfie and print it out. I encourage you to buy a small photo book to save your selfies in, or better yet, tape them in your bedroom where you can see them to keep your motivation strong. Below you'll find weekly spots for your selfie date, waist measurement, hip measurement, and hip-to-waist ratio, and weekly and daily spots for your weight. Use the tracker, so you can easily watch your progress improving over the next

12 weeks. You'll keep your drive and determination high by being able to see all your progress in one place. Be sure to pause as the weeks pass by to review each of the previous weeks. By taking notice of the inches and pounds that melt off your body, you'll create a natural reward. It's true, research shows that just pausing to take notice of positive experiences will stimulate the reward centers of your brain, which will inherently drive you to keep making healthy choices.

Feel free to jot notes in the white spaces on the pages below. It's a great opportunity to take notice of positive changes. Write down what works for you in the coming weeks, record circumstances where you successfully overcome obstacles and stick to your Tiny and Full™ plan, and be sure to take note as your clothes get roomier and as tasks such as carrying groceries or running up the stairs gets easier. It all counts—and the more you write, the more you remember.

The Success Contract

I, _____

commit to following the Tiny and Full™ menus and principles

for the next 12 weeks, starting on _____,

because I am worth it. I know that I deserve to be Tiny and

Full™. By tracking my progress in photos, weighing myself daily,

and measuring my waist weekly, I am committing to loving

myself, my body, and my life. By signing my name below, I am

acknowledging that I deserve radiance, energy, health, and

vitality. I promise myself to live in accordance with the rules of

Tiny and Full™. By following the eating plan to the letter, I am

creating what I deserve—epic health and happiness. I deserve a

Full Life. So be it.

Sign _____

Date _____

Congratulations! You've done all the prep work necessary to get started. You now know how to jump-start your day and to set the stage for getting your Tiny Waist and feeling Full all day. You've learned the strategies you need to plan healthy eating that will keep you satisfied and Full, never ravenous or deprived. You've taken the time to track your weight, waist, hips, waist-to-hip ratio, and your progress photos. You've created a team of support and signed a contract of commitment. With this strong foundation, you can't fail!

In the next chapter, you'll find detailed meal planners that I've created for you. Here you'll get a plan so automated that you can save all your brainpower for staying positive and powerful. I've even included weekly shopping lists so that you never have to wonder what to buy when you grocery shop. And, if you ever find yourself stuck without your planners, you can easily stay on the Tiny and Full™ plan by remembering the following rules:

1. Keep calorie density low.

2. Eat plant-based in the morning.

3. Keep all meals to 400 calories.

4. Keep all snacks to 100 calories, unless you fall into a higher calorie level.

5. Stay within your personalized calorie allotment.

That's it. You're now ready to get started. You've got this. It's simple. Fruits and veggies are your go-to friends. All your foods fall into a level, and it's always easy to find the calorie density of a given food by taking calories per serving and dividing by grams per serving (refer to page 24 in Chapter 2).

Week 1

Day 1:

Selfie	Waist	Hips	Waist-to-Hip Ratio	Weight

Day 2:   **Weight:**

Day 3:   **Weight:**

Day 4:   **Weight:**

Day 5:   **Weight:**

Day 6:   **Weight:**

Day 7:   **Weight:**

Week 2

Day 8:

Selfie	Waist	Hips	Waist-to-Hip Ratio	Weight

Day 9:   **Weight:**

Day 10:   **Weight:**

Day 11:   **Weight:**

Day 12:   **Weight:**

Day 13:   **Weight:**

Day 14:   **Weight:**

Week 3

Day 15:

Selfie	Waist	Hips	Waist-to-Hip Ratio	Weight

Day 16:   **Weight:**

Day 17:   **Weight:**

Day 18:   **Weight:**

Day 19:   **Weight:**

Day 20:   **Weight:**

Day 21:   **Weight:**

Week 4

Day 22:

Selfie	Waist	Hips	Waist-to-Hip Ratio	Weight

Day 23:   **Weight:**

Day 24:   **Weight:**

Day 25:   **Weight:**

Day 26:   **Weight:**

Day 27:   **Weight:**

Day 28:   **Weight:**

Week 5

Day 29:

Selfie	Waist	Hips	Waist-to-Hip Ratio	Weight

Day 30:   Weight:

Day 31:   Weight:

Day 32:   Weight:

Day 33:   Weight:

Day 34:   Weight:

Day 35:   Weight:

Week 6

Day 36:

Selfie	Waist	Hips	Waist-to-Hip Ratio	Weight

Day 37:   Weight:

Day 38:   Weight:

Day 39:   Weight:

Day 40:   Weight:

Day 41:   Weight:

Day 42:   Weight:

Week 7

Day 43:

Selfie	Waist	Hips	Waist-to-Hip Ratio	Weight

Day 44:   Weight:

Day 45:   Weight:

Day 46:   Weight:

Day 47:   Weight:

Day 48:   Weight:

Day 49:   Weight:

Week 8

Day 50:

Selfie	Waist	Hips	Waist-to-Hip Ratio	Weight

Day 51:   Weight:

Day 52:   Weight:

Day 53:   Weight:

Day 54:   Weight:

Day 55:   Weight:

Day 56:   Weight:

Week 9

Day 57:

Selfie	Waist	Hips	Waist-to-Hip Ratio	Weight

Day 58:   Weight:

Day 59:   Weight:

Day 60:   Weight:

Day 61:   Weight:

Day 62:   Weight:

Day 63:   Weight:

Week 10

Day 64:

Selfie	Waist	Hips	Waist-to-Hip Ratio	Weight

Day 65:   Weight:

Day 66:   Weight:

Day 67:   Weight:

Day 68:   Weight:

Day 69:   Weight:

Day 70:   Weight:

Week 11

Day 71:

Selfie	Waist	Hips	Waist-to-Hip Ratio	Weight

Day 72: Weight:

Day 73: Weight:

Day 74: Weight:

Day 75: Weight:

Day 76: Weight:

Day 77: Weight:

Week 12

Day 78:

Selfie	Waist	Hips	Waist-to-Hip Ratio	Weight

Day 79: Weight:

Day 80: Weight:

Day 81: Weight:

Day 82: Weight:

Day 83: Weight:

Day 84: Weight:

Part Two

How to Be Tiny and Full™

4 Your 12-Week Meal Planners

Now that you understand how *Tiny and Full*™ works, it's time to get started! I have provided you with a 12-week eating plan and a thyroid boost meal planner to guide you toward the types of food you should eat. Over the years, my clients have said that they like to have a consistent meal planner to follow so there are no surprises.

The meal planners all start at 1,200 calories with three main meals—breakfast, lunch, and dinner—as well as snacks and treats. The meals are all around 400 calories, and the snacks and treats are around 200 calories.

If your calorie goal is higher than 1,200 calories, you can increase the portions of your meals or increase your snacks. If you find you aren't losing weight or you're losing weight too quickly, adjust your caloric intake accordingly to find the right balance for you.

You'll notice that the meal planners include some of the recipes from Chapters 8–12, as well as some quick, toss-together meals. I recommend not making any substitutions to the meal planners to ensure your success. However, if you do decide to make substitutions, keep an eye out for the calories and adjust accordingly.

Turn the page, and let's eat!

When You're in a Pinch

On-the-go? In a pinch? I get it, I've been there. In fact, I'm probably there right now! I travel a lot for work, and even when I'm home, I'm running around with my kids or dashing off to the office. If you're constantly on the run as well, my go-to option is the Tiny and Full™ Fiber Bar (you can find these at TinyandFull.com).

Do you have any Tiny and Full™ on-the-go options you like? Tag @TinyandFull or use #TinyandFull on Instagram to share with me.

Week 1

Day 1

Breakfast

6 oz. plain coconut yogurt with 1 cup of blackberries and 1 tbsp. of plain granola (252 calories)

Snack

1 cup of sliced celery with 1 tbsp. sunflower seed butter (106 calories)

Lunch

Kale Caesar salad (page 242) with a 3 oz. grilled chicken breast (271 calories)

Snack

2 cups of air popped popcorn with fresh pepper (62 calories)

Dinner

Sauté 3 oz. large shrimp and 1 cup of asparagus in 1 tbsp. of coconut oil, season with salt and pepper. Serve with 2 cups of romaine lettuce tossed in 1 tsp. of balsamic vinegar, topped with 1 tbsp. of Parmesan cheese and 1 tbsp. of chopped pecans (260 calories)

Treat

4 strawberries dipped in 1 oz. melted 85% dark cacao (176 calories)

1,127 Total Calories

Day 2

Breakfast

1 cup of plain old fashioned oats cooked with water, topped with 1 cup of Silk unsweetened almond milk and 1 small sliced banana (244 calories)

Snack

1 large grapefruit (53 calories)

Lunch

AB & J Sandwich (page 238) with a half of a sliced apple (296 calories)

Snack

Sliced tomato with 1 oz. of goat cheese, seasoned with paprika and oregano. Add 1 tsp. of pepitas (108 calories)

Dinner

3 oz. of grilled filet mignon. Top with 1 cup of sliced cremini mushrooms and 2 tbsp. of sea beans, sautéed in vegetable stock. Serve with one cup of steamed green beans and Cauliflower Mashed Potatoes (page 296) (313 calories)

Treat

Blend ½ cup frozen pineapple and ½ cup of banana with ¼ cup of unsweetened almond milk, until smooth. Enjoy right away or freeze for 30 minutes (97 calories)

1,111 Total Calories

Day 3

Breakfast

6 oz. plain coconut yogurt with 1 cup of blackberries and 1 tbsp. of plain granola (252 calories)

Snack

1 cup of sliced celery with 1 tbsp. sunflower seed butter (106 calories)

Lunch

Hollywood Beet Salad (page 234) (306 calories)

Snack

2 cups of air popped popcorn with fresh pepper (62 calories)

Dinner

Grilled portobello mushroom on a bun, with slices of tomato, onion, and avocado, lettuce and chopped cilantro. Serve with 1 cup shredded cabbage tossed in apple cider vinegar (221 calories)

Treat

4 strawberries dipped in 1 oz. melted 85% dark cacao (176 calories)

1,061 Total Calories

Day 4

Breakfast

1 cup of plain old fashioned oats cooked with water, topped with 1 cup of Silk unsweetened almond milk and 1 small sliced banana (244 calories)

Snack

1 large grapefruit (53 calories)

Lunch

Kale Caesar salad (page 242) with a 3 oz. grilled chicken breast (271 calories)

Snack

Sliced tomato with 1 oz. of goat cheese, seasoned with paprika and oregano. Add 1 tsp. of pepitas (108 calories)

Dinner

Sauté 3 oz. large shrimp and 1 cup of asparagus in 1 tbsp. of coconut oil, season with salt and pepper. Serve with 2 cups of romaine lettuce tossed in 1 tsp. of balsamic vinegar, topped with 1 tbsp. of Parmesan cheese and 1 tbsp. of chopped pecans (260 calories)

Treat

Blend ½ cup frozen pineapple and ½ cup of banana with ¼ cup of unsweetened almond milk, until smooth. Enjoy right away or freeze for 30 minutes (97 calories)

1,033 Total Calories

Day 5

Breakfast

6 oz. plain coconut yogurt with 1 cup of blackberries and 1 tbsp. of plain granola (252 calories)

Snack

1 cup of sliced celery with 1 tbsp. sunflower seed butter (106 calories)

Lunch

AB & J Sandwich (page 238) with half of a sliced apple (296 calories)

Snack

2 cups of air popped popcorn with fresh pepper (62 calories)

Dinner

Grilled portobello mushroom on a bun, with slices of tomato, onion, and avocado, lettuce and chopped cilantro. Serve with 1 cup shredded cabbage tossed in apple cider vinegar (221 calories)

Treat

5 oz. glass of Merlot (124 calories)

1,061 Total Calories

Day 6

Breakfast

1 cup of plain old fashioned oats cooked with water, topped with 1 cup of Silk unsweetened almond milk and 1 small sliced banana (244 calories)

Snack

1 large grapefruit (53 calories)

Lunch

Hollywood Beet Salad (page 234) (306 calories)

Snack

Sliced tomato with 1 oz. of goat cheese, seasoned with paprika and oregano. Add 1 tsp. of pepitas (108 calories)

Dinner

3 oz. of grilled filet mignon. Top with 1 cup of sliced cremini mushrooms and 2 tbsp. of sea beans, sautéed in vegetable stock. Serve with one cup of steamed green beans and Cauliflower Mashed Potatoes (page 296) (313 calories)

Treat

Blend ½ cup frozen pineapple and ½ cup of banana with ¼ cup of unsweetened almond milk, until smooth. Enjoy right away or freeze for 30 minutes (97 calories)

1,121 Total Calories

Week 1

Day 7

Breakfast

6 oz. plain coconut yogurt with 1 cup of blackberries and 1 tbsp. of plain granola (252 calories)

Snack

1 cup of sliced celery with 1 tbsp. sunflower seed butter (106 calories)

Lunch

Kale Caesar salad (page 242) with a 3 oz. grilled chicken breast (271 calories)

Snack

2 cups of air popped popcorn with fresh pepper (62 calories)

Dinner

Grilled portobello mushroom on a bun, with slices of tomato, onion, and avocado, lettuce and chopped cilantro. Serve with 1 cup shredded cabbage tossed in apple cider vinegar (221 calories)

Treat

4 strawberries dipped in 1 oz. melted 85% dark cacao (176 calories)

1,088 Total Calories

Week 2

Day 8

Breakfast

1 toasted slice of bread with 2 tbsp. of plain hummus and 1 cup sliced strawberries (263 calories)

Snack

1 oz. Brazil nuts (95 calories)

Lunch

Creamy Spinach Quesadilla (page 221) (256 calories)

Snack

Santa Monica Kale Chips (page 295) (93 calories)

Dinner

3 oz. grilled chicken with fresh squeezed orange juice, 1 tsp. of soy sauce, minced garlic, grated ginger, salt, and pepper. Serve with ½ cup of brown rice and 2 cups of steamed baby broccoli (310 calories)

Treat

6 oz. container of coconut yogurt (120 calories)

1,029 Total Calories

Shopping List for Week 1

Produce:

- [ ] Celery – 4 cups
- [ ] Cabbage
- [ ] Asparagus – 2 cups
- [ ] Avocado – 2
- [ ] Romaine lettuce – 5 cups
- [ ] Kale – 2 bunches
- [ ] Beets
- [ ] Tomatoes – 4
- [ ] Onion
- [ ] Garlic
- [ ] Chives
- [ ] Cilantro
- [ ] Green beans – 2 cups
- [ ] Cauliflower – 1 head
- [ ] Portobello mushrooms – 3
- [ ] Cremini mushrooms – 2 cups
- [ ] Sea beans – 4 tbsp.
- [ ] Blackberries – 4 cups
- [ ] Strawberries – 12
- [ ] Banana – 4 small
- [ ] Apple – 2
- [ ] Grapefruit – 3
- [ ] Lemon

Meat:

- [ ] Chicken breast – 12 oz.
- [ ] Shrimp – 6 oz.
- [ ] Anchovies – 4
- [ ] Filet mignon – two 3 oz. pieces

Etc.:

- [ ] Parmesan cheese – 6 tbsp.
- [ ] Goat cheese
- [ ] Coconut yogurt – 12 oz.
- [ ] Light sour cream – 4 tbsp.
- [ ] Silk unsweetened almond milk – 5 cups
- [ ] Plain granola – 4 tbsp.
- [ ] Old fashioned oats – 3 cups
- [ ] Bread (Udi's, Rudi's, Ezekiel 4:9)
- [ ] Sunflower seed butter - 4 tbsp.
- [ ] Almond butter
- [ ] Sugar-free jelly
- [ ] Popcorn – 8 cups
- [ ] Pecans – 2 tbsp.
- [ ] Pepitas – 3 tsp.
- [ ] Coconut oil
- [ ] 85% dark cacao – 3 oz.
- [ ] Oregano
- [ ] Paprika
- [ ] Garlic salt
- [ ] Vegetable stock
- [ ] Balsamic vinegar
- [ ] Red wine vinegar
- [ ] Apple cider vinegar
- [ ] EVOO
- [ ] Dijon mustard
- [ ] Frozen pineapple
- [ ] Merlot – 5 oz.

Day 9

Breakfast

Blend 2 cups spinach, 1 cup peaches, 1 scoop of vanilla pea protein, 2 tbsp. chia seeds with 1 cup of ice water (244 calories)

Snack

1 toasted slice of bread with 1 tsp. of coconut oil and ½ cup of strawberry slices (167 calories)

Lunch

Brentwood BLT (page 229) (295 calories)

Snack

One sliced cucumber with 2 tbsp. of cream cheese mixed with ¼ cup of dried seaweed (51 calories)

Dinner

On one baking sheet, roast 3 oz. salmon filet with lemon and capers, and a sliced baby eggplant, zucchini, and carrot. Serve with ½ cup of sautéed cauliflower rice mixed with chopped spinach (253 calories)

Treat

Frozen half of banana dipped in 1 oz. melted 85% dark cacao (198 calories)

1,208 Total Calories

Day 10

Breakfast

1 toasted slice of bread with 2 tbsp. of plain hummus and 1 cup sliced strawberries (263 calories)

Snack

1 oz. Brazil nuts (95 calories)

Lunch

Creamy Spinach Quesadilla (page 221) (256 calories)

Snack

Santa Monica Kale Chips (page 295) (93 calories)

Dinner

3 oz. grilled chicken with fresh squeezed orange juice, 1 tsp. of soy sauce, minced garlic, grated ginger, salt, and pepper. Serve with ½ cup of brown rice and 2 cups of steamed baby broccoli (310 calories)

Treat

6 oz. container of coconut yogurt (120 calories)

1,137 Total Calories

Day 11

Breakfast

Blend 2 cups spinach, 1 cup peaches, 1 scoop of vanilla pea protein, 2 tbsp. chia seeds with 1 cup of ice water (244 calories)

Snack

1 toasted slice of bread with 1 tsp. of coconut oil and ½ cup of strawberry slices (167 calories)

Lunch

Herb Chicken Salad Sandwich (page 213) (275 calories)

Snack

One sliced cucumber with 2 tbsp. of cream cheese mixed with ¼ cup of dried seaweed (51 calories)

Dinner

Boil one lobster tail with 3 small red potatoes and 1 cup of green beans. Serve with green salad tossed in lemon juice (313 calories)

Treat

Frozen half of banana dipped in 1 oz. melted 85% dark cacao (198 calories)

1,248 Total Calories

Day 12

Breakfast

1 toasted slice of bread with 2 tbsp. of plain hummus and 1 cup sliced strawberries (263 calories)

Snack

1 oz. Brazil nuts (95 calories)

Lunch

Creamy Spinach Quesadilla (page 221) (256 calories)

Snack

Santa Monica Kale Chips (page 295) (93 calories)

Dinner

3 oz. grilled chicken with fresh squeezed orange juice, 1 tsp. of soy sauce, minced garlic, grated ginger, salt, and pepper. Serve with ½ cup of brown rice and 2 cups of steamed baby broccoli (310 calories)

Treat

6 oz. container of coconut yogurt (120 calories)

1,137 Total Calories

Day 13

Breakfast

Blend 2 cups spinach, 1 cup peaches, 1 scoop of vanilla pea protein, 2 tbsp. chia seeds with 1 cup of ice water (244 calories)

Snack

1 toasted slice of bread with 1 tsp. of coconut oil and ½ cup of strawberry slices (167 calories)

Lunch

Brentwood BLT (page 229) (295 calories)

Snack

One sliced cucumber with 2 tbsp. of cream cheese mixed with ¼ cup of dried seaweed (51 calories)

Dinner

On one baking sheet, roast 3 oz. salmon filet with lemon and capers, and a sliced baby eggplant, zucchini, and carrot. Serve with ½ cup of sautéed cauliflower rice mixed with chopped spinach (253 calories)

Treat

Sparkling Citrus Berry Sangria (page 348) (160 calories)

1,170 Total Calories

Day 14

Breakfast

1 toasted slice of bread with 2 tbsp. of plain hummus and 1 cup sliced strawberries (263 calories)

Snack

1 oz. Brazil nuts (95 calories)

Lunch

Herb Chicken Salad Sandwich (page 213) (275 calories)

Snack

Santa Monica Kale Chips (page 295) (93 calories)

Dinner

Boil one lobster tail with 3 small red potatoes and 1 cup of green beans. Serve with green salad tossed in lemon juice (313 calories)

Treat

6 oz. container of coconut yogurt (120 calories)

1,159 Total Calories

Shopping List for Week 2

Produce:

- [ ] Celery
- [ ] Baby broccoli – 6 cups
- [ ] Lettuce
- [ ] Tomato
- [ ] Baby eggplant
- [ ] Zucchini
- [ ] Carrot
- [ ] Cauliflower rice
- [ ] Red potatoes – 6
- [ ] Green beans – 2 cups
- [ ] Spinach – 8 cups
- [ ] Kale
- [ ] Cucumber – 3
- [ ] Red onion
- [ ] Garlic
- [ ] Ginger
- [ ] Rosemary
- [ ] Banana – 2
- [ ] Strawberries – 6 cups
- [ ] Peaches – 4 cups
- [ ] Lemon
- [ ] Orange – 3
- [ ] Blueberries – 1 cup
- [ ] Raspberries – 1 cup

Meat:

- [ ] Chicken breast – 13 oz.
- [ ] Extra lean turkey bacon – 2 slices
- [ ] Deli turkey – 6 slices
- [ ] Salmon – two 3 oz. pieces
- [ ] Lobster – 2 tails

Etc.:

- [ ] Parmesan cheese
- [ ] Nonfat mozzarella cheese
- [ ] Low fat plain Greek yogurt
- [ ] Coconut yogurt – four 6 oz. containers
- [ ] Cream cheese – 6 tbsp.
- [ ] Tortillas (Mission, Udi's, La Tortilla Factory)
- [ ] Bread (Udi's, Rudi's, Ezekiel 4:9)
- [ ] Brown rice – 1 1/2 cups
- [ ] Garlic powder
- [ ] Coconut oil
- [ ] Olive oil
- [ ] Soy sauce
- [ ] Hummus – 8 tbsp.
- [ ] Brazil nuts – 4 oz.
- [ ] Artichoke hearts
- [ ] Vanilla pea protein powder
- [ ] Chia seeds – 6 tbsp.
- [ ] Dried seaweed – 3/4 cup
- [ ] Capers
- [ ] 85% dark cacao – 3 oz.
- [ ] Vodka – 8 oz.
- [ ] Sparkling water
- [ ] Sparkling white wine or Brut Champagne

Day 15

Breakfast

Sweet Potato Waffles (page 197). Enjoy two waffles with ½ cup of sliced strawberries. **Save remaining waffles for breakfast and treat for the rest of the week** (245 calories)

Snack

1 cup of unsweetened applesauce sprinkled with cinnamon (100 calories)

Lunch

2 cups of spinach tossed with 2 strips of chopped turkey bacon, 1 oz. grated cheddar cheese, ½ diced tomato, and diced onion, with a squeeze of lemon and fresh ground pepper (219 calories)

Snack

1 medium banana (105 calories)

Dinner

Skewer 3 oz. of halloumi, sliced yellow squash, 10 cherry tomatoes, sliced beet, 3 oz. cubed steak, and green bell pepper. Season with salt, pepper, and thyme. Grill until steak is to desired doneness (301 calories)

Treat

Fiber Snack Bar - Dark Chocolate Coconut (150 calories)

1,120 Total Calories

Day 16

Breakfast

1 cup of old fashioned oatmeal cooked with water, topped with 1 cup of unsweetened almond milk and 1 cup of blackberries (258 calories)

Snack

6 oz. container of coconut yogurt (120 calories)

Lunch

Mix 1 cup of black beans with ¼ cup of corn, 1 diced tomato, chopped cilantro, and lime juice. Slice 1 cup jicama and use to scoop bean salsa (327 calories)

Snack

1 roasted artichoke with 1 tbsp. of Greek yogurt mixed with lemon and garlic for dipping (72 calories)

Dinner

Bake 1 sweet potato rubbed with coconut oil, and 3 oz. pork chop seasoned with salt, pepper, garlic, and rosemary at 350 degrees for 30 minutes. Serve with 2 cups of sautéed collard greens with 1 grated carrot (305 calories)

Treat

Sweet Potato Waffle (109 calories)

1,191 Total Calories

Day 17

Breakfast

Sweet Potato Waffles (page 197). Enjoy two waffles with ½ cup of sliced strawberries (245 calories)

Snack

1 cup of unsweetened applesauce sprinkled with cinnamon (100 calories)

Lunch

2 cups of spinach tossed with 2 strips of chopped turkey bacon, 1 oz. grated cheddar cheese, ½ diced tomato, and diced onion, with a squeeze of lemon and fresh ground pepper (219 calories)

Snack

1 medium banana (105 calories)

Dinner

Spiralize 2 zucchini and sauté with 1 tsp. of olive oil, garlic, and 5 cherry tomatoes, 1 cup of spinach, lemon juice, and 3 oz of shrimp. Once shrimp is cooked, top with ¼ cup of mozzarella cheese, 1 tbsp. of Parmesan cheese, and chopped parsley (316 calories)

Treat

Fiber Snack Bar - Dark Chocolate Coconut (150 calories)

1,135 Total Calories

Day 18

Breakfast

1 cup of old fashioned oatmeal cooked with water, topped with 1 cup of unsweetened almond milk and 1 cup of blackberries (258 calories)

Snack

6 oz. container of coconut yogurt (120 calories)

Lunch

Layer 3 slices of deli ham, 1 slice of provolone cheese, 1 tbsp. of sauerkraut, ½ diced tomato, sliced onion, and grated carrot in a romaine lettuce leaf (263 calories)

Snack

1 roasted artichoke with 1 tbsp. of Greek yogurt mixed with lemon and garlic for dipping (72 calories)

Dinner

Skewer 3 oz. of halloumi, sliced yellow squash, 10 cherry tomatoes, sliced beet, 3 oz. cubed steak, and green bell pepper. Season with salt, pepper and thyme. Grill until steak is to desired doneness (301 calories)

Treat

Sweet Potato Waffle (109 calories)

1,123 Total Calories

Day 19

Breakfast

Sweet Potato Waffles (page 197). Enjoy two waffles with ½ cup of sliced strawberries (245 calories)

Snack

1 cup of unsweetened applesauce sprinkled with cinnamon (100 calories)

Lunch

2 cups of spinach tossed with 2 strips of chopped turkey bacon, 1 oz. grated cheddar cheese, ½ diced tomato, and diced onion, with a squeeze of lemon and fresh ground pepper (219 calories)

Snack

1 medium banana (105 calories)

Dinner

Bake 1 sweet potato rubbed with coconut oil, and 3 oz. pork chop seasoned with salt, pepper, garlic, and rosemary at 350 degrees for 30 minutes. Serve with 2 cups of sautéed collard greens with 1 grated carrot (305 calories)

Treat

Fiber Snack Bar - Dark Chocolate Coconut (150 calories)

1,124 Total Calories

Day 20

Breakfast

1 cup of old fashioned oatmeal cooked with water, topped with 1 cup of unsweetened almond milk and 1 cup of blackberries (258 calories)

Snack

6 oz. container of coconut yogurt (120 calories)

Lunch

Layer 3 slices of deli ham, 1 slice of provolone cheese, 1 tbsp. of sauerkraut, ½ diced tomato, sliced onion, and grated carrot in a romaine lettuce leaf (263 calories)

Snack

1 roasted artichoke with 1 tbsp. of Greek yogurt mixed with lemon and garlic for dipping (72 calories)

Dinner

Spiralize 2 zucchini and sauté with 1 tsp. of olive oil, garlic, and 5 cherry tomatoes, 1 cup of spinach, lemon juice, and 3 oz. of shrimp. Once shrimp is cooked, top with ¼ cup of mozzarella cheese, 1 tbsp. of Parmesan cheese, and chopped parsley (316 calories)

Treat

Sweet Potato Waffle (109 calories)

1,138 Total Calories

Week 3

Day 21

Breakfast

Sweet Potato Waffles (page 197).
Enjoy two waffles with ½ cup of
sliced strawberries (245 calories)

Snack

1 cup of unsweetened applesauce
sprinkled with cinnamon (100
calories)

Lunch

Mix 1 cup of black beans with
¼ cup of corn, 1 diced tomato,
chopped cilantro, and lime juice.
Slice 1 cup jicama and use to
scoop bean salsa (327 calories)

Snack

1 medium banana (105 calories)

Dinner

Skewer 3 oz. of halloumi, sliced
yellow squash, 10 cherry tomatoes,
sliced beet, 3 oz. cubed steak, and
green bell pepper. Season with
salt, pepper, and thyme. Grill until
steak is to desired doneness (301
calories)

Treat

Fiber Snack Bar - Dark Chocolate
Coconut (150 calories)

1,228 Total Calories

Week 4

Day 22

Breakfast

1 slice of toasted bread topped with
1 tbsp. of almond butter and sliced
baby banana (289 calories)

Snack

6 oz. coconut yogurt (120 calories)

Lunch

Two cups of romaine lettuce with 3
oz. smoked salmon, red onion, ½
cup snap peas, 1 oz. of chopped
brie, tossed with lemon juice
and topped with 4 croutons (282
calories)

Snack

1 large orange (86 calories)

Dinner

Cut a zucchini lengthwise and
scoop out seeds. Puree a whole
tomato with one clove of garlic,
oregano, basil, salt, and pepper.
Fill the zucchini boats with the
tomato sauce, and top with ¼ cup
of grated mozzarella cheese and 2
oz. of mini pepperonis, then bake at
425 degrees until cheese is melted
and browned (264 calories)

Treat

One Minute Mug Cake (page 317)
(100 calories)

1,141 Total Calories

Shopping List for Week 3

Produce:

- [ ] Sweet potatoes – 3
- [ ] Romaine lettuce
- [ ] Collard greens – 4 cups
- [ ] Carrot – 3
- [ ] Green bell pepper
- [ ] Spinach – 6 cups
- [ ] Tomatoes – 5
- [ ] Yellow squash – 2
- [ ] Zucchini – 4
- [ ] Corn – 1/2 cup
- [ ] Cherry tomatoes – 40
- [ ] Beet
- [ ] Onion
- [ ] Garlic
- [ ] Thyme
- [ ] Rosemary
- [ ] Cilantro
- [ ] Parsley
- [ ] Jicama
- [ ] Artichoke – 3
- [ ] Banana – 3
- [ ] Strawberries – 2 cups
- [ ] Blackberries – 3 cups
- [ ] Lemon

Meat:

- [ ] Pork chop – two 3 oz. pieces
- [ ] Turkey bacon – 6 strips
- [ ] Steak – 9 oz.
- [ ] Shrimp – 6 oz.
- [ ] Deli ham – 6 slices

Etc.:

- [ ] Parmesan cheese – 2 tbsp.
- [ ] Cheddar cheese – 3 oz.
- [ ] Halloumi cheese – 9 oz.
- [ ] Mozzarella cheese – 1/2 cup
- [ ] Provolone cheese – 2 slices
- [ ] Coconut yogurt – 18 oz.
- [ ] Greek yogurt – 3 tbsp.
- [ ] Silk unsweetened almond milk
- [ ] Old fashioned oatmeal – 3 cups
- [ ] Buckwheat flour – 1 cup
- [ ] Cornstarch – 1/4 cup
- [ ] Baking powder – 2 tsp.
- [ ] Cinnamon – 2 tsp.
- [ ] Brazil nuts – 2
- [ ] Coconut oil
- [ ] Olive oil
- [ ] Vanilla extract
- [ ] White vinegar
- [ ] Stevia
- [ ] Nonstick cooking spray
- [ ] Unsweetened applesauce
- [ ] Black beans – 2 cups
- [ ] Sauerkraut
- [ ] Pea protein powder
- [ ] Fiber Snack Bar – Dark Chocolate Coconut

Day 23

Breakfast

6 oz. of coconut yogurt with 1 cup of sliced peaches and 2 tbsp. of chia seeds (318 calories)

Snack

1 cup of blueberries (84 calories)

Lunch

Plate a third of a head of iceberg lettuce and top with 2 tbsp. of blue cheese dressing, one slice of crumbled bacon, ¼ cup of grated carrots, and 1/3 cup of halved cherry tomatoes (239 calories)

Snack

Skinny Mint Chip (page 209) (140 calories)

Dinner

Soak ½ cup of shredded cabbage in 1 tsp. of vinegar, 1 tsp. of lemon juice, ½ tsp. of salt, and 1 tsp. of low sodium soy sauce. Cut half of a carrot and a cucumber, and 2 green onions into long strips. Chop 2 oz. of firm tofu into small cubes and season with pepper. Wet rice paper and layer all ingredients and top with 1 tsp. of chopped peanuts, then roll rice paper into a wrap. Enjoy spring roll with 1 tsp. of soy sauce for dipping (259 calories)

Treat

1 baby banana with 1 tbsp. chocolate chips (128 calories)

1,168 Total Calories

Day 24

Breakfast

1 slice of toasted bread topped with 1 tbsp. of almond butter and sliced baby banana (289 calories)

Snack

6 oz. coconut yogurt (120 calories)

Lunch

Add 1 tomato, ¼ onion, basil, garlic, 1 tsp. of extra-virgin olive oil, 1 tsp. of balsamic vinegar into food processor, and pulse, keeping mixture chunky. Top a toasted slice of bread with bruschetta mixture, then add 1 tsp. Parmesan cheese and fresh cracked pepper (243 calories)

Snack

1 large orange (86 calories)

Dinner

Cut a zucchini lengthwise and scoop out seeds. Puree a whole tomato with one clove of garlic, oregano, basil, salt, and pepper. Fill the zucchini boats with the tomato sauce, and top with ¼ cup of grated mozzarella cheese and 2 oz. of mini pepperonis, then bake at 425 degrees until cheese is melted and browned (264 calories)

Treat

One Minute Mug Cake (page 317) (100 calories)

1,102 Total Calories

Day 25

Breakfast

6 oz. of coconut yogurt with 1 cup of sliced peaches and 2 tbsp. of chia seeds (318 calories)

Snack

1 cup of blueberries (84 calories)

Lunch

Two cups of romaine lettuce with 3 oz. smoked salmon, red onion, ½ cup snap peas, 1 oz. of chopped brie, tossed with lemon juice and topped with 4 croutons (282 calories)

Snack

Skinny Mint Chip (page 209) (140 calories)

Dinner

3 oz. grilled halibut with 1 cup asparagus, seasoned with fresh dill and pepper. Serve with ½ cup quinoa cooked with lemon zest (271 calories)

Treat

1 baby banana with 1 tbsp. chocolate chips (128 calories)

1,223 Total Calories

Day 26

Breakfast

1 slice of toasted bread topped with 1 tbsp. of almond butter and sliced baby banana (289 calories)

Snack

6 oz. coconut yogurt (120 calories)

Lunch

Plate a third of a head of iceberg lettuce and top with 2 tbsp. of blue cheese dressing, one slice of crumbled bacon, ¼ cup of grated carrots, and 1/3 cup of halved cherry tomatoes (239 calories)

Snack

1 large orange (86 calories)

Dinner

Cut a zucchini lengthwise and scoop out seeds. Puree a whole tomato with one clove of garlic, oregano, basil, salt, and pepper. Fill the zucchini boats with the tomato sauce, and top with ¼ cup of grated mozzarella cheese and 2 oz. of mini pepperonis, then bake at 425 degrees until cheese is melted and browned (264 calories)

Treat

One Minute Mug Cake (page 317) (100 calories)

1,098 Total Calories

Week 4

Day 27

Breakfast

6 oz. of coconut yogurt with 1 cup of sliced peaches and 2 tbsp. of chia seeds (318 calories)

Snack

1 cup of blueberries (84 calories)

Lunch

Add 1 tomato, ¼ onion, basil, garlic, 1 tsp. of extra-virgin olive oil, 1 tsp. of balsamic vinegar into food processor, and pulse, keeping mixture chunky. Top a toasted slice of bread with bruschetta mixture, then add 1 tsp. Parmesan cheese and fresh cracked pepper (243 calories)

Snack

Skinny Mint Chip (page 209) (140 calories)

Dinner

3 oz. grilled halibut with 1 cup asparagus, seasoned with fresh dill and pepper. Serve with ½ cup quinoa cooked with lemon zest (271 calories)

Treat

1 baby banana with 1 tbsp. chocolate chips (128 calories)

1,184 Total Calories

Day 28

Breakfast

1 slice of toasted bread topped with 1 tbsp. of almond butter and sliced baby banana (289 calories)

Snack

6 oz. coconut yogurt (120 calories)

Lunch

Two cups of romaine lettuce with 3 oz smoked salmon, red onion, ½ cup snap peas, 1 oz of chopped brie, tossed with lemon juice and topped with 4 croutons (282 calories)

Snack

1 large orange (86 calories)

Dinner

Soak ½ cup of shredded cabbage in 1 tsp. of vinegar, 1 tsp. of lemon juice, ½ tsp. of salt, and 1 tsp. of low sodium soy sauce. Cut half of a carrot and a cucumber, and 2 green onions into long strips. Chop 2 oz. of firm tofu into small cubes and season with pepper. Wet rice paper and layer all ingredients and top with 1 tsp. of chopped peanuts, then roll rice paper into a wrap. Enjoy spring roll with 1 tsp. of soy sauce for dipping (259 calories)

Treat

One Minute Mug Cake (page 317) (100 calories)

1,136 Total Calories

Shopping List for Week 4

Produce:

- [ ] Kale – 2 cups
- [ ] Lettuce – 6 cups
- [ ] Iceberg lettuce
- [ ] Asparagus – 2 cups
- [ ] Red onion
- [ ] Garlic
- [ ] Oregano
- [ ] Basil
- [ ] Dill
- [ ] Snap peas – 1 1/2 cups
- [ ] Carrots – 3
- [ ] Cabbage – 1 cup
- [ ] Zucchini – 3
- [ ] Tomato – 3
- [ ] Cherry tomatoes – 2/3 cup
- [ ] Bananas – 8
- [ ] Peaches – 3 cups
- [ ] Blueberries – 3 cups
- [ ] Lemon
- [ ] Orange – 4

Meat:

- [ ] Smoked salmon – 9 oz.
- [ ] Mini pepperoni – 6 oz.
- [ ] Bacon – 2 slices
- [ ] Halibut – two 3 oz. pieces

Etc.:

- [ ] Silk unsweetened almond milk
- [ ] Firm tofu – 4 oz.
- [ ] Coconut yogurt – 42 oz.
- [ ] Brie – 3 oz.
- [ ] Parmesan cheese – 2 tsp.
- [ ] Mozzarella cheese
- [ ] Bread (Udi's, Rudi's, Ezekiel 4:9)
- [ ] Quinoa – 1 cup
- [ ] Rice paper
- [ ] Unsweetened cocoa powder
- [ ] Peppermint extract
- [ ] Vanilla extract
- [ ] Baking powder
- [ ] Peanuts – 2 tsp.
- [ ] Chocolate chips – 3 tbsp.
- [ ] Almond flour – 8 tbsp.
- [ ] Coconut oil
- [ ] Extra-virgin olive oil
- [ ] Balsamic vinegar
- [ ] Almond butter
- [ ] Chia seeds – 6 tbsp.
- [ ] Blue cheese dressing
- [ ] Nonstick cooking spray
- [ ] Vinegar
- [ ] Low sodium soy sauce
- [ ] Chocolate pea protein

Day 29

Breakfast

1 cup of old fashioned oatmeal cooked with water, and topped with 1 cup of almond milk and 2 sliced almonds. Serve with 1 large grapefruit (263 calories)

Snack

1 tbsp. of pistachios (81 calories)

Lunch

Sauté 3 oz. of cubed chicken in a saucepan, then add 1 cup of chicken stock, 1 small diced red chili, and ½ tsp. of grated ginger. Bring to a boil, then add 2 tbsp. of coconut milk, 1 sliced green onion, ½ cup of sliced cremini mushrooms, and chopped cilantro (269 calories)

Snack

1 cup of unsweetened applesauce with cocoa powder (102 calories)

Dinner

Asian Turkey Lettuce Cups (page 281). Serve with corn on the cob (253 calories)

Treat

1 oz. of cacao (145 calories)

1,113 Total Calories

Day 30

Breakfast

Top a slice of toasted bread with 2 tbsp. of avocado slices, 1 tbsp. of microgreens, and 2 tbsp. of chopped Brazil nuts (290 calories)

Snack

1 large banana (121 calories)

Lunch

Gooey Grilled Cheese (page 218) (297 calories)

Snack

2 cups of air popped popcorn with 1 tbsp. Parmesan cheese and fresh cracked pepper (84 calories)

Dinner

Wrap six spears of asparagus with a slice of bacon, and bake at 400 degrees for 15-20 minutes or until desired crispness (294 calories)

Treat

2 cups of diced watermelon (92 calories)

1,178 Total Calories

Day 31

Breakfast

1 cup of old fashioned oatmeal cooked with water, and topped with 1 cup of almond milk and 2 sliced almonds. Serve with 1 large grapefruit (263 calories)

Snack

1 tbsp. of pistachios (81 calories)

Lunch

Sauté 3 oz. of cubed chicken in a saucepan, then add 1 cup of chicken stock, 1 small diced red chili, and ½ tsp. of grated ginger. Bring to a boil, then add 2 tbsp. of coconut milk, 1 sliced green onion, ½ cup of sliced cremini mushrooms, and chopped cilantro (269 calories)

Snack

1 cup of unsweetened applesauce with cocoa powder (102 calories)

Dinner

Zoodle Linguine with Garlic Shrimp (page 273). Serve with 1 cup of spinach tossed with balsamic vinegar (209 calories)

Treat

1 oz. of cacao (145 calories)

1,069 Total Calories

Day 32

Breakfast

Top a slice of toasted bread with 2 tbsp. of avocado slices, 1 tbsp. of microgreens, and 2 tbsp. of chopped Brazil nuts (290 calories)

Snack

1 large banana (121 calories)

Lunch

Toss 2 cups of arugula with 3 slices of salami, 3 oz of mozzarella cheese, 10 cherry tomatoes, basil, and 1 tsp. of balsamic vinegar (279 calories)

Snack

2 cups of air popped popcorn with 1 tbsp. Parmesan cheese and fresh cracked pepper (84 calories)

Dinner

Asian Turkey Lettuce Cups (page 281). Serve with corn on the cob (253 calories)

Treat

2 cups of diced watermelon (92 calories)

1,119 Total Calories

Day 33

Breakfast

1 cup of old fashioned oatmeal cooked with water, and topped with 1 cup of almond milk and 2 sliced almonds. Serve with 1 large grapefruit (263 calories)

Snack

1 tbsp. of pistachios (81 calories)

Lunch

Sauté 3 oz. of cubed chicken in a saucepan, then add 1 cup of chicken stock, 1 small diced red chili, and ½ tsp. of grated ginger. Bring to a boil, then add 2 tbsp. of coconut milk, 1 sliced green onion, ½ cup of sliced cremini mushrooms, and chopped cilantro (269 calories)

Snack

1 cup of unsweetened applesauce with cocoa powder (102 calories)

Dinner

Zoodle Linguine with Garlic Shrimp (page 273). Serve with 1 cup of spinach tossed with balsamic vinegar (209 calories)

Treat

1 oz. of cacao (145 calories)

1,069 Total Calories

Day 34

Breakfast

Top a slice of toasted bread with 2 tbsp. of avocado slices, 1 tbsp. of microgreens, and 2 tbsp. of chopped Brazil nuts (290 calories)

Snack

1 large banana (121 calories)

Lunch

Gooey Grilled Cheese (page 218) (297 calories)

Snack

2 cups of air popped popcorn with 1 tbsp. Parmesan cheese and fresh cracked pepper (84 calories)

Dinner

Wrap six spears of asparagus with a slice of bacon, and bake at 400 degrees for 15–20 minutes or until desired crispness (294 calories)

Treat

2 cups of diced watermelon (92 calories)

1,178 Total Calories

Week 5

Day 35

Breakfast

1 cup of old fashioned oatmeal cooked with water, and topped with 1 cup of almond milk and 2 sliced almonds. Serve with 1 large grapefruit (263 calories)

Snack

1 tbsp. of pistachios (81 calories)

Lunch

Toss 2 cups of arugula with 3 slices of salami, 3 oz. of mozzarella cheese, 10 cherry tomatoes, basil, and 1 tsp. of balsamic vinegar (279 calories)

Snack

1 cup of unsweetened applesauce with cocoa powder (102 calories)

Dinner

Asian Turkey Lettuce Cups (page 281). Serve with corn on the cob (253 calories)

Treat

1 oz. of cacao (145 calories)

1,123 Total Calories

Week 6

Day 36

Breakfast

Promenade Protein Pancakes (page 201). Serve 1 pancake with 1 cup of sliced strawberries and 1 tbsp. of maple syrup. **Double recipe and save 3 pancakes for breakfast throughout the week** (265 calories)

Snack

1 large apple sliced with 1 tsp. of almond butter (93 calories)

Lunch

2 cups of romaine lettuce topped with 3 slices of salami, 1 slice of provolone, 2 tbsp. of giardiniera, sliced red onion, ½ sliced tomato tossed in 1 tbsp. of red wine vinegar (261 calories)

Snack

1 oz. of cheddar cheese (113 calories)

Dinner

Slice one tomato into thick slices, and 4 oz. of mozzarella cheese into thick slices. Layer a tomato slice, cheese, and top with basil leaves and a drizzle of balsamic vinegar. Sprinkle with pepper (246 calories)

Treat

5 oz. glass of Zinfandel (132 calories)

1,110 Total Calories

Shopping List for Week 5

Produce:

- [ ] Spinach – 2 cups
- [ ] Arugula – 4 cups
- [ ] Asparagus – 12 spears
- [ ] Microgreens – 3 tbsp.
- [ ] Bibb lettuce
- [ ] Scallions
- [ ] Carrots
- [ ] Zucchini – 4
- [ ] Tomatoes – 4
- [ ] Cherry tomatoes – 20
- [ ] Corn – 3 ears
- [ ] Onion
- [ ] Garlic
- [ ] Cilantro
- [ ] Basil
- [ ] Red chili
- [ ] Ginger
- [ ] Parsley
- [ ] Cremini mushrooms – 1 1/2 cup
- [ ] Avocado – 2
- [ ] Grapefruit – 4
- [ ] Banana – 3
- [ ] Watermelon

Meat:

- [ ] Shrimp – 10
- [ ] Ground lean turkey – 9 oz.
- [ ] Chicken – 9 oz.
- [ ] Bacon – 12 slices
- [ ] Salami – 6 slices

Etc.:

- [ ] Low fat cheddar cheese
- [ ] Mozzarella cheese – 6 oz.
- [ ] Parmesan cheese
- [ ] Silk unsweetened almond milk
- [ ] Coconut milk – 6 tbsp.
- [ ] Bread (Udi's, Rudi's, Ezekiel 4:9)
- [ ] Old fashioned oatmeal
- [ ] Almonds – 8
- [ ] Brazil nuts – 6 tbsp.
- [ ] Pistachios – 4 tbsp.
- [ ] Unsweetened applesauce – 4 cups
- [ ] Cocoa powder
- [ ] Cacao – 4 oz.
- [ ] Coconut oil
- [ ] Olive oil
- [ ] Chicken stock – 3 cups
- [ ] Red pepper flakes
- [ ] White wine
- [ ] Popcorn – 6 cups
- [ ] Water chestnuts – 3/4 cup
- [ ] Reduced sodium soy sauce
- [ ] Balsamic vinegar
- [ ] Sesame oil
- [ ] Wine vinegar

Day 37

Breakfast

Cafe Morning Mocha (page 206) (246 calories)

Snack

6 oz. of coconut yogurt (120 calories)

Lunch

3 oz. ground turkey with 2 cups of romaine lettuce, grated beet, sliced radish, grated zucchini, and 1 oz. of Cotija cheese with a squeeze of lime (272 calories)

Snack

½ cup of cubed avocado topped with cracked pepper and a pinch of salt (120 calories)

Dinner

Sauté 1 oz. of pancetta, ½ diced onion, and garlic in 1 tbsp. chicken stock until fragrant. Then add 1 sliced carrot and celery and cook until soft. Add ½ cup of navy beans and 1–2 cups of chicken stock, and let cook on low for 15 minutes. Before serving, throw in ½ cup of sliced kale and parsley (268 calories)

Treat

1 large apple, sliced and sprinkled with cinnamon (124 calories)

1,150 Total Calories

Day 38

Breakfast

Promenade Protein Pancakes (page 201). Serve 1 pancake with 1 cup of sliced strawberries and 1 tbsp. of maple syrup (265 calories)

Snack

1 large apple sliced with 1 tsp. of almond butter (93 calories)

Lunch

3 oz. shredded chicken with 2 cups of arugula, grated carrot, sliced celery, 1 tbsp. of black olives, 2 tbsp. of artichoke hearts, and 1 oz. of feta cheese tossed in lemon juice (253 calories)

Snack

1 oz. of cheddar cheese (113 calories)

Dinner

Slice one tomato into thick slices, and 4 oz. of mozzarella cheese into thick slices. Layer a tomato slice and cheese, and top with basil leaves and a drizzle of balsamic vinegar. Sprinkle with pepper (246 calories)

Treat

1 large apple, sliced and sprinkled with cinnamon (124 calories)

1,094 Total Calories

Day 39

Breakfast

Cafe Morning Mocha (page 206)
(246 calories)

Snack

6 oz. of coconut yogurt (120
calories)

Lunch

3 oz. ground turkey with 2 cups of
romaine lettuce, grated beet, sliced
radish, grated zucchini, and 1 oz.
of Cotija cheese with a squeeze of
lime (272 calories)

Snack

½ cup of cubed avocado topped
with cracked pepper and a pinch of
salt (120 calories)

Dinner

Mix ¾ cup of black beans with
½ cup of corn, ½ cup of diced
tomatoes, salt, pepper, and lime
juice, and cook on high in a skillet
until beans crisp. Fill warm corn
tortilla with mixture and top with
chopped cilantro (303 calories)

Treat

1 large apple, sliced and sprinkled
with cinnamon (124 calories)

1,185 Total Calories

Day 40

Breakfast

Promenade Protein Pancakes (page
201). Serve 1 pancake with 1 cup
of sliced strawberries and 1 tbsp. of
maple syrup (265 calories)

Snack

1 large apple sliced with 1 tsp. of
almond butter (93 calories)

Lunch

2 cups of romaine lettuce topped
with 3 slices of salami, 1 slice of
provolone, 2 tbsp. of giardiniera,
sliced red onion, ½ sliced tomato
tossed in 1 tbsp. of red wine
vinegar (261 calories)

Snack

1 oz. of cheddar cheese (113
calories)

Dinner

Slice one tomato into thick slices,
and 4 oz. of mozzarella cheese into
thick slices. Layer a tomato slice,
cheese, and top with basil leaves
and a drizzle of balsamic vinegar.
Sprinkle with pepper (246 calories)

Treat

5 oz. glass of Zinfandel (132
calories)

1,110 Total Calories

Day 41

Breakfast

Cafe Morning Mocha (page 206) (246 calories)

Snack

6 oz. of coconut yogurt (120 calories)

Lunch

3 oz. shredded chicken with 2 cups of arugula, grated carrot, sliced celery, 1 tbsp. of black olives, 2 tbsp. of artichoke hearts, and 1 oz. of feta cheese tossed in lemon juice (253 calories)

Snack

½ cup of cubed avocado topped with cracked pepper and a pinch of salt (120 calories)

Dinner

Mix ¾ cup of black beans with ½ cup of corn, ½ cup of diced tomatoes, salt, pepper, and lime juice, and cook on high in a skillet until beans crisp. Fill warm corn tortilla with mixture and top with chopped cilantro (303 calories)

Treat

5 oz. glass of Zinfandel (132 calories)

1,174 Total Calories

Day 42

Breakfast

Promenade Protein Pancakes (page 201). Serve 1 pancake with 1 cup of sliced strawberries and 1 tbsp. of maple syrup (265 calories)

Snack

1 large apple sliced with 1 tsp. of almond butter (93 calories)

Lunch

3 oz. ground turkey with 2 cups of romaine lettuce, grated beet, sliced radish, grated zucchini, and 1 oz. of Cotija cheese with a squeeze of lime (272 calories)

Snack

1 oz. of cheddar cheese (113 calories)

Dinner

Sauté 1 oz. of pancetta, ½ diced onion, and garlic in 1 tbsp. chicken stock until fragrant. Then add 1 sliced carrot and celery and cook until soft. Add ½ cup of navy beans and 1–2 cups of chicken stock, and let cook on low for 15 minutes. Before serving, throw in ½ cup of sliced kale and parsley (268 calories)

Treat

1 large apple, sliced and sprinkled with cinnamon (124 calories)

1,135 Total Calories

Shopping List for Week 6

Produce:

- ☐ Romaine lettuce
- ☐ Arugula – 4 cups
- ☐ Kale – 1 cup
- ☐ Tomatoes – 5
- ☐ Beet
- ☐ Radish
- ☐ Red onion
- ☐ Avocado
- ☐ Zucchini
- ☐ Carrot
- ☐ Corn – 1 cup
- ☐ Celery
- ☐ Basil
- ☐ Parsley
- ☐ Cilantro
- ☐ Onion
- ☐ Garlic
- ☐ Bananas – 4
- ☐ Strawberries – 4 cups
- ☐ Apples – 8
- ☐ Lime
- ☐ Lemon

Meat:

- ☐ Salami – 6 slices
- ☐ Ground turkey – 9 oz.
- ☐ Pancetta – 2 oz.
- ☐ Chicken – 6 oz.

Etc.:

- ☐ Mozzarella cheese – 12 oz.
- ☐ Cotija cheese – 3 oz.
- ☐ Provolone cheese – 2 slices
- ☐ Cheddar cheese – 4 oz.
- ☐ Feta cheese – 2 oz.
- ☐ Silk unsweetened almond milk
- ☐ Coconut yogurt – 18 oz.
- ☐ Corn tortilla – 2
- ☐ Rolled oats
- ☐ Coffee 1 1/2 cups
- ☐ Almond butter – 4 tsp.
- ☐ Cinnamon
- ☐ Chocolate/ vanilla pea protein powder
- ☐ Mini dark chocolates – 3 tsp.
- ☐ Nonstick cooking spray
- ☐ Maple syrup – 4 tbsp.
- ☐ Navy beans – 1 cup
- ☐ Black beans – 1 1/2 cup
- ☐ Black olives
- ☐ Artichoke hearts – 4 tbsp.
- ☐ Giardiniera
- ☐ Balsamic vinegar
- ☐ Chicken stock
- ☐ Red wine vinegar
- ☐ Zinfandel – 15 oz.

Day 43

Breakfast

Cook 1 cup of old fashioned oatmeal with water, then top with 1 tbsp. coconut milk and 1 cup of sliced strawberries (255 calories)

Snack

2 cups of cantaloupe (108 calories)

Lunch

Margherita Tortilla Pizza (page 253) (205 calories)

Snack

15 almonds (105 calories)

Dinner

Sauté 3 oz. shrimp in 1 tbsp. of unsalted butter and 2 minced cloves of garlic. Add ¼ cup of noodles and top with chopped parsley and 1 tsp. of Parmesan cheese (274 calories)

Treat

6 oz. coconut yogurt (120 calories)

1,067 Total Calories

Day 44

Breakfast

Toast 1 slice of bread and spread 1 tsp. of coconut oil and top with a sliced banana and 1 tbsp. of chopped walnuts (254 calories)

Snack

1 medium pear (103 calories)

Lunch

Three Minute Zucchini Pasta (page 246) (301 calories)

Snack

1 oz. of Brazil nuts (102 calories)

Dinner

Grill 3 oz. skirt steak seasoned with chili pepper, salt, and pepper. Serve with 2 cups of wilted spinach, ½ cup of sautéed mushrooms, and 1 tbsp. of bleu cheese (243 calories)

Treat

Green tea with steamed almond milk and a blood orange (91 calories)

1,094 Total Calories

Day 45

Breakfast

Cook 1 cup of old fashioned oatmeal with water, then top with 1 tbsp. coconut milk and 1 cup of sliced strawberries (255 calories)

Snack

2 cups of cantaloupe (108 calories)

Lunch

Downtown Pita Pizza (page 265) (321 calories)

Snack

15 almonds (105 calories)

Dinner

Sauté 3 oz. shrimp in 1 tbsp. of unsalted butter and 2 minced cloves of garlic. Add to ¼ cup of noodles and top with chopped parsley and 1 tsp. of Parmesan cheese (274 calories)

Treat

6 oz. coconut yogurt (120 calories)

1,183 Total Calories

Day 46

Breakfast

Toast 1 slice of bread and spread 1 tsp. of coconut oil and top with a sliced banana and 1 tbsp. of chopped walnuts (254 calories)

Snack

1 medium pear (103 calories)

Lunch

Three Minute Zucchini Pasta (page 246) (301 calories)

Snack

1 oz. of Brazil nuts (102 calories)

Dinner

One chicken sausage with ½ cup of sauerkraut, diced onion, and 1 tsp. of mustard in a bun. Serve with 1 cup of spinach tossed with 1 tsp. of apple cider vinegar in the bun or on the side (280 calories)

Treat

Green tea with steamed almond milk and a blood orange (91 calories)

1,131 Total Calories

Day 47

Breakfast

Cook 1 cup of old fashioned oatmeal with water, then top with 1 tbsp. coconut milk and 1 cup of sliced strawberries (255 calories)

Snack

2 cups of cantaloupe (108 calories)

Lunch

Margherita Tortilla Pizza (page 253) (205 calories)

Snack

15 almonds (105 calories)

Dinner

Sauté 3 oz. shrimp in 1 tbsp. of unsalted butter and 2 minced cloves of garlic. Add ¼ cup of noodles and top with chopped parsley and 1 tsp. of Parmesan cheese (274 calories)

Treat

6 oz. coconut yogurt (120 calories)

1,067 Total Calories

Day 48

Breakfast

Toast 1 slice of bread and spread 1 tsp. of coconut oil and top with a sliced banana and 1 tbsp. of chopped walnuts (254 calories)

Snack

1 medium pear (103 calories)

Lunch

Downtown Pita Pizza (page 265) (321 calories)

Snack

1 oz. of Brazil nuts (102 calories)

Dinner

One chicken sausage with ½ cup of sauerkraut, diced onion, and 1 tsp. of mustard in a bun. Serve with 1 cup of spinach tossed with 1 tsp. of apple cider vinegar in the bun or on the side (280 calories)

Treat

Green tea with steamed almond milk and a blood orange (91 calories)

1,151 Total Calories

Week 7

Day 49

Breakfast

Cook 1 cup of old fashioned oatmeal with water, then top with 1 tbsp. coconut milk and 1 cup of sliced strawberries (255 calories)

Snack

2 cups of cantaloupe (108 calories)

Lunch

Three Minute Zucchini Pasta (page 246) (301 calories)

Snack

15 almonds (105 calories)

Dinner

Grill 3 oz. skirt steak seasoned with chili pepper, salt, and pepper. Serve with 2 cups of wilted spinach, ½ cup of sautéed mushrooms, and 1 tbsp. of bleu cheese (243 calories)

Treat

6 oz. coconut yogurt (120 calories)

1,132 Total Calories

Week 8

Day 50

Breakfast

1 grapefruit with 1 slice of toasted bread topped with 1 tbsp. of almond butter (294 calories)

Snack

1 cup of unsweetened applesauce with cocoa powder (102 calories)

Lunch

Grill a 3 oz. filet of cod coated with pepper and lemon juice. Serve with sautéed 1/3 cup of diced tomatoes, 1/3 cup of grated zucchini, and 2 sliced green onions mixed with ½ cup of brown rice (230 calories)

Snack

1 cup of blueberries (85 calories)

Dinner

Cook a 3 oz. ground turkey patty seasoned with Worcestershire and ground pepper. Lightly grill two portobello mushrooms with the stems and gills removed. Assemble burger with portobello mushroom buns, a tsp. of mustard, a slice of tomato, a leaf of lettuce, and a slice of red onion (231 calories)

Treat

Three Ingredient Chocolate Ice Cream (page 309) (143 calories)

1,085 Total Calories

Shopping List for Week 7

Produce:

- ☐ Zucchini – 3
- ☐ Tomatoes
- ☐ Basil
- ☐ Parsley
- ☐ Kale
- ☐ Garlic
- ☐ Onion
- ☐ Spinach – 4 cups
- ☐ Mushrooms – 1 cup
- ☐ Strawberries – 4 cups
- ☐ Cantaloupe – 8 cups
- ☐ Banana – 3
- ☐ Pear – 3
- ☐ Blood orange – 3

Meat:

- ☐ Chicken breast – 9 oz.
- ☐ Deli turkey – 4oz
- ☐ Pepperoni
- ☐ Shrimp – 9 oz.
- ☐ Steak – two 3 oz. pieces
- ☐ Chicken sausage – 2

Etc.:

- ☐ Mozzarella cheese – 2 cups
- ☐ Parmesan cheese – 7 tbsp.

- ☐ Bleu cheese – 2 tbsp.
- ☐ Coconut yogurt – 24 oz.
- ☐ Butter – 3 tbsp.
- ☐ Coconut milk – 4 tbsp.
- ☐ Silk unsweetened almond milk
- ☐ Extra-virgin olive oil
- ☐ Coconut oil
- ☐ Old fashioned oatmeal
- ☐ Tortilla (Mission, Udi's, or La Tortilla Factory)
- ☐ Bun (Udi's, Rudi's)
- ☐ Bread (Udi's, Rudi's, Ezekiel 4:9)
- ☐ Noodles (Barilla, Ancient Harvest)
- ☐ Pita (Udi's, Joseph's, Simply Balanced, Ezekiel 4:9)
- ☐ Almonds – 60
- ☐ Walnuts – 3 tbsp.
- ☐ Brazil nuts – 3 oz.
- ☐ Marinara sauce
- ☐ Mustard
- ☐ Apple cider vinegar
- ☐ Black olives
- ☐ Sauerkraut – 1 cup
- ☐ Green tea

Week 8

Day 51

Breakfast

Beverly Banana Split (page 193) (313 calories)

Snack

6 oz. coconut yogurt with cinnamon (122 calories)

Lunch

3 oz. grilled chicken breast, 1 cup cooked green beans seasoned with salt and pepper, and ¼ cup brown rice (238 calories)

Snack

1 cup of cherries (87 calories)

Dinner

Fill a romaine lettuce leaf with ½ cup of black beans and 3 oz. of cooked ground beef seasoned with cayenne pepper, then ¼ cup of chopped tomatoes, ¼ diced red onion, ¼ diced jalapeño, and 1 tsp. of lime juice (299 calories)

Treat

20 raspberries filled with mini chocolate chips, enjoy right away or freeze (90 calories)

1,149 Total Calories

Day 52

Breakfast

1 grapefruit with 1 slice of toasted bread topped with 1 tbsp. of almond butter (294 calories)

Snack

1 cup of unsweetened applesauce with cocoa powder (102 calories)

Lunch

Grill a 3 oz. filet of cod coated with pepper and lemon juice. Serve with sautéed 1/3 cup of diced tomatoes, 1/3 cup of grated zucchini, and 2 sliced green onions mixed with ½ cup of brown rice (230 calories)

Snack

1 cup of blueberries (85 calories)

Dinner

3 oz. roasted chicken with 2 cups roasted vegetables, 1/3 cup cooked brown rice, and ½ baked sweet potato (372 calories)

Treat

Three Ingredient Chocolate Ice Cream (page 309) (143 calories)

1,226 Total Calories

Day 53

Breakfast

Beverly Banana Split (page 193) (313 calories)

Snack

6 oz. coconut yogurt with cinnamon (122 calories)

Lunch

Wrap a slice of deli turkey with a slice of deli cheese, 1 cup of spinach, and a slice of tomato in a tortilla with a smear of 1 tsp. of cream cheese (287 calories)

Snack

1 cup of cherries (87 calories)

Dinner

Cook a 3 oz. ground turkey patty seasoned with Worcestershire and ground pepper. Lightly grill two portobello mushrooms with the stems and gills removed. Assemble burger with portobello mushroom buns, a tsp. of mustard, a slice of tomato, a leaf of lettuce, and a slice of red onion (231 calories)

Treat

20 raspberries filled with mini chocolate chips, enjoy right away or freeze (90 calories)

1,130 Total Calories

Day 54

Breakfast

1 grapefruit with 1 slice of toasted bread topped with 1 tbsp. of almond butter (294 calories)

Snack

1 cup of unsweetened applesauce with cocoa powder (102 calories)

Lunch

Grill a 3 oz. filet of cod coated with pepper and lemon juice. Serve with sautéed 1/3 cup of diced tomatoes, 1/3 cup of grated zucchini, and 2 sliced green onions mixed with ½ cup of brown rice (230 calories)

Snack

1 cup of blueberries (85 calories)

Dinner

3 oz. roasted chicken with 2 cups roasted vegetables, 1/3 cup cooked brown rice, and ½ baked sweet potato (372 calories)

Treat

Three Ingredient Chocolate Ice Cream (page 309) (143 calories)

1,226 Total Calories

Day 55

Breakfast

Beverly Banana Split (page 193) (313 calories)

Snack

6 oz. coconut yogurt with cinnamon (122 calories)

Lunch

3 oz. grilled chicken breast, 1 cup cooked green beans seasoned with salt and pepper, and ¼ cup brown rice (238 calories)

Snack

1 cup of cherries (87 calories)

Dinner

Fill a romaine lettuce leaf with ½ cup of black beans and 3 oz. of cooked ground beef seasoned with cayenne pepper, then ¼ cup of chopped tomatoes, ¼ diced red onion, ¼ diced jalapeño, and 1 tsp. of lime juice (299 calories)

Treat

20 raspberries filled with mini chocolate chips, enjoy right away or freeze (90 calories)

1,149 Total Calories

Day 56

Breakfast

1 grapefruit with 1 slice of toasted bread topped with 1 tbsp. of almond butter (294 calories)

Snack

1 cup of unsweetened applesauce with cocoa powder (102 calories)

Lunch

Wrap a slice of deli turkey with a slice of deli cheese, 1 cup of spinach, and a slice of tomato in a tortilla with a smear of 1 tsp. of cream cheese (287 calories)

Snack

1 cup of blueberries (85 calories)

Dinner

Cook a 3 oz. ground turkey patty seasoned with Worcestershire and ground pepper. Lightly grill two portobello mushrooms with the stems and gills removed. Assemble burger with portobello mushroom buns, a tsp. of mustard, a slice of tomato, a leaf of lettuce, and a slice of red onion (231 calories)

Treat

Three Ingredient Chocolate Ice Cream (page 309) (143 calories)

1,142 Total Calories

Produce:

☐ Lettuce

☐ Spinach

☐ Tomatoes

☐ Zucchini

☐ Green beans – 1 cup

☐ Green onions

☐ Sweet potato

☐ Jalapeño

☐ Onion

☐ Mint

☐ Portobello mushrooms – 6

☐ Bananas – 7

☐ Blueberries – 4 cups

☐ Blackberries – 1 1/2 cups

☐ Raspberries – 3 cups

☐ Grapefruit – 4

☐ Cherries – 3 cups

☐ Lemon

☐ Lime

Meat:

☐ Cod – three 3 oz. pieces

☐ Ground turkey – three 3 oz. patties

☐ Ground beef – 6 oz.

☐ Chicken breast – 12 oz.

☐ Deli turkey – 2 slices

Etc.:

☐ Deli cheese – 2 slices

☐ Cream cheese – 2 tsp.

☐ Coconut yogurt – 30 oz.

☐ Silk unsweetened almond milk

☐ Bread (Udi's, Rudi's, Ezekiel 4:9)

☐ Tortilla (Mission, Udi's, or La Tortilla Factory)

☐ Brown rice – 3 cups

☐ Almond butter

☐ Unsweetened applesauce

☐ Cocoa powder

☐ Cinnamon

☐ Mini dark chocolate chips – 7 tbsp.

☐ Granola

☐ Black beans – 1 cup

☐ Worcestershire sauce

☐ Mustard

Day 57

Breakfast

Blend half of a red bell pepper with 1 cup of strawberries, 1 cup of spinach, ½ tbsp. of cashews, and 2 tbsp. of almond milk. Add water and ice for desired consistency (233 calories)

Snack

1 medium apple (95 calories)

Lunch

Mix 1 cup of cooked quinoa with ½ cup of grated beet, 1 cup of shredded spinach, 2 tbsp. of feta cheese, and 1 tbsp. of dried seaweed. Serve with 3 oz. of turkey breast (293 calories)

Snack

1 cup of baby carrots with 2 tbsp. of tzatziki (110 calories)

Dinner

Roast one small butternut squash until fork tender, then remove skin. Sauté onions and garlic, add chopped squash with 2 cups of vegetable stock. Add salt, pepper, thyme, and 2 tbsp. of Greek yogurt, let simmer for 15 minutes. Puree or leave chunky. Stir in 1 oz. cheddar cheese, and serve once cheese has melted. Serve with 1 cup of romaine lettuce tossed with balsamic vinegar (254 calories)

Treat

Banana Berry Ice Cream (page 310) (96 calories)

1,081 Total Calories

Day 58

Breakfast

6 oz. of coconut yogurt with 1 cup of blackberries and 1 oz. of sliced Brazil nuts (277 calories)

Snack

1 large banana (121 calories)

Lunch

1 slice of bread with 2 slices of deli ham, 1 slice of deli cheese, mustard, and 1 cup of kale with a drizzle of balsamic vinegar (294 calories)

Snack

1 roasted artichoke with 1 tbsp. of Greek yogurt mixed with lemon and garlic for dipping (72 calories)

Dinner

Stir fry 3 oz. of chicken with ½ cup peas, carrots, corn, and broccoli seasoned with 1 tbsp. of soy sauce, garlic, and red chili flakes. Serve with ½ cup brown rice and 1 cup of spinach (313 calories)

Treat

Banana Berry Ice Cream (page 310) (96 calories)

1,083 Total Calories

Day 59

Breakfast

Blend half of a red bell pepper with 1 cup of strawberries, 1 cup of spinach, ½ tbsp. of cashews, and 2 tbsp. of almond milk. Add water and ice for desired consistency (233 calories)

Snack

1 medium apple (95 calories)

Lunch

Mix 1 cup of cooked quinoa with ½ cup of grated beet, 1 cup of shredded spinach, 2 tbsp. of feta cheese, and 1 tbsp. of dried seaweed. Serve with 3 oz. of turkey breast (293 calories)

Snack

1 cup of baby carrots with 2 tbsp. of tzatziki (110 calories)

Dinner

Grill 3 oz. of grass-fed steak, seasoned with salt, pepper, and sage. Serve with 3 baked baby red potatoes and 1 cup of steamed Swiss chard (257 calories)

Treat

Banana Berry Ice Cream (page 310) (96 calories)

1,084 Total Calories

Day 60

Breakfast

6 oz. of coconut yogurt with 1 cup of blackberries and 1 oz. of sliced Brazil nuts (277 calories)

Snack

1 large banana (121 calories)

Lunch

2 cups shredded romaine lettuce tossed in 2 tbsp. Caesar dressing and topped with 5 grilled shrimp, 1 tbsp. grated Parmesan cheese, and ¼ cup croutons (271 calories)

Snack

1 roasted artichoke with 1 tbsp. of Greek yogurt mixed with lemon and garlic for dipping (72 calories)

Dinner

Roast one small butternut squash until fork tender, then remove skin. Sauté onions and garlic, add chopped up squash with 2 cups of vegetable stock. Add salt, pepper, thyme, and 2 tbsp. of Greek yogurt, let simmer for 15 minutes. Puree or leave chunky. Stir in 1 oz. cheddar cheese, and serve once cheese has melted. Serve with 1 cup of romaine lettuce tossed with balsamic vinegar (254 calories)

Treat

Banana Berry Ice Cream (page 310) (96 calories)

1,091 Total Calories

Day 61

Breakfast

Blend half of a red bell pepper with 1 cup of strawberries, 1 cup of spinach, ½ tbsp. of cashews, and 2 tbsp. of almond milk. Add water and ice for desired consistency (233 calories)

Snack

1 medium apple (95 calories)

Lunch

Mix 1 cup of cooked quinoa with ½ cup of grated beet, 1 cup of shredded spinach, 2 tbsp. of feta cheese, and 1 tbsp. of dried seaweed. Serve with 3 oz. of turkey breast (293 calories)

Snack

1 cup of baby carrots with 2 tbsp. of tzatziki (110 calories)

Dinner

Stir fry 3 oz. of chicken with ½ cup peas, carrots, corn, and broccoli seasoned with 1 tbsp. of soy sauce, garlic, and red chili flakes. Serve with ½ cup brown rice and 1 cup of spinach (313 calories)

Treat

Tiny Sparkling Margarita (page 344) (76 calories)

1,120 Total Calories

Day 62

Breakfast

6 oz. of coconut yogurt with 1 cup of blackberries and 1 oz. of sliced Brazil nuts (277 calories)

Snack

1 large banana (121 calories)

Lunch

1 slice of bread with 2 slices of deli ham, 1 slice of deli cheese, mustard, and 1 cup of kale with a drizzle of balsamic vinegar (294 calories)

Snack

1 roasted artichoke with 1 tbsp. of Greek yogurt mixed with lemon and garlic for dipping (72 calories)

Dinner

Grill 3 oz. of grass-fed steak, seasoned with salt, pepper, and sage. Serve with 3 baked baby red potatoes and 1 cup of steamed Swiss chard (257 calories)

Treat

Tiny Sparkling Margarita (page 344) (76 calories)

1,097 Total Calories

Day 63

Breakfast

Blend half of a red bell pepper with 1 cup of strawberries, 1 cup of spinach, ½ tbsp. of cashews, and 2 tbsp. of almond milk. Add water and ice for desired consistency (233 calories)

Snack

1 medium apple (95 calories)

Lunch

2 cups shredded romaine lettuce tossed in 2 tbsp. Caesar dressing and topped with 5 grilled shrimp, 1 tbsp. grated Parmesan cheese, and ¼ cup croutons (271 calories)

Snack

1 cup of baby carrots with 2 tbsp. of tzatziki (110 calories)

Dinner

Roast one small butternut squash until fork tender, then remove skin. Sauté onions and garlic, add chopped up squash with 2 cups of vegetable stock. Add salt, pepper, thyme, and 2 tbsp. of Greek yogurt, let simmer for 15 minutes. Puree or leave chunky. Stir in 1 oz. cheddar cheese, and serve once cheese has melted. Serve with 1 cup of romaine lettuce tossed with balsamic vinegar (254 calories)

Treat

Banana Berry Ice Cream (page 310) (96 calories)

1,059 Total Calories

Day 64

Breakfast

Mix 2 tbsp. chia seeds with 1 cup of almond milk, let set in refrigerator for at least 30 minutes, or overnight. Top with 1 cup of sliced plums and 2 sliced almonds (259 calories)

Snack

2 tbsp. of toasted walnuts (84 calories)

Lunch

Toss 2 cups of spinach with ¼ cup quinoa, ¼ cup cucumber, 3 oz. chopped grilled chicken, 1 tbsp. feta cheese, ¼ cup sliced red onion, and ½ cup cherry tomatoes. Drizzle with 1 tbsp. of balsamic vinegar (243 calories)

Snack

2 cups of air popped popcorn sprinkled with ½ tsp. cocoa powder and 1 tsp. unsweetened shredded coconut (101 calories)

Dinner

3 oz. grilled yellowtail tuna seasoned with pepper and fennel greens. Serve with sautéed fennel root, 1 cup green beans, and raw cucumber with a squeeze of lemon (246 calories)

Treat

Two 37 Calorie Brownie (page 325) and 1 cup of almond milk (104 calories)

1,037 Total Calories

Shopping List for Week 9

Produce:

- [ ] Romaine lettuce
- [ ] Kale – 2 cups
- [ ] Swiss chard – 2 cups
- [ ] Artichoke – 3
- [ ] Baby carrots – 4 cups
- [ ] Red bell pepper – 2
- [ ] Butternut squash – 3
- [ ] Baby red potatoes – 6
- [ ] Peas
- [ ] Carrots
- [ ] Corn
- [ ] Broccoli
- [ ] Onions
- [ ] Garlic
- [ ] Thyme
- [ ] Sage
- [ ] Beets
- [ ] Spinach – 9 cups
- [ ] Lime
- [ ] Blueberries – 9 oz.
- [ ] Blackberries – 3 cups
- [ ] Strawberries – 4 cups
- [ ] Apple – 4
- [ ] Banana – 3
- [ ] Lemon

Meat:

- [ ] Turkey breast – three 3 oz. pieces
- [ ] Deli ham – 4 slices
- [ ] Chicken – 6 oz.
- [ ] Grass-fed steak – two 3 oz. pieces
- [ ] Shrimp – 10

Etc.:

- [ ] Deli cheese – 2 slices
- [ ] Parmesan cheese – 2 tbsp.
- [ ] Cheddar cheese – 3 oz.
- [ ] Feta cheese – 6 oz.
- [ ] Fat free Greek yogurt – 16 oz.
- [ ] Coconut yogurt – 18 oz.
- [ ] Tzatziki – 8 tbsp.
- [ ] Silk unsweetened almond milk
- [ ] Bread (Udi's, Rudi's, Ezekiel 4:9)
- [ ] Brown rice – 1 cup
- [ ] Cashews – 2 tbsp.
- [ ] Brazil nuts – 3 oz.
- [ ] Dried seaweed – 3 tbsp.
- [ ] Quinoa – 3 cups
- [ ] Balsamic vinegar
- [ ] Mustard
- [ ] Caesar dressing
- [ ] Soy sauce
- [ ] Chili flakes
- [ ] Perrier (lime) – 6 oz.
- [ ] Tequila – 2 oz.

Day 65

Breakfast

Whisk ¼ cup of almond milk with 1 tsp. of agave nectar, ½ tsp. of vanilla extract, and 1 tsp. of cinnamon. Dip one slice of gluten-free bread into liquid and then onto a hot griddle. Grill French toast until crisp and top with two sliced strawberries (310 calories)

Snack

2 tbsp. of dried apricots (68 calories)

Lunch

Assemble 2 oz. of smoked salmon, 1 oz. of brie, 1 tbsp. of diced red onion, 1/3 cup of arugula, 5 almonds, and 5 crackers. Serve on a tray and mix and match ingredients (289 calories)

Snack

½ cup of cottage cheese topped with fresh ground pepper (81 calories)

Dinner

Halve a bell pepper and remove seeds and pith. Mix ¼ cup of cooked quinoa with ½ cup grated zucchini, ¼ cup chopped cauliflower, 2 chopped walnuts, and crushed sage. Fill bell pepper with mixture and sprinkle 1 tsp. of Parmesan cheese. Bake at 400 degrees until cheese is melted. Serve with 1 cup of chopped romaine lettuce tossed in lemon juice (296 calories)

Treat

Lemon Raspberry Belly Burning Sherbet (page 329) (101 calories)

1,145 Total Calories

Day 66

Breakfast

Mix 2 tbsp. chia seeds with 1 cup of almond milk, let set in refrigerator for at least 30 minutes, or overnight. Top with 1 cup of sliced plums and 2 sliced almonds (259 calories)

Snack

2 tbsp. of toasted walnuts (84 calories)

Lunch

Toss 2 cups of spinach with ¼ cup quinoa, ¼ cup cucumber, 3 oz. chopped grilled chicken, 1 tbsp. feta cheese, ¼ cup sliced red onion, and ½ cup cherry tomatoes. Drizzle with 1 tbsp. of balsamic vinegar (243 calories)

Snack

2 cups of air popped popcorn sprinkled with ½ tsp. cocoa powder and 1 tsp. unsweetened shredded coconut (101 calories)

Dinner

In a saucepan, sauté ½ cup of diced onion, one clove of minced garlic, 1/3 cup of diced bell pepper, and half of a diced jalapeno. Then add 3 oz. of ground turkey and brown. Stir in ½ cup of pinto beans, ½ cup of diced tomatoes, and 1–2 cups of chicken stock. Serve with 1 tsp. of sour cream and 1 tbsp. of sliced chives (304 calories)

Treat

Two 37 Calorie Brownie (page 325) and 1 cup of almond milk (104 calories)

1,095 Total Calories

Day 67

Breakfast

Whisk ¼ cup of almond milk with 1 tsp. of agave nectar, ½ tsp. of vanilla extract, and 1 tsp. of cinnamon. Dip one slice of bread into liquid and then onto a hot griddle. Grill French toast until crisp and top with two sliced strawberries (310 calories)

Snack

2 tbsp. of dried apricots (68 calories)

Lunch

Toss 2 oz. diced chicken with ¼ cup marinara sauce, ½ cup spinach, 1 tbsp. grated Parmesan, and 1 oz. goat cheese. Then assemble grilled cheese with 1 slice of bread. Grill until crispy and cheese is melted (332 calories)

Snack

½ cup of cottage cheese topped with fresh ground pepper (81 calories)

Dinner

Halve a bell pepper and remove seeds and pith. Mix ¼ cup of cooked quinoa with ½ cup grated zucchini, ¼ cup chopped cauliflower, 2 chopped walnuts, and crushed sage. Fill bell pepper with mixture and sprinkle 1 tsp. of Parmesan cheese. Bake at 400 degrees until cheese is melted. Serve with 1 cup of chopped romaine lettuce tossed in lemon juice (296 calories)

Treat

Lemon Raspberry Belly Burning Sherbet (page 329) (101 calories)

1,188 Total Calories

Day 68

Breakfast

Mix 2 tbsp. chia seeds with 1 cup of almond milk, let set in refrigerator for at least 30 minutes, or overnight. Top with 1 cup of sliced plums and 2 sliced almonds (259 calories)

Snack

2 tbsp. of toasted walnuts (84 calories)

Lunch

Toss 2 cups of spinach with ¼ cup quinoa, ¼ cup cucumber, 3 oz. chopped grilled chicken, 1 tbsp. feta cheese, ¼ cup sliced red onion, and ½ cup cherry tomatoes. Drizzle with 1 tbsp. of balsamic vinegar (243 calories)

Snack

2 cups of air popped popcorn sprinkled with ½ tsp. cocoa powder and 1 tsp. unsweetened shredded coconut (101 calories)

Dinner

3 oz. grilled yellowtail tuna seasoned with pepper and fennel greens. Serve with sautéed fennel root, 1 cup green beans, raw cucumber, and a squeeze of lemon (246 calories)

Treat

Two 37 Calorie Brownie (page 325) and 1 cup of almond milk (104 calories)

1,037 Total Calories

Day 69

Breakfast

Whisk ¼ cup of almond milk with 1 tsp. of agave nectar, ½ tsp. of vanilla extract, and 1 tsp. of cinnamon. Dip one slice of gluten-free bread into liquid and then onto a hot griddle. Grill French toast until crisp and top with two sliced strawberries (310 calories)

Snack

2 tbsp. of dried apricots (68 calories)

Lunch

Assemble 2 oz. of smoked salmon, 1 oz. of brie, 1 tbsp. of diced red onion, 1/3 cup of arugula, 5 almonds, and 5 crackers. Serve on a tray and mix and match ingredients (289 calories)

Snack

½ cup of cottage cheese topped with fresh ground pepper (81 calories)

Dinner

In a saucepan, sauté ½ cup of diced onion, one clove of minced garlic, 1/3 cup of diced bell pepper, and half of a diced jalapeño. Then add 3 oz. of ground turkey and brown. Stir in ½ cup of pinto beans, ½ cup of diced tomatoes, and 1–2 cups of chicken stock. Serve with 1 tsp. of sour cream and 1 tbsp. of sliced chives (304 calories)

Treat

Lemon Raspberry Belly Burning Sherbet (page 329) (101 calories)

1,153 Total Calories

Day 70

Breakfast

Mix 2 tbsp. chia seeds with 1 cup of almond milk, let set in refrigerator for at least 30 minutes, or overnight. Top with 1 cup of sliced plums and 2 sliced almonds (259 calories)

Snack

2 tbsp. of toasted walnuts (84 calories)

Lunch

Toss 2 oz. diced chicken with ¼ cup marinara sauce, ½ cup spinach, 1 tbsp. grated Parmesan, and 1 oz. goat cheese. Then assemble grilled cheese with 1 slice of bread. Grill until crispy and cheese is melted (332 calories)

Snack

2 cups of air popped popcorn sprinkled with ½ tsp. cocoa powder and 1 tsp. unsweetened shredded coconut (101 calories)

Dinner

Halve a bell pepper and remove seeds and pith. Mix ¼ cup of cooked quinoa with ½ cup grated zucchini, ¼ cup chopped cauliflower, 2 chopped walnuts, and crushed sage. Fill bell pepper with mixture and sprinkle 1 tsp. of Parmesan cheese. Bake at 400 degrees until cheese is melted. Serve with 1 cup of chopped romaine lettuce tossed in lemon juice (296 calories)

Treat

Two 37 Calorie Brownie (page 325) with 1 cup of almond milk (104 calories)

1,176 Total Calories

Produce:

- [ ] Spinach
- [ ] Romaine lettuce
- [ ] Arugula
- [ ] Cucumber
- [ ] Zucchini
- [ ] Cauliflower
- [ ] Red onion
- [ ] Onion
- [ ] Garlic
- [ ] Bell pepper – 3
- [ ] Jalapeño
- [ ] Cherry tomatoes
- [ ] Fennel
- [ ] Sage
- [ ] Chives
- [ ] Green beans – 2 cups
- [ ] Lemon
- [ ] Strawberries – 6
- [ ] Raspberries – 12 oz.
- [ ] Plums – 4 cups

Meat:

- [ ] Chicken – 13 oz.
- [ ] Yellowtail tuna – two 3 oz. pieces
- [ ] Smoked salmon – 4 oz.
- [ ] Ground turkey – 6 oz.

Etc.:

- [ ] Feta cheese – 3 tbsp.
- [ ] Brie – 2 oz.
- [ ] Parmesan cheese

- [ ] Goat cheese – 2 oz.
- [ ] Nonfat Greek yogurt
- [ ] Cottage cheese – 1 1/2 cups
- [ ] Sour cream
- [ ] Coconut milk
- [ ] Silk unsweetened almond milk
- [ ] Cocoa powder
- [ ] Old fashioned rolled oats
- [ ] Bread (Udi's, Rudi's, Ezekiel 4:9)
- [ ] Crackers
- [ ] Stevia
- [ ] Egg – 1
- [ ] Vanilla extract
- [ ] Baking powder
- [ ] Quinoa – 1 1/4 cup
- [ ] Chia seeds – 8 tbsp.
- [ ] Almonds – 18
- [ ] Walnuts – 9 tbsp.
- [ ] Honey
- [ ] Agave nectar
- [ ] Vanilla extract
- [ ] Cinnamon
- [ ] Dried apricots – 6 tbsp.
- [ ] Pinto beans – 1 cup
- [ ] Diced tomatoes
- [ ] Chicken stock
- [ ] Marinara sauce
- [ ] Balsamic vinegar
- [ ] Popcorn – 8 cups
- [ ] Cocoa powder
- [ ] Unsweetened shredded coconut – 4 tsp.

Day 71

Breakfast

Blend 1 cup almond milk, ½ frozen medium banana, 1 cup frozen mixed berries, and 1 tbsp. coconut yogurt. Pour into a bowl and top with ¼ cup blueberries, ¼ cup raspberries, and 1 tsp. pepitas (256 calories)

Snack

1 cup of grapes (104 calories)

Lunch

Mix 2 cups of romaine lettuce with ¼ cup grated carrot, ¼ cup beets, and ¼ cup radishes. Add 3 oz. of chopped chicken and a squeeze of lemon (268 calories)

Snack

2 cups of sugar snap peas (52 calories)

Dinner

Stuff a sweet potato with a mixture of a cup of kale, 1 tbsp. of grated cheese, and ¼ cup of diced bell pepper, and bake for 20–30 minutes at 375 degrees. Serve with a 3 oz. piece of pork loin (263 calories)

Treat

1 wedge of watermelon with 1 tbsp. of Greek yogurt spread across, a squeeze of lemon, and topped with torn mint leaves (84 calories)

1,027 Total Calories

Day 72

Breakfast

Toast 1 slice of bread and top with 1 tbsp. hummus, ¼ diced tomato, ¼ diced bell pepper, ¼ grated beet, 1 tsp. of lemon juice, salt, and pepper. Drizzle balsamic vinegar on top (276 calories)

Snack

1 medium pear (103 calories)

Lunch

California English Muffin (page 198). Enjoy both halves of the English muffin (268 calories)

Snack

1 cup strawberry kefir (140 calories)

Dinner

Preheat the oven to 500°F. Toss 5 large shrimp, ½ cup cannellini beans, ½ cup halved cherry tomatoes, ½ cup green beans, and ¼ cup sliced red bell peppers with ½ tbsp. olive oil and ½ tsp. lemon zest. Place on a baking sheet, and bake for 15 minutes. Place all ingredients in a bowl and top with 1 tbsp. crumbled reduced fat feta cheese (253 calories)

Treat

Chocolate Avocado Cookie (page 322) (67 calories)

1,107 Total Calories

Day 73

Breakfast

Blend 1 cup almond milk, ½ frozen medium banana, 1 cup frozen mixed berries, and 1 tbsp. coconut yogurt. Pour into a bowl and top with ¼ cup blueberries, ¼ cup raspberries, and 1 tsp. pepitas (256 calories)

Snack

1 cup of grapes (104 calories)

Lunch

Mix 2 cups of romaine lettuce with ¼ cup grated carrot, ¼ cup beets, and ¼ cup radishes. Add 3 oz. of chopped chicken and a squeeze of lemon (268 calories)

Snack

2 cups of sugar snap peas (52 calories)

Dinner

Sauté ¼ diced onion, 1 cup of diced tomatoes, and a clove of minced garlic. Mix in 3 oz. of ground turkey and fresh parsley. Serve over noodles (290 calories)

Treat

1 wedge of watermelon with 1 tbsp. of Greek yogurt spread across, a squeeze of lemon, and topped with torn mint leaves (84 calories)

1,054 Total Calories

Day 74

Breakfast

Toast 1 slice of bread and top with 1 tbsp. hummus, ¼ diced tomato, ¼ diced bell pepper, ¼ grated beet, 1 tsp. of lemon juice, salt, and pepper. Drizzle balsamic vinegar on top (276 calories)

Snack

1 medium pear (103 calories)

Lunch

In a bowl, toss together 2 cups spinach, 3 oz. diced chicken, ½ cup halved cherry tomatoes, ¼ cup sliced red onions, ¼ cup diced cucumber, 2 tbsp. garbanzo beans, 1 tbsp. feta cheese, and 1 tbsp. Greek salad dressing (300 calories)

Snack

1 cup strawberry kefir (140 calories)

Dinner

Stuff a sweet potato with a mixture of a cup of kale, 1 tbsp. of grated cheese, and ¼ cup of diced bell pepper and bake for 20–30 minutes at 375 degrees. Serve with a 3 oz. piece of pork loin (263 calories)

Treat

Chocolate Avocado Cookie (page 322) (67 calories)

1,149 Total Calories

Day 75

Breakfast

Blend 1 cup almond milk, ½ frozen medium banana, 1 cup frozen mixed berries, and 1 tbsp. coconut yogurt. Pour into a bowl and top with ¼ cup blueberries, ¼ cup raspberries, and 1 tsp. pepitas (256 calories)

Snack

1 cup of grapes (104 calories)

Lunch

Mix 2 cups of romaine lettuce with ¼ cup grated carrot, ¼ cup beets, and ¼ cup radishes. Add 3 oz. of chopped chicken and a squeeze of lemon (268 calories)

Snack

2 cups of sugar snap peas (52 calories)

Dinner

Preheat the oven to 500°F. Toss 5 large shrimp, ½ cup cannellini beans, ½ cup halved cherry tomatoes, ½ cup green beans, and ¼ cup sliced red bell peppers with ½ tbsp. olive oil and ½ tsp. lemon zest. Place on a baking sheet, and bake for 15 minutes. Place all ingredients in a bowl and top with 1 tbsp. crumbled reduced fat feta cheese (253 calories)

Treat

1 wedge of watermelon with 1 tbsp. of Greek yogurt spread across, a squeeze of lemon, and topped with torn mint leaves (84 calories)

1,017 Total Calories

Day 76

Breakfast

Toast 1 slice of bread and top with 1 tbsp. hummus, ¼ diced tomato, ¼ diced bell pepper, ¼ grated beet, 1 tsp. of lemon juice, salt, and pepper. Drizzle balsamic vinegar on top (276 calories)

Snack

1 medium pear (103 calories)

Lunch

In a bowl, toss together 2 cups spinach, 3 oz. diced chicken, ½ cup halved cherry tomatoes, ¼ cup sliced red onions, ¼ cup diced cucumber, 2 tbsp. garbanzo beans, 1 tbsp. feta cheese, and 1 tbsp. Greek salad dressing (300 calories)

Snack

1 cup strawberry kefir (140 calories)

Dinner

Stuff a sweet potato with a mixture of a cup of kale, 1 tbsp. of grated cheese, and ¼ cup of diced bell pepper and bake for 20–30 minutes at 375 degrees. Serve with a 3 oz. piece of pork loin (263 calories)

Treat

Chocolate Avocado Cookie (page 322) (67 calories)

1,149 Total Calories

Week 11

Day 77

Breakfast

Blend 1 cup almond milk, ½ frozen medium banana, 1 cup frozen mixed berries, and 1 tbsp. coconut yogurt. Pour into a bowl and top with ¼ cup blueberries, ¼ cup raspberries, and 1 tsp. pepitas (256 calories)

Snack

1 cup of grapes (104 calories)

Lunch

California English Muffin (page 198). Enjoy both halves of the English muffin (268 calories)

Snack

2 cups of sugar snap peas (52 calories)

Dinner

Sauté ¼ diced onion, 1 cup of diced tomatoes, and a clove of minced garlic. Mix in 3 oz. of ground turkey and fresh parsley. Serve over noodles (290 calories)

Treat

1 wedge of watermelon with 1 tbsp. of Greek yogurt spread across, a squeeze of lemon, and topped with torn mint leaves (84 calories)

1,052 Total Calories

Week 12

Day 78

Breakfast

Combine 2 tbsp. coconut milk, ¼ tsp. vanilla extract, ¼ tsp. almond extract, and ¼ tsp. cinnamon. Mix with 2 tbsp. chia seeds and let soak 4 hours to overnight. Once pudding is set, mix in 6 toasted pecans (244 calories)

Snack

1 large banana (121 calories)

Lunch

Scoop out a half of an avocado and mash the meat with salt and pepper, set aside. Lay a slice of prosciutto in the avocado shell and fill the rest with one egg, bake for 15–20 minutes at 350 degrees. Top baked egg with mashed avocado and chopped parsley (289 calories)

Snack

1 sliced cucumber with 2 tbsp. of green pitted olives and 2 tbsp. of crumbled feta cheese topped with ground pepper (115 calories)

Dinner

Grill 4 oz. of mahimahi seasoned with salt and pepper. Remove fish from pan and sauté one clove of minced garlic, one inch of grated ginger, and minced green chili until aromatic. Add 1 cup of spinach and cook until wilted. Plate mahimahi on bed of brown rice and top with spinach mixture (259 calories)

Treat

Vanilla Chai Spice (page 205) (175 calories)

1,203 Total Calories

Shopping List for Week 11

Produce:

- [ ] Spinach
- [ ] Cucumber
- [ ] Romaine lettuce
- [ ] Carrot
- [ ] Beet
- [ ] Bell pepper
- [ ] Radishes
- [ ] Tomatoes
- [ ] Cherry tomatoes – 1 cup
- [ ] Onion
- [ ] Red onion
- [ ] Garlic
- [ ] Green beans – 1 cup
- [ ] Sugar snap peas – 8 cups
- [ ] Sweet potatoes – 3
- [ ] Kale – 3 cups
- [ ] Mint
- [ ] Parsley
- [ ] Avocado
- [ ] Lemon
- [ ] Banana
- [ ] Blueberries – 1 cup
- [ ] Raspberries – 1 cup
- [ ] Grapes – 4 cups
- [ ] Watermelon
- [ ] Pear – 3

Meat:

- [ ] Chicken – 15 oz.
- [ ] Pork loin – three 3 oz. pieces
- [ ] Shrimp – 10
- [ ] Ground turkey – 6 oz.

Etc.:

- [ ] Feta cheese – 3 tbsp.
- [ ] Grated cheese – 3 tbsp.
- [ ] Parmesan cheese
- [ ] Nonfat Greek yogurt
- [ ] Strawberry kefir – 3 cups
- [ ] Coconut yogurt
- [ ] Coconut milk
- [ ] Coconut oil
- [ ] Olive oil
- [ ] Unsweetened cocoa powder
- [ ] Dark chocolate chunks
- [ ] Baking soda
- [ ] Silk unsweetened almond milk
- [ ] English muffin – 2 (Ener-G, Udi's, Ezekiel 4:9)
- [ ] Bread (Udi's, Rudi's, Ezekiel 4:9)
- [ ] Noodles – 1 cup
- [ ] Stevia
- [ ] Pepitas – 4 tsp.
- [ ] Cannellini beans – 1 cup
- [ ] Garbanzo beans – 4 tbsp.
- [ ] Greek salad dressing
- [ ] Hummus – 3 tbsp.
- [ ] Balsamic vinegar
- [ ] Frozen mixed berries

Day 79

Breakfast

Melrose Blueberry Muffins (page 194). Enjoy two muffins with 1 cup of blackberries tossed with 1 tbsp. unsweetened shredded coconut (252 calories)

Snack

1 cup of peaches with 5 almonds (95 calories)

Lunch

Sauté ½ cup of diced bell peppers, ¼ cup of onions, and ½ cup of grated zucchini and mix into 1 cup of quinoa. Top with 3 oz. of seared scallops (320 calories)

Snack

½ cup of sliced carrots with 1 tbsp. of sunflower seed butter (117 calories)

Dinner

Grill 3 oz. chicken breast coated in 1 tsp. of honey and spicy mustard. Serve with 1 cup shredded cabbage, collard greens, and carrots soaked in apple cider vinegar. Also, 1 baked sweet potato (261 calories)

Treat

1 oz. of cacao (145 calories)

1,190 Total Calories

Day 80

Breakfast

Combine 2 tbsp. coconut milk, ¼ tsp. vanilla extract, ¼ tsp. almond extract, and ¼ tsp. cinnamon. Mix with 2 tbsp. chia seeds and let soak 4 hours to overnight. Once pudding is set, mix in 6 toasted pecans (244 calories)

Snack

1 large banana (121 calories)

Lunch

In a bowl, mix together 2 cups cooked spaghetti squash, ¼ cup pesto sauce, and 1 cup raw spinach. Top with 3 oz. chopped chicken breast and 1 tsp. Parmesan cheese (263 calories)

Snack

1 sliced cucumber with 2 tbsp. of green pitted olives and 2 tbsp. of crumbled feta cheese topped with ground pepper (115 calories)

Dinner

Grill 4 oz. of mahimahi seasoned with salt and pepper. Remove fish from pan and sauté one clove of minced garlic, one inch of grated ginger, and minced green chili until aromatic. Add 1 cup of spinach and cook until wilted. Plate mahimahi on bed of brown rice and top with spinach mixture (259 calories)

Treat

Vanilla Chai Spice (page 205) (175 calories)

1,177 Total Calories

Day 81

Breakfast

Melrose Blueberry Muffins (page 194). Enjoy two muffins with 1 cup of blackberries tossed with 1 tbsp. unsweetened shredded coconut (252 calories)

Snack

1 cup of peaches with 5 almonds (95 calories)

Lunch

Sauté ½ cup of diced bell peppers, ¼ cup of onions, and ½ cup of grated zucchini and mix into 1 cup of quinoa. Top with 3 oz. of seared scallops (320 calories)

Snack

½ cup of sliced carrots with 1 tbsp. of sunflower seed butter (117 calories)

Dinner

Steam 1 cup of cauliflower with vegetable stock. Mix ¼ cup of grated cheddar cheese and 1 tbsp. of Greek yogurt and stir in hot cauliflower then top with Parmesan cheese. Sauté asparagus with lemon zest as a side (304 calories)

Treat

1 oz. of cacao (145 calories)

1,233 Total Calories

Day 82

Breakfast

Combine 2 tbsp. coconut milk, ¼ tsp. vanilla extract, ¼ tsp. almond extract, and ¼ tsp. cinnamon. Mix with 2 tbsp. chia seeds and let soak 4 hours to overnight. Once pudding is set, mix in 6 toasted pecans (244 calories)

Snack

1 large banana (121 calories)

Lunch

Scoop out a half of an avocado and mash the meat with salt and pepper, set aside. Lay a slice of prosciutto in the avocado shell and fill the rest with one egg, bake for 15–20 minutes at 350 degrees. Top baked egg with mashed avocado and chopped parsley (289 calories)

Snack

1 sliced cucumber with 2 tbsp. of green pitted olives and 2 tbsp. of crumbled feta cheese topped with ground pepper (115 calories)

Dinner

Grill 4 oz. of mahimahi seasoned with salt and pepper. Remove fish from pan and sauté one clove of minced garlic, one inch of grated ginger, and minced green chili until aromatic. Add 1 cup of spinach and cook until wilted. Plate mahimahi on bed of brown rice and top with spinach mixture (259 calories)

Treat

Vanilla Chai Spice (page 205) (175 calories)

1,203 Total Calories

Day 83

Breakfast

Melrose Blueberry Muffins (page 194). Enjoy two muffins with 1 cup of blackberries tossed with 1 tbsp. unsweetened shredded coconut (252 calories)

Snack

1 cup of peaches with 5 almonds (95 calories)

Lunch

In a bowl, mix together 2 cups cooked spaghetti squash, ¼ cup pesto sauce, and 1 cup raw spinach. Top with 3 oz. chopped chicken breast and 1 tsp. Parmesan cheese (263 calories)

Snack

½ cup of sliced carrots with 1 tbsp. of sunflower seed butter (117 calories)

Dinner

Grill 3 oz. chicken breast coated in 1 tsp. of honey and spicy mustard. Serve with 1 cup shredded cabbage, collard greens, and carrots soaked in apple cider vinegar. Also, 1 baked sweet potato (261 calories)

Treat

1 oz. of cacao (145 calories)

1,133 Total Calories

Day 84

Breakfast

Combine 2 tbsp. coconut milk, ¼ tsp. vanilla extract, ¼ tsp. almond extract, and ¼ tsp. cinnamon. Mix with 2 tbsp. chia seeds and let soak 4 hours to overnight. Once pudding is set, mix in 6 toasted pecans (244 calories)

Snack

1 large banana (121 calories)

Lunch

Sauté ½ cup of diced bell peppers, ¼ cup of onions, and ½ cup of grated zucchini and mix into 1 cup of quinoa. Top with 3 oz. of seared scallops (320 calories)

Snack

1 sliced cucumber with 2 tbsp. of green pitted olives and 2 tbsp. of crumbled feta cheese topped with ground pepper (115 calories)

Dinner

Steam 1 cup of cauliflower with vegetable stock. Mix ¼ cup of grated cheddar cheese and 1 tbsp. of Greek yogurt and stir in hot cauliflower then top with Parmesan cheese. Sauté asparagus with lemon zest as a side (304 calories)

Treat

Vanilla Chai Spice (page 205) (175 calories)

1,279 Total Calories

Shopping List for Week 12

Produce:

- ☐ Spinach
- ☐ Asparagus
- ☐ Cabbage – 2 cups
- ☐ Cauliflower
- ☐ Collard greens – 2 cups
- ☐ Sweet potato – 2
- ☐ Spaghetti squash
- ☐ Cucumber
- ☐ Bell pepper
- ☐ Avocado
- ☐ Carrots
- ☐ Ginger
- ☐ Garlic
- ☐ Onion
- ☐ Zucchini
- ☐ Green chili
- ☐ Parsley
- ☐ Lemon
- ☐ Blueberries
- ☐ Banana – 6
- ☐ Blackberries – 3 cups
- ☐ Peaches – 3 cups

Meat:

- ☐ Chicken – 12 oz.
- ☐ Ground turkey – 6 oz.
- ☐ Prosciutto – 2 slices
- ☐ Mahimahi – three 4 oz. pieces
- ☐ Scallops – 9 oz.

Etc.:

- ☐ Feta cheese – 8 tbsp.
- ☐ Cheddar cheese – 1/2 cup

- ☐ Parmesan cheese – 4 tsp.
- ☐ Greek yogurt – 2 tbsp.
- ☐ Coconut milk
- ☐ Coconut oil
- ☐ Baking soda
- ☐ Buckwheat flour
- ☐ Silk unsweetened almond milk
- ☐ Brown rice
- ☐ Quinoa – 3 cups
- ☐ Unsweetened shredded coconut
- ☐ Eggs – 2
- ☐ Almonds – 15
- ☐ Green olives
- ☐ Stevia
- ☐ Cinnamon
- ☐ Cardamom
- ☐ Clove
- ☐ Nutmeg
- ☐ Brazil nuts
- ☐ Pecans – 24
- ☐ Vanilla extract
- ☐ Almond extract
- ☐ Sunflower seed butter – 3 tbsp.
- ☐ Chia seeds – 8 tbsp.
- ☐ Apple cider vinegar
- ☐ Balsamic vinegar
- ☐ Honey – 2 tsp.
- ☐ Spicy mustard – 2 tsp.
- ☐ Pesto
- ☐ Vegetable stock
- ☐ Nonstick cooking spray
- ☐ Cacao – 3 oz.
- ☐ Muffin cups
- ☐ Pea protein

Thyroid Boost Week Meal Planner

Day 1

Breakfast

1 cup plain oatmeal cooked with water, topped with 1 cup almond milk, ½ cup sliced strawberries, and 1 chopped Brazil nut (256 calories)

Snack

1 tbsp. of Brazil nuts with 1 tbsp. of dried cranberries (139 calories)

Lunch

3 oz. of shredded chicken breast mixed with 1 diced celery, ½ grated cucumber, ½ diced jalapeño, 1 oz. grated cheddar cheese, and 2 tbsp. of Greek yogurt. Season with ground mustard, garlic, salt, and pepper. Fill romaine lettuce leaf with mixture (288 calories)

Snack

Hard-boiled egg (78 calories)

Dinner

3 oz. of grilled halibut seasoned with fennel and celery seeds topped with one diced tomato, parsley, and capers. Serve with ½ cup of brown rice and 5 spears of asparagus (273 calories)

Treat

1 cup of strawberries with ½ oz. melted dark chocolate (131 calories)

1,165 Total Calories

Day 2

Breakfast

Blend 2 cups of spinach with 1 cup cranberries, 6 oz. coconut yogurt, 2 Brazil nuts, and 1 tsp. of acai powder with 8 oz. water and 1 cup of ice (265 calories)

Snack

2 cups of strawberries (92 calories)

Lunch

2 cups of spinach tossed with 1 sliced hard-boiled egg, 2 slices of chopped turkey bacon, ½ cup sliced mushrooms, sliced red onion, and 2 tbsp. of mashed avocado with lemon zest and pepper (262 calories)

Snack

1 cup each of sliced carrots and celery with 2 tbsp. cream cheese mixed with 1 tbsp. of dried seaweed and fresh dill (91 calories)

Dinner

3 oz. of roasted turkey breast with one baked sweet potato rubbed with coconut oil. Serve with ½ cup of navy beans mixed with sauteed collard greens and 1 tbsp. of dried cranberries seasoned with ground mustard, lemon zest, rosemary, and cayenne pepper (299 calories)

Treat

6 oz. of Greek yogurt with ½ cup of raspberries and 1 tsp. of unsweetened shredded coconut (119 calories)

1,128 Total Calories

Day 3

Breakfast

1 cup plain oatmeal cooked with water, topped with 1 cup almond milk, ½ cup sliced strawberries, and 1 chopped Brazil nut (256 calories)

Snack

1 tbsp. of Brazil nuts with 1 tbsp. of dried cranberries (139 calories)

Lunch

1 cup of spinach and 1 cup of romaine lettuce tossed with 3 oz. of tuna, 1 diced baked red potato, ¼ cup of grated carrot, ½ diced bell pepper, topped with lemon juice (242 calories)

Snack

Hard-boiled egg (78 calories)

Dinner

3 oz. of grass-fed beef sautéed with 1 diced tomato, ½ grated beet, diced onion, and garlic. Add 1 tsp. of tomato paste to thicken sauce, then add 1 large spiralized zucchini and 1 oz. of grated Parmesan cheese. Top with parsley and serve with 1 cup of romaine lettuce tossed with balsamic vinegar (293 calories)

Treat

1 cup of strawberries with ½ oz. melted dark chocolate (131 calories)

1,139 Total Calories

Day 4

Breakfast

Blend 2 cups of spinach with 1 cup cranberries, 6 oz. coconut yogurt, 2 Brazil nuts, and 1 tsp. of acai powder with 8 oz. water and 1 cup of ice (265 calories)

Snack

2 cups of strawberries (92 calories)

Lunch

2 cups of spinach tossed with 1 sliced hard-boiled egg, 2 slices of chopped turkey bacon, ½ cup sliced mushrooms, sliced red onion, and two tablespoons of mashed avocado with lemon zest and pepper (262 calories)

Snack

1 cup each of sliced carrots and celery with 2 tbsp. cream cheese mixed with 1 tbsp. of dried seaweed and fresh dill (91 calories)

Dinner

3 oz. of grilled halibut seasoned with fennel and celery seeds topped with 1 diced tomato, parsley, and capers. Serve with ½ cup of brown rice and 5 spears of asparagus (273 calories)

Treat

6 oz. of Greek yogurt with ½ cup of raspberries and 1 tsp. of unsweetened shredded coconut (119 calories)

1,102 Total Calories

Day 5

Breakfast

1 cup plain oatmeal cooked with water, topped with 1 cup almond milk, ½ cup sliced strawberries, and 1 chopped Brazil nut (256 calories)

Snack

1 tbsp. of Brazil nuts with 1 tbsp. of dried cranberries (139 calories)

Lunch

3 oz. of shredded chicken breast mixed with 1 diced celery, ½ grated cucumber, ½ diced jalapeño, 1 oz. grated cheddar cheese, and 2 tbsp. of Greek yogurt. Season with ground mustard, garlic, salt, and pepper. Fill romaine lettuce leaf with mixture (288 calories)

Snack

Hard-boiled egg (78 calories)

Dinner

3 oz. of grass-fed beef sautéed with 1 diced tomato, ½ grated beet, diced onion, and garlic. Add 1 tsp. of tomato paste to thicken sauce, then add 1 large spiralized zucchini and 1 oz. of grated Parmesan cheese. Top with parsley and serve with 1 cup of romaine lettuce tossed with balsamic vinegar (293 calories)

Treat

1 cup of strawberries with ½ oz. melted dark chocolate (131 calories)

1,185 Total Calories

Day 6

Breakfast

Blend 2 cups of spinach with 1 cup cranberries, 6 oz. coconut yogurt, 2 Brazil nuts, and 1 tsp. of acai powder with 8 oz. water and 1 cup of ice (265 calories)

Snack

2 cups of strawberries (92 calories)

Lunch

1 cup of spinach and 1 cup of romaine lettuce tossed with 3 oz. of tuna, one diced baked red potato, ¼ cup of grated carrot, ½ diced bell pepper, topped with lemon juice (242 calories)

Snack

1 cup each of sliced carrots and celery with 2 tbsp. of cream cheese mixed with 1 tbsp. of dried seaweed and fresh dill (91 calories)

Dinner

3 oz. of roasted turkey breast with 1 baked sweet potato rubbed with coconut oil. Serve with ½ cup of navy beans mixed with sautéed collard greens and 1 tbsp. of dried cranberries seasoned with ground mustard, lemon zest, rosemary, and cayenne pepper (299 calories)

Treat

6 oz. of Greek yogurt with ½ cup of raspberries and 1 tsp. of unsweetened shredded coconut (119 calories)

1,108 Total Calories

Day 7

Breakfast

1 cup plain oatmeal cooked with water, topped with 1 cup almond milk, ½ cup sliced strawberries, and 1 chopped Brazil nut (256 calories)

Snack

1 tbsp. of Brazil nuts with 1 tbsp. of dried cranberries (139 calories)

Lunch

3 oz. of shredded chicken breast mixed with 1 diced celery, ½ grated cucumber, ½ diced jalapeño, 1 oz. grated cheddar cheese, and 2 tbsp. of Greek yogurt. Season with ground mustard, garlic, salt, and pepper. Fill romaine lettuce leaf with mixture (288 calories)

Snack

Hard-boiled egg (78 calories)

Dinner

3 oz. of grilled halibut seasoned with fennel and celery seeds topped with 1 diced tomato, parsley, and capers. Serve with ½ cup of brown rice and 5 spears of asparagus (273 calories)

Treat

1 cup of strawberries with ½ oz. melted dark chocolate (131 calories)

1,165 Total Calories

Shopping List for Thyroid Boost Meal Planner

Produce:

- [ ] Celery
- [ ] Spinach
- [ ] Carrots
- [ ] Asparagus
- [ ] Collard greens
- [ ] Romaine lettuce
- [ ] Bell pepper
- [ ] Beet
- [ ] Tomatoes – 6
- [ ] Mushrooms
- [ ] Red onions
- [ ] Zucchini – 2
- [ ] Avocado
- [ ] Parsley
- [ ] Rosemary
- [ ] Dill
- [ ] Garlic
- [ ] Cucumber
- [ ] Sweet potatoes – 2
- [ ] Red potatoes – 2
- [ ] Jalapeño
- [ ] Strawberries
- [ ] Cranberries – 3 cups
- [ ] Raspberries
- [ ] Lemon

Meat:

- [ ] Chicken – 9 oz.
- [ ] Halibut – three 3 oz. pieces
- [ ] Turkey bacon – 4 slices
- [ ] Turkey breast – two 3 oz. pieces
- [ ] Tuna – 6 oz.
- [ ] Grass-fed ground beef – 6 oz.

Etc.:

- [ ] Cheddar cheese – 3 oz.
- [ ] Parmesan cheese – 2 oz.
- [ ] Greek yogurt
- [ ] Coconut yogurt – 18 oz.
- [ ] Cream cheese
- [ ] Silk unsweetened almond milk
- [ ] Egg – 6
- [ ] Oatmeal
- [ ] Brown rice
- [ ] Brazil nuts
- [ ] Dried cranberries
- [ ] Ground mustard
- [ ] Fennel seeds
- [ ] Celery seeds
- [ ] Coconut oil
- [ ] Balsamic vinegar
- [ ] Capers
- [ ] Dark chocolate – 2 oz.
- [ ] Acai powder
- [ ] Dried seaweed
- [ ] Navy beans
- [ ] Unsweetened shredded coconut

5 Your 12-Week Fitness Guide

As a celebrity fitness trainer, I know the stigmas that come with working out. People often picture gym memberships and personal trainers, spending mindless hours on the elliptical, crunches upon crunches…the list could go on. While there are those who enjoy this type of exercise, it's not for everyone. It's also not required for true health and fitness.

In fact, working out can be short—and fun! And more importantly, the exercise I'm about to introduce to you comes from absolute, unequivocal evidence that you can—and will—trigger your body's most aggressive belly fat-burning mechanisms.

Here's a brief chemistry lesson: To burn off fat, your body creates an enzyme called hormone-sensitive lipase (HSL). HSL breaks down fat and tells your body to burn it up as fuel. If your body isn't making a whole lot of HSL, you're not going to break down much fat. If HSL is high, your body becomes a fat-burning furnace. A whole bunch of hormones have an effect on HSL—testosterone, cortisol, estrogen, and human growth hormone—but the most distinctive are catecholamines.

Catecholamines are a group of hormones, including dopamine, histamine, adrenaline, and more, that unleash HSL like nothing else. The most important of these for our fat-burning purposes is adrenaline, which is the main hormone released when we are triggered by a threat, surprise, or danger—often referred to as the fight or flight response. During this reaction, adrenaline is released, speeding the heart rate, slowing digestion, shunting blood flow to major muscle groups, and changing various other nervous system functions. When this happens, it gives your body a burst of energy and strength. It's this reaction that pushes your body into a state where fat stores start breaking down so that they can be used for fuel.

Here's the scenario: Your body believes it's in danger, it's stressed, and it knows that it has to do everything possible to protect and save itself. So what does it do? Your body releases all the fat possible so it can start using it as fuel and keep you going even if you don't have the energy to do it for yourself.

That very same adrenaline makes it possible to spot-reduce your abdominal area because your belly region is loaded with more catecholamine receptors than any other part of your body. In other words, you have your own personal army of fat burners living right there in the place they're needed the most. But if you're used to doing cardio on cruise control—or not exercising at all—your army has been doing a lot more snoozing than fighting. So how do we wake it up without actually putting you in grave danger? Catecholamines respond most to one type of exercise technique, which is the very basis for the exercise routines here. This type of exercise is called High-Intensity Interval Training (HIIT). According to a groundbreaking study published in the *Journal of Obesity*, at the University of South Wales, women who performed HIIT just three times a week lost more subcutaneous and abdominal fat than those who did low-impact exercise. **They spot-reduced their belly fat**, which isn't supposed to be possible according to older research, but now we know that HIIT stimulates the catecholamine receptors in your abdominal muscles. You turn on the receptors and the adrenaline, which mobilizes the fat in your belly and burns it up during your workout.

HIIT is more often referred to as intense interval training, which is simply a workout made up of alternating short intense anaerobic exercise with less intense recovery periods. I've designed these workouts to do just this. You'll simply perform

Why Most Exercise Fails at Burning Fat

Many health experts recommend that you get an hour or more of moderate-level exercise each day. But did you know that hour is really intended to maintain weight and health, not to lose fat or inches and not to fight disease? There is actually no research that backs up using this type of exercise specifically for weight loss. I'm not saying that exercising for an hour a day is bad for you—it's certainly not. Any time you move, your mental and physical health will benefit. But your belly fat will still be there.

the 4 circuit exercises for 7 minutes, take a quick rest, then perform the other 4 circuit exercises for another 7 minutes, rest, and repeat the entire workout a second time. By doing this just three times a week, you'll burn belly fat, boost your heart rate, and condition every muscle in your body. This is all it takes to set off catecholamines, especially adrenaline, and start burning belly fat.

Do these moves three times a week on nonconsecutive days (Monday, Wednesday, Friday, or Tuesday, Thursday, and Saturday). These workouts are all you need to activate the powerful fat-mobilizing catecholamines and burn off belly fat in a way that's far more effective than working out every single day. Plus, because of the intense nature of your workout, you need a day off in between workouts. If you're working as hard as you should be during these 28 minutes, three times a week, your body will need time to recover. Remember that muscle is built when you're resting, not when you're working out.

Be active on rest days

I want to be clear that I'm not suggesting that you should do this routine and then settle into your sofa until the next workout time rolls around. Before obesity and being overweight were an issue for us humans, we walked about 10 miles per day— that was the status quo! While I'm not suggesting that you block out three hours a day to stroll, I am suggesting that you move more and sit less. It's good for your circulation, stabilizes your mood, helps reduce cravings, and increases impulse control. On page 155 in this chapter, you'll find several suggestions for what to do on your active rest days to keep your mind and body feeling its best.

Exercise before you eat

With Tiny and Full™ Fitness, our goal is blasting away belly fat—and body fat in general—as fast as possible. So we're going to do everything we can to make each exercise session as efficient as possible at fat burning. Exercising first thing in the morning—before eating—allows you to accomplish this (and it's a technique that's been practiced by the bodybuilding community for decades).

Because you'll be working at such an intense level, I can tell you that you definitely won't be able to do so on anywhere near a full stomach. Besides, you'll burn more fat if you make sure to not eat for three hours before your workout.

In a study published in the *International Journal of Obesity,* researchers found that women who ate three hours before exercising burned more fat than a second group of women who ate one hour before an identical exercise session. Each participant performed two separate workout sessions on nonconsecutive days (exactly like you will be with these workouts), and all women ate identical meals and burned the same amount of calories.

Focus on Form

When you get tired and your muscles start burning, you may curse every single rep you have left to do. Pay attention! This is when your form starts to suffer. Shoulders roll forward, knees dip where they're not supposed to dip. Bad form can cause bad injuries, so be sure to follow these tips:

- Follow exercise descriptions carefully.

- Look in a wall mirror, or invest in a freestanding one (stores like Target have these for $5—they're lightweight and don't even need to be mounted). Use it every time you work out, or find a buddy to work out with you. You can be each other's mirrors.

- While you should be moving as fast as you can to make sure you're reaching the correct level of intensity, it's better to do fewer proper reps than many sloppy ones. As you get stronger and more accustomed to the moves, your pace will pick up.

- If you absolutely must rest to regain proper form, do it. As the weeks fly by, you'll be able to skip rest periods.

What you'll need for the Tiny and Full™ workouts

Make sure you are set up with the following:

- Good fitness shoes

- A room with space to move

- Your favorite music

Warming up and cooling down

Before and after every workout, take a few minutes to move your body around to get it ready for your workout and to transition back down when you are done. Walk in place, jog gently, circle your arms, lift and lower your shoulders, lift and lower your knees, or dance around—any sort of movement will do.

Let's start!

I have outlined 9 different workouts that you will use for the 12 weeks. There is a calendar that organizes the workouts so you'll know exactly what to do each week. Remember, each workout consists of 2 cycles of 4 moves.

Here's how each workout should play out:

Warm Up

Cycle 1
Rest 30–60 seconds

Cycle 2
Rest 30–60 seconds

Cycle 1
Rest 30–60 seconds

Cycle 2
Rest 30–60 seconds

Cool Down

It's time to get your move on!

Workout 1

Cycle 1

Jump rope
100 reps

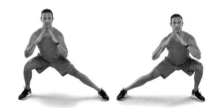

Stand up straight with a slight bend in your knees and hands by your sides. Pretend you're holding a jump rope, and make small circle movements with your hands while quickly jumping up and down on your toes, as you would if you were using a real jump rope.

Side-to-side lunge
30 reps (15 per side)

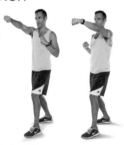

Stand with your feet hip-width apart. Take a giant step out to your right with your right leg and bend your knee to a 90-degree angle. You want to land with your heel first, followed by your forefoot. Press into your foot to return to starting position.

Power punch
60 reps
(30 per side)

Stand with feet shoulder-width apart, and right leg slightly in front of the left. Raise your fists up and keep your elbows in and pointing down. Punch your left fist out and across your body, while rotating your torso. Keep your chest lifted. Switch arm and leg stance after 10 punches. Punch as fast and furiously as you can.

Hip hinger
20 reps

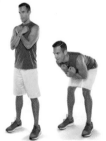

Stand with your feet shoulder-width apart. Shift your weight to your heels and push your hips back as you hinge forward at the hips, keeping your knees slightly bent, until your torso is at about a 45-degree angle. Keep your head, neck, shoulders, chest, and torso in one line, abs engaged and tight. Contract your butt muscles as you lift back up from your hips. Repeat.

Cycle 2

High knees
50 reps

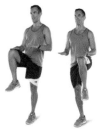

Stand with your feet hip-width apart, chest lifted, shoulders back and down. Place your hands out in front of you with your arms bent at 90 degrees. Drive your right knee toward your chest and quickly place it back on the ground. Immediately drive your left knee toward your chest. Continue alternating quickly.

Wide squats
15 reps

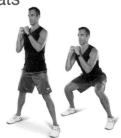

Stand with your feet wider than shoulder width. "Sit down," pushing your buttocks back and keeping your chest up, until your thighs are parallel to the floor. Make sure your knees stay behind your toes. Pause for a second, and then stand up quickly. Repeat, and try to get lower with each squat.

Side steps
30 reps
(15 per side)

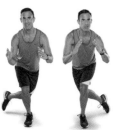

Start off with your feet shoulder-width apart, and body lowered as if you're doing a slight squat. Stay at this height during the entire move (instead of popping up and down). Shuffle feet from side to side by taking one foot out and putting all of your weight on it. Step back and then take the other foot out. Alternate legs.

Russian twists
30 reps (15 per side)

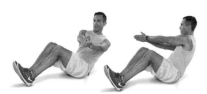

Sit with knees bent and feet together on the floor. Keeping your head, shoulders, and chest all in one line, engage your abs and lean back about 45 degrees, lifting your feet a few inches off the floor. Twist your torso and arms as one unit from side to side, keeping your abdominal muscles engaged. Continue moving side to side.

Cycle 1

Bicycle
40 reps

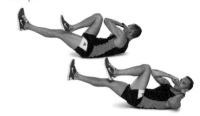

Lie down on your back with knees in toward your chest and hands behind your head. Bring your right elbow toward the left knee while right leg straightens. Alternate sides just like you're pedaling on a bike. Move as quickly as possible, making sure to keep abs braced and tight throughout the movement.

Plank row
1 minute

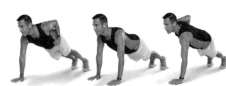

Start in push-up position. Draw right elbow up so that hand comes to rib cage. Lower to starting position, and repeat on left side. Alternate sides, dropping to knees when necessary.

Slalom
40 reps
(20 per side)

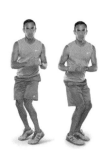

Start with both feet together and your hands in front of you (elbows at your side), as if you're holding ski poles. Jump and twist your upper body to the right and your feet to the left. Then jump up and twist your upper body to the left and your feet to the right. Repeat.

Military press
30 reps

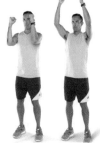

Stand with your feet shoulder-width apart. Make fists and put your elbows at 90 degrees. Raise your arms up above your head. Lower your arms back to 90 degrees. Repeat.

Cycle 2

Cross jacks
30 reps

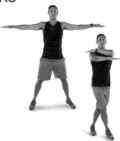

Stand tall with your feet shoulder-width apart and extend your arms straight out to either side with palms facing down. Jump and cross your right arm over your left and your right foot over your left. Jump back to the starting position, then cross with the opposite arm and foot. Continue alternating sides without rest.

Deep overhead squat
30 reps

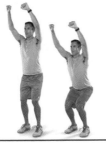

Stand with your feet shoulder-width apart and hands above your head. Bend your knees and squat. Repeat. Keep your hands above your head the whole time.

Running in place
1 minute

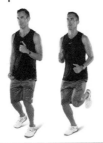

Start jogging in place as fast as you can. Lift your knees up to increase intensity—your thighs can go as high as being parallel to the ground. Remember to move your arms back and forth to boost your heart rate even more. Keep your chest lifted and your head and neck in line with your shoulders.

Squats
20 reps

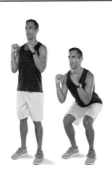

Stand with your feet shoulder-width apart, toes pointed out slightly. Bend your knees to sit back, lowering yourself until your thighs are parallel to the floor. Make sure that your knees stay behind your toes, and keep your chest lifted and your head in line with your neck and shoulders. Pause for a second, and then stand back up to starting position. Repeat.

Cycle 1

Side steps
30 reps
(15 per side)

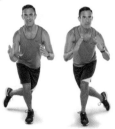

Start off with your feet shoulder-width apart, body lowered as if you're doing a slight squat. Stay at this height during the entire move (instead of popping up and down). Shuffle feet from side to side by taking one foot out and putting all of your weight on it. Step back and then take the other foot out. Alternate legs.

Curtsy lunge
20 (10 per side)

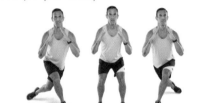

Stand with feet hip-width apart. Take a giant step with your left leg and cross it behind your right. Bend your knees until your right thigh is nearly parallel to the floor. Make sure that your front knee doesn't jut out over your front toes. Press back up to starting position. Step back with other leg. Alternate sides.

Walking lunges
30 reps
(15 per side)

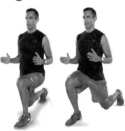

Stand with feet together. Take a giant step forward with your right foot and align knee over ankle. Bend your back knee down close to the floor, heel lifted. Before your back knee touches the floor, push up with your back left leg, simultaneously bringing your left foot together with your right. Alternate sides without pausing.

Push-up to knee tuck
10 reps (5 per side)

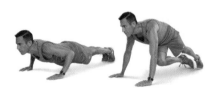

Start in standard push-up position. As you lower your body, bring your right knee up into a tucked position. As you raise your body, bring the leg back out so it's straight and toes are on floor again. Alternate sides.

Workout 3

Power punch
60 reps
(30 per side)

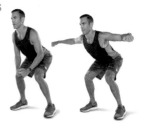

Stand with feet shoulder-width apart, and right leg slightly in front of the left. Raise your fists up and keep your elbows in. Punch your left fist out and across your body, while rotating your torso. Keep your chest lifted and abs tight. Switch arm and leg stance after 10 punches. Punch as fast and furiously as you can.

Bent over lateral raise
15 reps

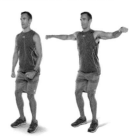

Stand with your legs shoulder-width apart and your knees slightly bent. Lean forward from your hips, keeping your head in line with your shoulders. Let your arms hang. Begin to raise arms to a horizontal position. Pause and contract the shoulder and back muscles. Return to starting position. Repeat.

Lateral shoulder raises
20 reps

Stand with your feet shoulder-width apart and arms at your side. With your back straight, raise arms out to shoulder height with elbows leading the movement. Stop lifting when your arms are at shoulder height. Your upper body should resemble a T. Lower arms toward the starting position in a slow and controlled manner.

Side-to-side lunge
30 reps (15 per side)

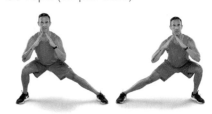

Stand with your feet hip-width apart. Take a giant step out to your right with your right leg and bend your knee to a 90-degree angle. You want to land with your heel first, followed by your forefoot. Press into your foot to return to starting position.

141

Your 12-Week Fitness Guide

Cycle 1

Lateral shuffle
50 reps

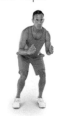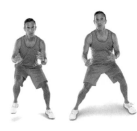

Stand with feet a little wider than hip-distance apart. Shuffle sideways to the right, pretending that you are stepping into a ladder on the floor. Step both feet into the first square of the ladder, staying on the balls of your feet. Move your arms to mimic a running motion. After 4 seconds, switch directions and shuffle to the left.

Plank row
1 minute

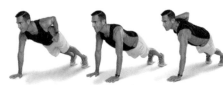

Start in push-up position. Draw right elbow up so that hand comes to rib cage. Lower to starting position, and repeat on left side. Alternate sides, dropping to knees when necessary.

Jump and butt kick
20 reps

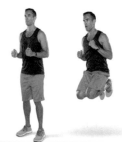

Start by standing up tall. Jump up as high as you can and kick your heels back to your butt so that the two make contact. Land on both feet. Jump back up into the same movement immediately after hitting the ground.

Lateral shoulder raises
20 reps

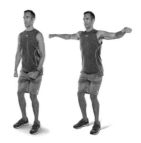

Stand with your feet shoulder-width apart and arms at your side. With your back straight, raise arms out to shoulder height with elbows leading the movement. Stop lifting when your arms are at shoulder height. Your upper body should resemble a T. Lower arms toward the starting position in a slow and controlled manner.

Workout 4

Cycle 2

Ski jumps
24 reps
(12 per side)

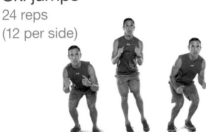

Stand with feet slightly apart, elbows bent as if you were holding ski poles. Jump to the right with both feet. Without pausing, jump back to starting position, and immediately jump again, this time to the other side. Continue alternating, swinging your elbows back and forth to help with your momentum. Keep your chest lifted.

Russian twists
30 reps (15 per side)

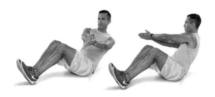

Sit with knees bent and feet together on the floor. Keeping your head, shoulders, and chest all in one line, engage your abs and lean back about 45 degrees, lifting your feet a few inches off the floor. Twist your torso and arms as one unit from side to side, keeping your abdominal muscles engaged. Continue moving side to side.

Burpees
15 reps

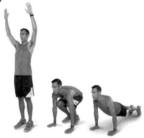

Stand tall with your feet shoulder-width apart. Squat until your hips are lower than your knees. Place your hands on the floor in between your feet and jump your feet back so you're in a push-up position. Jump your feet back up to your hands and stand up tall, finishing by tensing your butt. Repeat.

Deep overhead squat
30 reps

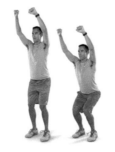

Stand with your feet shoulder-width apart and hands above your head. Bend your knees and squat. Repeat. Keep your hands above your head the whole time.

Workout 5

Cycle 1

Wall sit
1 minute

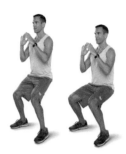

Stand about 2 feet in front of a wall, and lean against it. Slide down until your knees are at 90-degree angles and hold, keeping the abs contracted, for a full minute.

Squats
20 reps

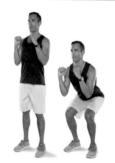

Stand with your feet shoulder-width apart. Bend your knees to sit back, lowering yourself until your thighs are parallel to the floor. Make sure that your knees stay behind your toes, and keep your chest lifted. Pause for a second, and then stand back up to starting position. Repeat.

Curtsy lunge
20 reps (10 per side)

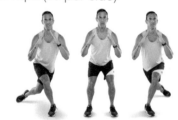

Stand with feet hip-width apart. Take a giant step with your left leg and cross it behind your right. Bend your knees until your right thigh is nearly parallel to the floor. Make sure that your front knee doesn't jut out over your front toes. Press back up to starting position. Step back with other leg. Alternate sides.

Knee kicks
40 reps
(20 per side)

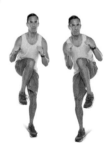

Stand tall with knees slightly bent and fists staggered in front of your face. Drive your right knee up as high as you can and then kick the leg out, extending from the knee out. Add a hop to the movement so that you're jumping each time you raise your knee. Alternate legs. Do not lower arms or rest between kicks.

Workout 5

Cycle 2

Shoulder bridges
30 reps

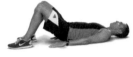
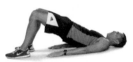

Lie on your back with your knees bent, feet flat on the floor. Lean into your hands and lift your hips, rolling your feet so that they are flat on the ground. Your body should form a straight line and your arms should be directly below your shoulders. Hold for a count of 2 and gently drop your hips. Repeat.

Crab kicks
20 reps (10 per side)

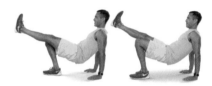

Sit on the floor with the bottom of your feet flat on the floor. Place your hands about one foot behind you, palms flat. Make sure your chest is lifted. Lean into your hands and lift your butt off the floor. Kick right leg up and then lower. Repeat with left. Alternate legs with no rest in between kicks.

Jump rope
100 reps

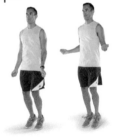

Stand up straight with a slight bend in your knees and hands by your sides. Pretend you're holding a jump rope, and make small circle movements with your hands while quickly jumping up and down on your toes, as you would if you were using a real jump rope.

Wide squats
15 reps

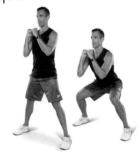

Stand with your feet wider than shoulder width and toes slightly pointed out. "Sit down," pushing your buttocks back and keeping your chest up, until your thighs are parallel to the floor. Look straight ahead, and make sure your knees stay behind your toes. Pause for a second, and then stand up quickly. Repeat, and try to get lower with each squat.

Cycle 1

High knees
50 reps

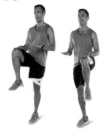

Stand with your feet hip-width apart, chest lifted, and look straight ahead. Place your hands out in front of you with your arms bent at 90 degrees. Drive your right knee toward your chest and quickly place it back on the ground. Immediately drive your left knee toward your chest. Continue alternating knees quickly.

Hip hinger
20 reps

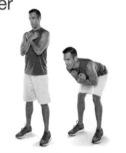

Stand with your feet shoulder-width apart. Shift your weight to your heels and push your hips back as you hinge forward at the hips, until your torso is at about a 45-degree angle. Keep your head, neck, and torso in one line, abs engaged and tight. Contract your butt muscles as you lift back up from your hips. Repeat.

Butt kicks
60 reps

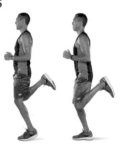

Standing with feet in line with your hips, chest lifted, and looking straight ahead, begin to jog, kicking up your heels behind you. Let your arms move naturally, as they do when you are running. Really exaggerate your back stride, bringing your heels up to your butt. Continue alternating your legs quickly.

Standing leg raise
40 reps
(20 per side)

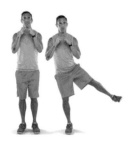

Stand with feet together. If need be, place one hand on the back of a chair to help you balance. Keeping your right leg on the floor, lift your left leg out to the side as high as you can manage. Keep your extended leg straight. Hold this position for a count of 6, and then lower your leg back to the starting position. Now repeat on the opposite side.

Cycle 2

Burpees
15 reps

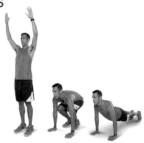

Stand tall with your feet shoulder-width apart. Squat until your hips are lower than your knees. Place your hands on the floor in between your feet and jump your feet back so you're in a push-up position. Jump your feet back up to your hands and stand up tall, finishing by tensing your butt. Repeat.

Wall sit
1 minute

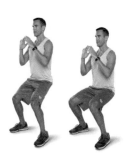

Stand about 2 feet in front of a wall, and lean against it. Slide down until your knees are at 90-degree angles and hold, keeping the abs contracted, for a full minute.

Slalom
40 reps
(20 per side)

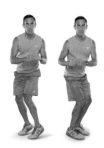

Start with both feet together and your hands in front of you (elbows at your side), as if you're holding ski poles. Jump and twist your upper body to the right and your feet to the left. Then jump up and twist your upper body to the left and your feet to the right. Repeat.

Frog push-ups
15 reps

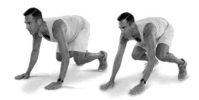

Start in normal push-up position with hands directly under shoulders and fingers pointing forward. Bend your knees at a 90-degree angle and move them in closer to your hands. Bend your elbows and shift your weight forward. Lower your upper body down until your nose is close to the ground, then push back up.

Cycle 1

Ski jumps

24 reps
(12 per side)

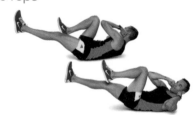

Stand with feet slightly apart, elbows bent as if you were holding ski poles. Jump to the right with both feet. Without pausing, jump back to starting position, and immediately jump again, this time to the other side. Continue alternating, swinging your elbows back and forth to help with your momentum. Keep your chest lifted.

Shoulder bridges

30 reps

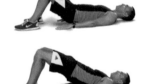

Lie on your back with your knees bent, feet flat on the floor. Lean into your hands and lift your hips, rolling your feet so that they are flat on the ground. Your body should form a straight line and your arms should be directly below your shoulders. Hold for a count of 2 and gently drop your hips. Repeat.

Bicycle

40 reps

Lie down on your back with knees in toward your chest and hands behind your head. Bring your right elbow toward the left knee while right leg straightens. Alternate sides just like you're pedaling on a bike. Move as quickly as possible, making sure to keep abs braced and tight throughout the movement.

Power lunges

20 reps

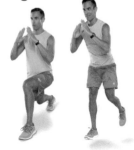

Stand with your feet together and hands on your hips. Bend your knees and hop your feet apart, landing with your right foot forward and your left foot back, knees bent, in a lowered lunge position. Press into your feet and jump back into the air, switching sides. Continue, alternating sides.

Workout 7

Running in place
1 minute

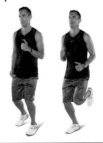

Start jogging in place as fast as you can. Lift your knees up to increase intensity—your thighs can go as high as being parallel to the ground. Remember to move your arms back and forth to boost your heart rate even more. Keep your chest lifted to keep your head and neck in line with your shoulders.

One-legged Romanian deadlift 20 reps (10 per side)

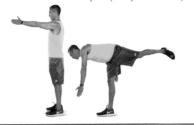

Stand with feet together and arms straight out. Lift leg back slightly so foot is just off floor. Lower your hands to floor while raising lifted leg back behind. Keep your back straight and the knee of supporting leg slightly bent. Once stretch is felt, raise torso and drop leg to return to starting position. Repeat.

Mountain climbers
40 reps

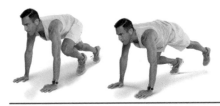

Start in push-up position on hands and toes. Keeping your hips low and your head in line with your spine, bring one knee toward chest and back, and then the other in a fluid motion, returning each foot to the starting position each time. Alternate sides as quickly as possible.

Military press
30 reps

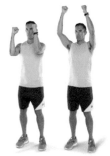

Stand with your feet shoulder-width apart. Make fists and put your elbows at 90 degrees. Raise your arms up above your head. Lower your arms back to 90 degrees. Repeat.

Cycle 1

Burpees

15 reps

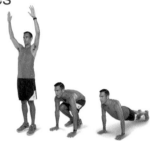

Stand tall with your feet shoulder-width apart. Squat until your hips are lower than your knees. Place your hands on the floor in between your feet and jump your feet back so you're in a push-up position. Jump your feet back up to your hands and stand up tall, finishing by tensing your butt. Repeat.

Walking lunges

30 reps
(15 per side)

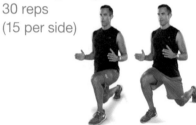

Stand with feet together. Take a giant step forward with your right foot and align knee over ankle. Bend your back knee down close to the floor, heel lifted. Before your back knee touches the floor, push up with your back left leg, simultaneously bringing your left foot together with your right. Alternate sides without pausing.

Knee kicks

40 reps
(20 per side)

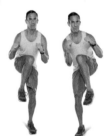

Stand tall with knees slightly bent and fists staggered in front of your face. Drive your right knee up as high as you can and then kick the leg out, extending from the knee out. Add a hop to the movement so that you're jumping each time you raise your knee. Alternate legs. Do not rest between kicks.

Bent over lateral raise

15 reps

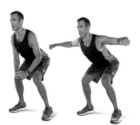

Stand with your legs shoulder-width apart and your knees slightly bent. Lean forward from your hips, keep your back straight, and keep your head in line with your shoulders. Let your arms hang. Begin to raise arms to a horizontal position. Pause and contract the shoulder and back muscles. Return to starting position. Repeat.

Cycle 2

Lateral shuffle
50 reps

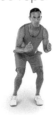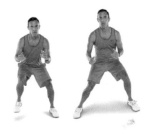

Stand with feet a little wider than hip-distance apart. Shuffle sideways to the right, pretending that you are stepping into a ladder on the floor. Step both feet into the first square of the ladder, staying on the balls of your feet. Move your arms to mimic a running motion. After 4 seconds, switch directions and shuffle to the left.

Standing leg raise
40 reps
(20 per side)

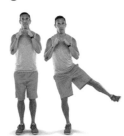

Stand with feet together. Keeping your right leg on the floor, lift your left leg out to the side as high as you can manage. Keep your extended leg straight. Hold this position for a count of 6, and then lower your leg back to the starting position. Now repeat on the opposite side.

Cross jacks
30 reps

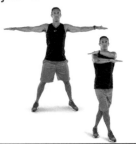

Stand tall with your feet shoulder-width apart and extend your arms straight out to either side with palms facing down. Jump and cross your right arm over your left and your right foot over your left. Jump back to the starting position, then cross with the opposite arm and foot. Continue alternating sides without rest.

Side lift and lunge
20 reps (10 per side)

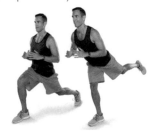

Stand with your feet hip-width apart. Do a side lunge to the right, and at the same time, punch your left hand down toward the floor. Return to standing position and raise both arms directly in front of you to shoulder level (so they're parallel with the floor). At the same time, slightly kick your right leg back. Alternate sides.

Cycle 1

Butt kicks
60 reps

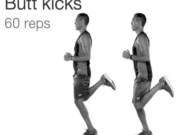

Standing with feet in line with your hips, chest lifted, begin to jog, kicking up your heels behind you. Let your arms move naturally, as they do when you are running. Exaggerate your back stride, bringing your heels up to your butt in an attempt to make contact between the two. Continue alternating your legs quickly.

Frog push-ups
15 reps

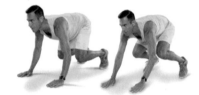

Start in normal push-up position with hands directly under shoulders and fingers pointing forward. Bend your knees at a 90-degree angle and move them in closer to your hands. Bend your elbows and shift your weight forward. Lower your upper body down until your nose is close to the ground, then push back up.

Mountain climbers
40 reps

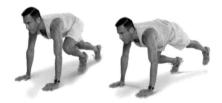

Start in push-up position on hands and toes. Keeping your hips low and your head in line with your spine, bring one knee toward chest and back, and then the other in a fluid motion, returning each foot to the starting position each time. Alternate sides as quickly as possible.

One-legged Romanian deadlift 20 reps (10 per side)

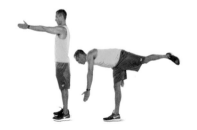

Stand with feet together and arms straight out. Lift leg back slightly so foot is just off floor. Lower your hands to floor while raising lifted leg back behind. Keep your back straight and the knee of supporting leg slightly bent. Once stretch is felt or your hands contacts floor, raise torso and drop leg to return to starting position. Repeat.

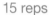

Cycle 2

Crab kicks
20 reps (10 per side)

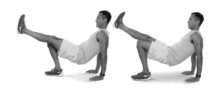

Sit with the bottom of your feet flat on the floor. Place your hands about one foot behind you, palms flat. Make sure your chest is lifted. Lean into your hands and lift your butt off the floor. Kick right leg up and then lower. Repeat with left. Alternate legs with no rest in between kicks.

Push-up to knee tuck
10 reps (5 per side)

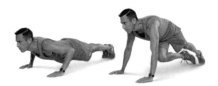

Start in standard push-up position. As you lower your body, bring your right knee up into a tucked position. As you raise your body, bring the leg back out so it's straight and toes are on floor again. Alternate sides.

Jump and butt kick
20 reps

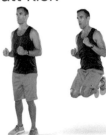

Start by standing up tall. Jump up as high as you can and kick your heels back to your butt so that the two make contact. Land on both feet. Jump back up into the same movement immediately after hitting the ground.

Power lunges
20 reps

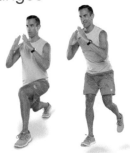

Stand with your feet together and hands on your hips. Bend your knees and hop your feet apart, landing with your right foot forward and your left foot back, knees bent, in a lowered lunge position. Press into your feet and jump back into the air, switching sides. Continue, alternating sides.

Workout Calendar

Week 1	Week 2	Week 3	Week 4
Day 1	Day 1	Day 1	Day 1
Workout 1	Workout 1	Workout 4	Workout 4
Day 2	Day 2	Day 2	Day 2
Workout 2	Workout 2	Workout 5	Workout 5
Day 3	Day 3	Day 3	Day 3
Workout 3	Workout 3	Workout 6	Workout 6

Week 5	Week 6	Week 7	Week 8
Day 1	Day 1	Day 1	Day 1
Workout 1	Workout 1	Workout 5	Workout 5
Day 2	Day 2	Day 2	Day 2
Workout 4	Workout 4	Workout 3	Workout 3
Day 3	Day 3	Day 3	Day 3
Workout 2	Workout 2	Workout 6	Workout 6

Week 9	Week 10	Week 11	Week 12
Day 1	Day 1	Day 1	Day 1
Workout 4	Workout 4	Workout 7	Workout 7
Day 2	Day 2	Day 2	Day 2
Workout 7	Workout 7	Workout 8	Workout 8
Day 3	Day 3	Day 3	Day 3
Workout 5	Workout 5	Workout 9	Workout 9

What to do on your active rest days

There's plenty of science to support that an active lifestyle will benefit your overall health. In fact, in a giant survey that followed the exercise habits and quality of health in more than 250,000 men and women ages 50 to 71 years old for nearly a decade, researchers found that the people who exercised vigorously for 20 minutes, three times a week were 32 percent less likely to die from any cause, and people who exercised moderately at least 30 minutes most days of the week were 27 percent less likely to die from any cause. Put these two together, and you should be living a long healthy and happy life. Can't think of an activity? Try one of these:

Go for a walk.

Taking a walk won't impede your body's recovery from your Tiny and Full™ workouts, and it provides multiple benefits beyond physical health. Some studies have found that walking can counter faltering memories in people over age 50. This makes perfect sense to me because when I walk, I think. It's an easy, natural movement that doesn't really engage our brains, but it does refresh and rejuvenate our minds. So we can reflect on a problem (and a solution) or even meditate in our own way. Consider taking a walk at a local park, at the beach, at a lake, or even in a pretty neighborhood. Research shows that any sort of a "green" or "nature" walk can boost mood, lower anxiety, improve willpower and impulse control, and increase overall energy. Walks are also a great activity to do with someone else because the easy pace lets you carry on a conversation—and the complete lack of distractions provides a focus we don't usually get in our hectic lives.

Ride a bike.

Leisure bike riding can provide all the benefits you get on a walk. No matter your age or fitness level, you can enjoy the scenery and feel the wind whip through your hair just like when you were a kid. Another benefit of pedaling is that it can help keep you feeling happy! In a survey conducted by Portland State University, respondents who biked to work reported the highest levels of well-being.

Say "Namaste."

A favorite "rest" day activity of one of my clients is yoga, often because it provides a great stretch for hardworking muscles. While flexibility improves, so does strength, as yoga incorporates movements such as the plank, which not only tones muscles but helps you become stronger. Other yoga benefits are wonderful too, like helping you get a better night's sleep! A study reported in *Medical Science Monitor* found that patients with sleep problems reported an improved quality of their sleep on days when they did yoga and meditation. Doing yoga also releases feel-good chemicals in your brain. Scientists at Boston University School of Medicine and McLean Hospital were able to see that people who did yoga for 30 minutes had a 27 percent increase of gamma-aminobutyric acid (GABA) in their brains. This feel-good chemical helps regulate nerve activity—it's reduced in people with mood and anxiety disorders, so the goal is to have more if you want to feel happier and more relaxed.

Take a hike.

Most of us live within driving distance to some truly beautiful nature. Get up close and personal with all of nature's splendor by taking a hike. It's one of my favorite ways to leave behind the hustle, bustle, and fast pace of everyday life. Make sure to take along your smartphone, not just to snap photos, but to make the most out of some helpful hiking apps, such as The Spot, a free GPS tracker that uploads real-time information on your location and condition. Bring a friend along too, especially if you're heading somewhere without a lot of foot traffic.

Put on your dancing shoes.

You can always just rock out at home to your favorite music, or take a jazz, tap, or hip-hop class at a local community college; many gyms also have Zumba. Or, if you have a willing partner, sign up for ballroom dance classes, or check out your local churches and community centers for line dancing, square dancing, contra dancing, salsa, or Zydeco dancing. Nobody to go with you? No problem. Many of the just-mentioned classes offer singles options, so just ask. This is a great way to get some social—or one-on-one—time and do it while moving your body. Besides being a fun activity on your "rest" days, I absolutely love this idea for date night—instead of going out for a heavy dinner and a movie, you can have a light dinner and get your move on.

My Tech Secret to Better Fitness

I am always searching for a smarter way to stay motivated with fitness. My top pick for myself, my family, and all my celebrity clients is the Apple Watch Series 2. It is probably the most valuable tool I use daily to track my fitness. If you follow me on Instagram (@JorgeCruise or @TinyandFull), you can probably tell that I always have my watch on. It takes fitness monitoring to a whole new level by encouraging healthier behaviors like sitting less, moving more, and getting brisk exercise. The secret to the Apple Watch Series 2 is the Activity App, which is critical in tracking three vital pieces of information. It reminds you to stand and allows you to visually see how many hours each day you've been on your feet. The second thing it tracks is when you move by showing you how many active calories you've burned throughout the day. Finally, it tracks your exercise by monitoring any brisk activity you've done throughout the day, such as the HIIT workouts in this book. It will tell you how many minutes you've done with a goal of 30 per day. The Apple Watch Series 2 truly tracks it all! With an emphasis on Stand, Move, and Exercise, you will constantly be reminded to sit less (such as when you're relaxing at the pool), move more (such as by taking a hike), and do 30 minutes of brisk activity (such as HIIT)!

Plus, the new Apple Watch Series 2 has some incredible health applications such as WaterMinder, Lose It, and Headspace. My favorite, Breathe, is installed by default in Apple watchOS 3 software. This app prompts you to focus on breathing for one minute every four hours, though you can change the time and frequency to suit your personal preferences. As you start your sessions, a blue-green mandala emerges and expands and contracts with your breath. (Cool, right?) If you want to close your eyes, the watch also gives you haptic feedback in the form of taps, to prompt you when to inhale and exhale. After your finish, your recorded heart rate during the session is shown along with how many breathe sessions you have completed that day. This really helps me de-stress and lowers my anxiety, making it by far my favorite app! The bottom line is that being more aware is key . . . and as we all know, knowledge is power. So don't just guess how many calories you've eaten or burned today . . . track them! You will know exactly where you stand with the Apple Watch Series 2 . . . no pun intended.

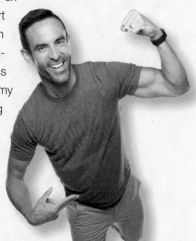

Part Three

Tiny and Full™ Forever

6 Beyond the 12 Weeks

Y ou did it!

If you are reading this chapter, you have hopefully completed the 12-week challenge. Congrats! If you are looking ahead and have yet to finish—or even start—the 12 weeks, that's okay! It's good to be prepared.

So here's what to do now that the initial 12 weeks are over. As you have been doing each week, it's time to take an "after" photo to capture your complete transformation. You will appreciate this in the months to come. I challenge you to share this photo with me and others. Visit Tiny and Full™ on Facebook, Instagram, or Twitter to share your story with me.

Now, you have a few options on how to proceed. Choose one of the following option paths to make this a sustainable lifestyle.

OPTION 1: Keep it simple.

Repeat this book. Simply return to the meal planners and workouts and keep following them. There is power in simplicity, and automation is the key to success. This option is great for those of you who enjoy a done-for-you, laid out plan that requires no thinking.

OPTION 2: Step out on your own.

If you are comfortable with the tools I have provided in this book but don't want to follow the meal planners or workouts again, feel free to step out on your own. You can use the food list in Chapter 7 to make your own menus. Use the recipes and meal planners as structure and inspiration. Just keep in mind your calorie goal and plan ahead. It's never any fun to get to dinner and realize you've eaten most of your calories. Planning ahead is key! You can also use the exercises found in Chapter 5 and mix and match the cycles to make your own workouts.

Quick tips for stepping out on your own:

- Use the food list.

- Use recipes and meal planners for ideas.

- Stick to Level 1 foods as much as possible. Make them the base of your meal.

- Think of Level 2 as the secondary part of your meal.

- Use Level 3 as condiments.

- Avoid Level 4 when possible or use in limited amounts.

- Use the workouts for ideas to create your own cycles.

OPTION 3: Let me help.

Visit me at TinyandFull.com for more meal planning options, recipes ideas, workout routines, and motivation. You can also join my Tiny and Full club where I become your one-on-one coach with live streamed videos, customized meal planners, workouts, support, and much more! You can also check out Tiny and Full™ on social media for inspiration, tips, recipes, and more.

Facebook.com/TinyandFull

Instagram/TinyandFull

Twitter/TinyandFull

#TinyandFull

So now you have the information you need to take this book beyond the 12 weeks and make it a sustainable routine. Remember to keep me updated on your progress and success, as well as get tips, recipes, and inspiration, by following Tiny and Full™ on Facebook, Instagram, and Twitter!

What to do when you reach your goal weight

When you reach your goal, feel free to switch to 1,800 or even 2,000 calories a day. Keep monitoring your weight and adjust accordingly.

7 Tiny and Full™ Foods

The following list of foods will help you if you are stepping out on your own and want to make your own meals and menu planners. The foods are organized alphabetically according to food categories. The four levels are color-coded to help you easily identify foods that are lowest in calorie density, as shown in the following legend:

Level 1: Minimal Calorie Density

Level 2: Low Calorie Density

Level 3: Medium Calorie Density

Level 4: High Calorie Density

Remember, when making meals, you want to make the base of your meal come from Level 1 foods. Add from Level 2 occasionally, dip into Level 3 as condiments, and try to minimize or avoid Level 4. Levels 2–4 are to be thought of as condiments to Level 1. You will notice that oils, such as olive oil, are a Level 4. While we definitely want to minimize the usage of oils due to their low calorie density, oils do help with cooking and baking. Just remember to use them in small amounts (check out the recipes in Chapter 8 for examples). Other Level 4 items such as sugary snacks and treats should be avoided.

Each food on the list will show you two things: the calorie density number and a real-life conversion. This real-life conversion will show you what 100 calories of that particular food looks like. For example, the energy density of watermelon (Level 1) is .26. But what does that mean? That is where this conversion comes into play to let you know that 100 calories of watermelon is about 2 cups, diced. Compare that to 100 calories of walnuts (Level 4), which is only 7 halves. This is meant to give you a visual example to help you understand what calorie density looks like.

Use this list to help pick lower-calorie-density foods as much as possible. If you want to calculate the calorie density of a food not on this list, simply look at the label and divide the number of calories in the food by the number of grams.

Calorie density = calories ÷ grams

Happy eating!

Tiny and Full™ Food List

Calorie Density Legend

Level 1: Minimal Calorie Density	From 0–0.59
Level 2: Low Calorie Density	From 0.6–1.5
Level 3: Medium Calorie Density	From 1.6–3.9
Level 4: High Calorie Density	From 4.0–9.0

Fruit

	Calorie Density	Real-Life Conversion
Acai berries, dried	0.70	5 oz.
Apple	0.56	1 medium
Applesauce, unsweetened	0.41	2 cups
Apricot	0.51	6 apricots

Fruit (continued)

	Calorie Density	Real-Life Conversion
Avocado	1.90	⅓ cup
Banana	0.90	1 7-inch banana
Banana, dried	3.71	1 oz.
Blackberries	0.60	1⅓ cups
Blueberries	0.57	1¼ cups
Boysenberry	0.50	1½ cups
Cantaloupe	0.34	2 cups cubed
Cherries	0.70	1 cup
Cherry tomatoes	0.18	32 cherry tomatoes
Currant	2.68	1.3 oz.
Date	1.17	3 dates
Date, dried	3.00	1 oz.
Dragon fruit	0.60	1¾ dragon fruit
Durian	1.47	¼ cup
Fig	0.73	2 figs
Fig, dried	2.47	2 figs
Gogi berry, dried	3.21	¼ cup
Grape	0.41	62 grapes
Guava	0.68	2 medium
Honeydew	0.33	¼ 5-inch melon
Kiwi	0.61	2 large
Kirkland Frozen Blueberries	0.50	1 cup
Kirkland Frozen Strawberries	0.36	2 cups
Kumquat	0.68	7 kumquats
Lemon	0.29	5 lemons
Lime	0.30	5 limes
Loquat	0.47	11 large
Mango	0.60	⅔ medium
Mulberry	0.43	1½ cups
Nectarine	0.64	1½ large nectarines
Olive	1.14	18 olives

Fruit (continued)

	Calorie Density	Real-Life Conversion
Orange	0.47	1¼ large orange
Papaya	0.43	½ medium papaya
Passion fruit	0.97	5 passion fruits
Peach	0.50	2½ medium peaches
Pear	0.51	1 medium pear
Persimmon, Japanese	0.70	¾ whole persimmon
Pineapple	0.56	1¼ cups of chunks
Plum	0.60	3 medium plums
Plum tomato	0.17	9½ plum tomatoes
Plum, prune	2.40	5 prunes
Pomegranate	0.83	1 medium pomegranate
Pumpkin	0.20	2 cups mashed
Raisin	3.25	2 miniature boxes
Raspberry	0.57	1½ cups
Red and pink grapefruit	0.42	1 4-inch grapefruit
Squash, all	0.20	3 cups sliced
Star fruit	0.31	2½ star fruits
Strawberry	0.32	25 medium
Tamarillo	0.33	5 tamarillos
Tiny and Full™ Power Fruits, with 8 oz. water	0.13	3 fruits and a 3-oz. shake
Tomato	0.17	4¾ medium tomatoes
Watermelon	0.26	2 cups diced

Vegetables

	Calorie Density	Real-Life Conversion
Alfalfa spouts	0.20	13 cups
Artichoke	0.53	1½ medium artichokes
Arugula	0.25	20 cups
Asparagus	0.22	30 spears ½-inch base
Bell pepper	0.20	5 medium bell peppers

My Go-To List for Costco

In order to save time and money, I am a Costco member. I love their Kirkland Signature brand foods for their quality and pricing.

Below is my go-to shopping list of my favorite kind of Kirkland Signature items that I always grab when I am at Costco. Check out the food list for their calorie density values.

Make sure to check out Costco.com for more Kirkland Signature products as well as follow Costco on Facebook (www.facebook.com/Costco) and Instagram (@Costco).

- ☐ Greek Yogurt
- ☐ Chicken Breast
- ☐ Rotisserie Chicken
- ☐ Sockeye Salmon Fillets
- ☐ Lean Ground Beef
- ☐ Chocolate Chip Oatmeal
- ☐ Cooked Quinoa
- ☐ Basmati Rice
- ☐ Multigrain Whole Wheat Grain Bread
- ☐ Frozen Strawberries
- ☐ Frozen Green Beans
- ☐ Frozen Mixed Vegetables
- ☐ Frozen Blueberries
- ☐ Unsweetened Tea
- ☐ Coffee Sumatra
- ☐ Coffee Costa Rica
- ☐ Coffee Guatemalan Lake Atitlan
- ☐ Coffee Rwanda
- ☐ Coffee Panama Geisha
- ☐ Bottled Water

Vegetables (continued)

	Calorie Density	Real-Life Conversion
Bok choy	0.14	10 cups
Broccoli	0.35	3 cups chopped
Brussels sprouts	0.36	1¾ cups
Cabbage	0.23	4½ cups chopped
Carrot	0.41	4 medium
Cauliflower	0.23	4 cups
Celery	0.15	16½ medium stalks
Chard	0.19	14 cups
Collard greens	0.26	9 cups
Corn, white	0.86	¾ cup
Corn, yellow	0.96	¾ cup
Cucumber	0.15	6⅓ cups sliced
Eggplant	0.33	¾ cup
Endive	0.16	12½ cups
Fennel	0.31	1⅓ bulbs
Green bean	0.35	60 beans 4 inches long
Green onion	0.33	20 medium 4 inches long
Jicama	0.38	2 cups
Kale	0.49	13 cups chopped
Kirkland Frozen Mixed Vegetables	0.33	2.5 cups
Kirkland Green Beans	0.17	2.5 tbsp.
Lettuce, iceberg	0.14	11 cups shredded
Lettuce, red leaf	0.16	22 cups shredded
Lettuce, romaine	0.17	12 cups shredded
Mint	0.43	8 oz.
Mushroom	0.26	26 medium
Mustard green	0.27	7 cups
Okra	0.23	2½ cups
Onion	0.43	2 medium onions
Pepper, jalapeño	0.29	25 peppers
Pepper, serrano	0.33	50 peppers

Vegetables (continued)

	Calorie Density	Real-Life Conversion
Pickle, dill	0.12	6 large pickles
Pickles, gherkin	0.14	20 pickles
Potato, baked	0.97	¾ small potato
Potato, french fries, fast food	3.07	¼ medium order
Potato, french fries, homemade	2.67	⅔ cup
Potato, mashed with whole milk and margarine	1.13	⅔ cup
Radicchio	0.23	50 radicchios
Radish	0.11	101 radishes
Rutabaga, cubed	0.39	2 cups
Seaweed, nori	4.00	10 sheets
Shallots	0.70	14 tbsp.
Spinach	0.23	14 cups
Sweet potato, baked	0.90	¾ medium potato
Tiny and Full™ Chocolate Pea Protein, with 8 oz. water	0.21	1 protein and a 7-oz. shake
Tiny and Full™ Essential Fiber	4.00	10 tsp.
Tiny and Full™ Power Greens	0.15	3 shakes
Tiny and Full™ Unflavored Pea Protein, with 8 oz. water	0.22	1 protein and a 6-oz. shake
Tiny and Full™ Vanilla Pea Protein, with 8 oz. water	0.21	1 protein and a 7-oz. shake
Turnip greens	0.20	5 cups
Turnip, cubed	0.22	3 cups
Vegetable blend, stir fry frozen	0.25	2½ cups
Watercress	0.20	20 cups chopped

Legumes

	Calorie Density	Real-Life Conversion
Baked beans, original, Bush's Best	1.19	⅓ cup
Black beans, cooked	1.32	⅓ cup
Chickpeas	1.19	⅓ cup

Legumes (continued)

	Calorie Density	Real-Life Conversion
Edamame, shelled	1.60	⅓ cup
Hummus	1.80	4 tbsp.
Kidney beans	1.27	⅓ cup
Lentils	1.14	⅓ cup
Peanut butter	5.88	1 tbsp.
Pinto beans	1.43	⅓ cup

Pasta

	Calorie Density	Real-Life Conversion
Brown rice pasta, any size, cooked	1.23	⅓ cup
Gluten-free pasta, any size, cooked	1.31	⅓ cup
Traditional, any size, cooked	1.58	⅓ cup
Whole-wheat, any size, cooked	1.24	½ cup

Fish & Seafood

	Calorie Density	Real-Life Conversion
Catfish	1.35	2½ oz.
Clams	1.48	2⅓ oz.
Cod	1.05	3⅓ oz.
Crab	1.11	3 oz.
Flounder	0.91	3¾ oz.
Halibut	0.94	3¾ oz.
Kirkland Sockeye Salmon Fillets	1.59	2.2 oz.
Lobster	0.90	3¾ oz.
Mahimahi	1.09	3¼ oz.
Orange roughy	1.05	3⅓ oz.
Oysters	0.51	14 medium
Salmon	1.32	2½ oz.
Sardines	1.64	2 oz.
Scallops	0.87	8 large or 20 small

Fish & Seafood (continued)

	Calorie Density	Real-Life Conversion
Shrimp	1.18	3 oz.
Sole	1.05	3⅓ oz.
Swordfish	1.55	2¼ oz.
Tilapia	0.96	3½ oz.
Trout	1.50	2⅓ oz.
Tuna, canned	1.16	3 oz.
Tuna, fresh	1.39	2½ oz.

Poultry

	Calorie Density	Real-Life Conversion
Chicken, breast, without skin	1.25	2¾ oz.
Chicken, leg, without skin	1.91	1¾ oz.
Chicken, thigh, without skin	1.41	2½ oz.
Chicken, wing, without skin	2.05	1¾ oz.
Duck, breast, without skin	1.29	2¾ oz.
Kirkland Chicken Breast	0.98	1 piece
Kirkland Rotisserie Chicken	1.65	2 oz.
Processed sandwich/ deli meats – chicken	1.15	3 oz.
Processed sandwich/ deli meats – turkey	1.13	3 oz.
Sausage, chicken	2.12	⅔ link
Sausage, turkey	1.61	¾ link
Turkey bacon	1.29	2¾ oz.
Turkey bacon, lean	1.29	2¾ oz.
Turkey breast	2.33	1½ oz.
Turkey burger	1.34	2½ oz.
Turkey leg with skin	2.08	1¾ oz.
Turkey thigh	1.25	2¾ oz.
Turkey, lean ground, 85% fat-free	2.14	1½ oz.
Turkey, lean ground, 99% fat-free	1.52	2¼ oz.

Tiny and Full™ Foods

Red Meat & Pork

	Calorie Density	Real-Life Conversion
Bacon	5.42	3 slices
Beef chuck	3.45	1 oz.
Beef flank	1.94	1.8 oz.
Beef jerky	4.10	1¼ pieces
Beef porterhouse	2.04	1.7 oz.
Beef rib	2.95	¼ rib
Beef round, sirloin	1.86	1.9 oz.
Beef rump roast	1.92	1.8 oz.
Beef T-bone steak	2.21	1.6 oz.
Beef tenderloin	2.11	1.6 oz.
Bison, ground	2.38	1.5 oz.
Bologna	3.11	1¼ slices
Canadian bacon	1.37	2½ oz.
Chorizo, beef	4.08	⅔ link
Chorizo, pork	2.71	½ sausage
Corned beef	1.89	1.8 oz.
Ground beef, 75% fat-free	2.54	1.3 oz.
Ground beef, 85% fat-free	2.27	1.5 oz.
Ground beef, 95% fat-free	1.64	2.15 oz.
Ham, extra lean	1.07	3⅓ oz.
Ham, regular	1.64	2 6-inch slices
Hot dog	3.09	¾ dog
Hot dog, 97% fat-free	1.01	2 dogs
Hot dog, vegan	1.32	2 dogs
Hot dog, veggie dog	1.25	2 dogs
Kirkland 9% Lean Ground Beef	.61	2.2 oz.
Lamb chop	2.83	1.25 oz.
Lamb leg	2.65	1.3 oz.
Lamb roast	2.65	1.3 oz.
Liverwurst	3.21	1 oz.
Pastrami	1.46	2½ oz.

Red Meat & Pork (continued)

	Calorie Density	Real-Life Conversion
Pastrami, 98% fat-free	0.95	3¾ oz.
Pepperoni	4.91	4 × 1³⁄₈ inch diameter slices
Pork center loin chop	2.02	1.7 oz.
Pork tenderloin	1.44	2½ oz.
Processed sandwich/ deli meats – ham	1.11	3 oz.
Processed sandwich/ deli meats – roast beef	1.19	3 oz.
Prosciutto	2.25	3 slices
Roast beef	1.11	3 oz.
Salami	2.61	1²⁄₃ slice
Sausage, breakfast	2.42	2 4-inch links
Sausage, polish	3.26	⅓ link
Veal loin chop or roast	1.75	2 oz.

Cereals & Grains

	Calorie Density	Real-Life Conversion
Basmati rice, cooked	1.20	½ cup
Brown rice, cooked	1.11	⅓ cup
Cereal, Cheerios	3.57	1 cup
Cereal, Ezekiel 4:9 sprouted whole grain	3.33	¼ cup
Cereal, Ezekiel 4:9 sprouted whole grain golden flax	3.15	¼ cup
Cereal, Post shredded wheat	3.47	⅔ cup
Cereal, Total	3.33	¾ cup
Cereal, Wheaties	3.70	¾ cup
Corn muffin, "Jiffy"	4.84	½ of a small muffin
Couscous, cooked	1.12	⅔ cup
Croutons	4.07	¾ cup
Granola, low-fat without raisins	3.80	¼ cup
Jasmine rice, cooked	1.03	½ cup

Cereals & Grains (continued)

	Calorie Density	Real-Life Conversion
Oatmeal, instant, apples and cinnamon, cooked	1.08	¼ cup
Oatmeal, instant, cooked	0.91	⅓ cup
Oatmeal, steel cut, cooked	0.71	⅔ cup
Quinoa, cooked	1.20	⅓ cup
Spanish rice, cooked	0.87	⅓ cup
White rice, cooked	1.30	½ cup

Breads & Tortillas

	Calorie Density	Real-Life Conversion
Bagels, honey whole-wheat	3.08	1¼ slices
Bread, sprouted whole-grain	2.35	1¼ slices
Bread, whole-wheat	2.44	1½ slices
Hamburger bun	2.62	1 bun
Hamburger bun, sprouted whole-grain	2.44	½ bun
Kirkland Multigrain 100% Whole Wheat Grain Bread	2.64	⅔ slice
Pancakes, plain frozen, ready-to-heat	2.31	1 pancake
Pita, whole-wheat	2.66	½ 6-inch pita
Roll, dinner	3.33	1 2-inch square roll
Tortilla, corn	2.14	2 6-inch tortillas
Tortilla, flour	2.86	1 6-inch tortilla
Waffles, frozen	2.00	1⅓ waffles
Wrap, whole-wheat	2.86	1¼ 6-inch tortillas

Dairy

	Calorie Density	Real-Life Conversion
Greek yogurt	0.97	½ container
Greek yogurt, fruit on the bottom	0.82	⅔ container
Greek yogurt, nonfat	0.57	1 container
Half-and-half	1.33	5 tbsp.

Dairy (continued)

	Calorie Density	Real-Life Conversion
Kirkland Greek Yogurt	0.57	¾ cup
Milk, 1%	0.42	8 oz.
Milk, 2%	0.50	7 oz.
Milk, fat-free	0.35	10 oz.
Milk, whole	0.63	5 oz.
Rice milk, plain	0.49	7 oz.
Sour cream	1.67	4 tbsp.
Soy milk, plain, Silk	0.54	6 oz.
Whipped cream, Cool-Whip	2.75	8 tbsp.
Whipped cream, Cool-Whip, fat-free	1.67	13 tbsp.
Whipped cream, extra creamy	4.00	10 tbsp.
Whipped cream, fat-free	1.00	40 tbsp.
Whipping cream	3.47	13 tbsp.
Yogurt, fat-free, plain	0.44	8 oz.
Yogurt, fat-free, strawberry	0.44	8 oz.
Yogurt, plain	0.61	⅔ container
Yogurt, strawberry	0.97	½ container

Cheese

	Calorie Density	Real-Life Conversion
American	2.38	1½ oz.
Asiago	3.57	1 oz.
Blue	3.57	1 oz.
Brick	3.57	1 oz.
Brie	3.35	1 oz.
Cheddar	4.04	¾ oz.
Colby	3.93	¾ oz.
Colby Jack	3.93	¾ oz.
Cottage cheese, 1% fat	0.72	⅔ cup
Cottage cheese, 2% fat	0.90	½ cup
Cottage cheese, 4% fat	0.93	⅓ cup

	Calorie Density	Real-Life Conversion
Cottage cheese, fat-free	0.62	⅔ cup
Cream cheese	2.58	1⅓ oz.
Cream cheese, fat-free	0.93	7 tbsp.
Cream cheese, strawberry light	2.17	5 tbsp.
Cream cheese, whipped	2.27	4 tbsp.
Edam	3.57	1 oz.
Farmer cheese	3.57	1 oz.
Feta	2.63	1⅓ oz.
Fontina	3.89	¾ oz.
Gorgonzola	3.36	1 oz.
Gouda	3.57	1 oz.
Gruyère	4.14	¾ oz.
Havarti	3.93	¾ oz.
Limburger	3.28	1 oz.
Mascarpone	4.64	¾ oz.
Monterey Jack	3.71	1 oz.
Mozzarella, part skim milk	2.54	1⅓ oz.
Mozzarella, whole milk	3.00	1 oz.
Muenster	3.57	1 oz.
Parmesan	3.92	¾ oz.
Pepper Jack	3.77	1 oz.
Provolone	3.50	1 oz.
Queso blanco	3.93	¾ oz.
Ricotta, part skim milk	1.38	⅓ cup
Ricotta, whole milk	1.74	¼ cup
Romano	3.89	¾ oz.
String cheese	2.86	1¼ oz.
String cheese, light	2.38	1½ oz.
Swiss	3.79	1 oz.

Eggs

	Calorie Density	Real-Life Conversion
Egg beaters	0.53	6 eggs
Egg, white	0.52	6 eggs
Egg, whole	1.44	1⅓ eggs
Avocado oil	8.99	3 tsp.

Fats

	Calorie Density	Real-Life Conversion
Barlean's Key Lime Omega Swirl To Go	6.00	1½ tsp.
Butter	7.20	1 tbsp.
Butter, substitute	4.93	1½ tbsp.
Butter, substitute, light	2.86	2½ tbsp.
Coconut oil	8.93	3 tsp.
Crisco	9.17	3 tsp.
Flaxseed oil	5.87	3 tsp.
Ghee	9.00	3 tsp.
Lard	8.98	3 tsp.
Olive oil	8.00	3 tsp.
Sesame oil	8.89	3 tsp.
Walnut oil	8.89	3 tsp.

Tiny and Full™ Foods

Nuts* & Seeds

	Calorie Density	Real-Life Conversion
Almond butter, unsweetened	6.15	1 tbsp.
Almond flour/meal	5.80	⅛ cup
Almonds	5.80	15 almonds
Brazil nuts	6.53	3 nuts
Cashews	6.28	25 halves
Coconut, flour	6.45	¼ cup

Nuts* & Seeds (continued)

	Calorie Density	Real-Life Conversion
Coconut, meat, dried	6.61	½ oz.
Coconut, meat, raw	3.53	⅓ cup shredded
Coconut, meat, sweetened	4.56	⅕ cup shredded
Macadamia nuts	6.28	5 nuts
Pecans	7.00	10 pieces
Pine nuts	5.71	⅛ cup
Pumpkin seeds	5.60	2 tbsp.
Sunflower seeds	5.85	⅛ cup without shells
Walnuts	6.54	7 halves

Herbs & Spices

	Calorie Density	Real-Life Conversion
Basil	0.17	1,470 leaves
Chives	0.33	100 tbsp.
Cilantro	0.20	25 cups
Garlic	1.33	25 cloves
Ginger	0.50	33 tbsp.
Oregano	3.00	20 tbsp.
Parsley	0.37	4 cups

Condiments & Dressings

	Calorie Density	Real-Life Conversion
Barbecue sauce	1.50	¼ cup
Blue cheese dressing	4.67	1½ tbsp.
Blue cheese dressing, fat-free	1.00	6 tbsp.
Cocktail sauce	0.91	¼ cup
Honey	3.05	1½ oz.
Hot sauce	0.36	25 tbsp.
Italian dressing	3.00	2 tbsp.
Italian dressing, fat-free	0.61	10 tbsp.

Condiments & Dressings (continued)

	Calorie Density	Real-Life Conversion
Ketchup	1.00	7 tbsp.
Mayo, Primal Kitchen	6.66	1½ tbsp.
Mayonnaise, light	2.33	3 tbsp.
Mayonnaise, omega light	3.33	2 tbsp.
Mayonnaise, real	6.92	1½ tbsp.
Mayonnaise, reduced-fat, olive oil	3.21	2 tbsp.
Miracle Whip	2.67	2½ tbsp.
Miracle Whip, light	1.31	5 tbsp.
Mustard	1.00	7 tbsp.
Ranch dressing	4.67	1½ tbsp.
Ranch dressing, fat-free	1.47	2½ tbsp.
Ranch dressing, light	2.33	2½ tbsp.
Salsa	0.36	1⅓ cups
Soy sauce	0.67	10 tbsp.
Teriyaki, ready-to-serve	0.89	6 tbsp.

Miscellaneous

	Calorie Density	Real-Life Conversion
Anchovy paste	1.80	3⅓ tbsp.
Baking flour, enriched	3.64	⅕ cup
Baking powder	1.50	33 tsp.
Balsamic vinegar	0.88	7 tbsp.
Chia flour	4.89	1 tbsp.
Chia seed	3.84	2 tbsp.
Chocolate chips, carob	5.33	2½ tbsp.
Chocolate chips, dark	4.93	1⅓ tbsp.
Chocolate chips, semi-sweet	4.93	1⅓ tbsp.
Chocolate chips, unsweetened	3.93	110 chips
Cocoa powder	2.22	½ cup
Coconut milk, canned	1.83	⅕ cup

Miscellaneous (continued)

	Calorie Density	Real-Life Conversion
Egg replacer	3.75	8½ tbsp.
Ground flaxseed	5.33	2 tbsp.
Kirkland Chocolate Chip Oatmeal	3.95	½ packet
Kirkland Cooked Quinoa	1.20	¼ cup
Kirkland Basmati Rice	3.64	⅛ cup
Sesame seeds	5.78	2 tbsp.
Shirataki Noodles, Miracle Noodle	0.00	Unlimited
Soy cheese	2.11	1⅓ slice
Sugar, white and brown	3.81	⅛ cup
Tempeh	1.96	½ serving
Tofu, firm	0.82	1½ slices
Tofu, light firm	0.51	2 slices
Veggie burger patties	1.27	⅔ patty
Vinegar	0.20	Unlimited

Frozen Foods

	Calorie Density	Real-Life Conversion
Amy's Enchilada Verde	1.41	¼ container
Amy's Indian Vegetable Korma	1.15	⅓ container
Amy's Soft Taco Fiesta, Light and Lean	0.97	½ container
Amy's Vegetable Pot Pie	1.98	¼ container
Lean Cuisine – Angel Hair Pomodoro	0.89	⅓ container
Lean Cuisine – Cheddar Bacon Chicken	0.88	½ container
Lean Cuisine – Cheese & Tomato Snack Pizza	1.88	½ flatbread
Lean Cuisine – Chicken Teriyaki Stir Fry	1.06	½ container
Lean Cuisine – Chicken, Spinach & Mushroom Panini	1.76	⅓ container
Lean Cuisine – Classic Macaroni & Beef	1.16	⅓ container
Lean Cuisine – Lasagna with Meat Sauce	1.04	⅓ container

Frozen Foods (continued)

	Calorie Density	Real-Life Conversion
Lean Cuisine – Macaroni & Cheese	1.06	⅓ container
Lean Cuisine – Pasta Romano with Bacon	0.92	⅓ container
Lean Cuisine – Pomegranate Chicken	0.85	½ container
Lean Cuisine – Ricotta Cheese and Spinach Ravioli	1.37	⅓ container
Lean Cuisine – Roasted Chicken and Garden Vegetables	0.74	½ container
Lean Cuisine – Roasted Turkey & Vegetables	0.88	½ container
Lean Cuisine – Roasted Turkey Breast	0.98	⅓ container
Lean Cuisine – Salisbury Steak with Mac & Cheese	0.97	⅓ container
Lean Cuisine – Salmon with Basil	0.92	⅓ container
Lean Cuisine – Spaghetti with Meatballs	0.95	⅓ container
Lean Cuisine – Steak Portobello	0.71	⅔ container
Lean Cuisine – Swedish Meatballs	1.12	⅓ container
Lean Cuisine – Sweet & Sour Chicken	1.06	⅓ container
Lean Cuisine – Vegetable Eggroll	1.25	⅓ container

Beverages

	Calorie Density	Real-Life Conversion
Almond milk, sweetened	0.25	14 oz.
Almond milk, unsweetened	0.13	3¼ cups
Apple juice	0.46	7 oz.
Beer, Coors Light	0.30	12 oz.
Beer, Michelob Ultra	0.28	12 oz.
Beer, Miller Lite	0.32	11 oz.
Beer, O'Doul's, nonalcoholic	0.19	18 oz.
Coconut milk, sweetened	0.33	10 oz.
Coconut milk, unsweetened	0.19	18 oz.
Coconut water	0.19	18 oz.

Beverages (continued)

	Calorie Density	Real-Life Conversion
Coffee, black	0.00	Unlimited
Coffee, with 2 tbsp. half & half	0.06	7⅓ cups
Coffee, with sweetened creamer	0.10	4⅓ cups
Espresso	0.00	Unlimited
Espresso, latte, 1% milk	0.37	9 oz.
Espresso, latte, 1% milk, caramel	0.50	7 oz.
Espresso, latte, 2% milk	0.42	8 oz.
Espresso, latte, 2% milk, caramel	0.55	6 oz.
Espresso, latte, half & half	0.97	3 oz.
Espresso, latte, half & half, caramel	1.03	3 oz.
Espresso, latte, skim milk	0.29	12 oz.
Espresso, latte, skim milk, caramel	0.35	10 oz.
Espresso, latte, whole milk	0.49	7 oz.
Espresso, latte, whole milk, caramel	0.61	5 oz.
Ginger ale, Schweppes	0.35	10 oz.
Grapefruit juice, light, Ocean Spray	0.50	7 oz.
Kirkland Bottled Water	0.00	Unlimited
Kirkland Coffee Costa Rica	0.00	Unlimited
Kirkland Coffee Guatemalan Lake Atitlan	0.00	Unlimited
Kirkland Coffee Panama Geisha	0.00	Unlimited
Kirkland Coffee Rwanda	0.00	Unlimited
Kirkland Coffee Sumatra	0.00	Unlimited
Kirkland Unsweetened Tea	0.00	Unlimited
Sports drink, Gatorade, lemonade	0.22	16 oz.
Tea, unsweetened plain, hot or iced	0.01	44 cups
Vegetable juice, V8 100%	0.22	16 oz.
Wine, dessert	1.60	2 oz.
Wine, red	0.85	4 oz.
Wine, white	0.84	4 oz.

Snacks & Treats

	Calorie Density	Real-Life Conversion
Cheetos, crunchy	5.46	14 pieces
Cheetos, jumbo cheese puffs	5.43	9 pieces
Cheez-its	4.76	17 crackers
Doritos, Cool Ranch	5.36	8 chips
Granola bar, 25% less sugar	4.17	1 bar
Granola bar, chocolate chunk	3.75	1 bar
Green and Black's, organic dark 72% chocolate	3.77	5 pieces
Green and Black's, organic dark 85% chocolate	6.25	5 pieces
Hershey's, milk chocolate	3.71	½ bar
Ice cream, soft serve, vanilla	1.33	⅓ cup
Kettle chips, lightly salted	5.28	9 chips
Nabisco Ritz Crackers, original	5.03	6 crackers
Nabisco Ritz Crackers, reduced-fat	4.67	7 crackers
Newman's Own, chocolate crème cookies	4.44	1½ cookies
Oreo	4.74	2 cookies
Oreo, thin crisps	4.35	1 package
Pepperidge Farm goldfish crackers	4.67	40 pieces
Pirate's Booty	4.64	¾ oz.
Popchips, original	4.30	1 small bag
Popcorn, air popped	3.88	3 cups
Popcorn, kettle corn	4.15	1½ cups
Quaker rice cakes, lightly salted	3.89	3 cakes
Trail mix	4.84	⅛ cup
Wasa Original Crispbread	4.00	1½ slices
Wheat Thins	4.33	11 crackers
Wheat Thins, reduced fat	4.48	12 crackers

Recipe Icons

In this recipe section you will find delicious recipes with powerful plant-based ingredients that can help you fast-track your weight loss and remedy certain health issues. Use the recipe icons below to learn what each recipe can do for you other than just being tasty.

 contains ingredients that turn off hunger

 contains ingredients that boost your thyroid

 contains phytochemical ingredients that burn belly fat

 contains low sugar and low sodium ingredients

* Please note some recipes have more than one icon. If your recipe has more than one icon, it contains additional ingredients that will further benefit your weight loss.

8 Tiny and Full™ Breakfast Recipes

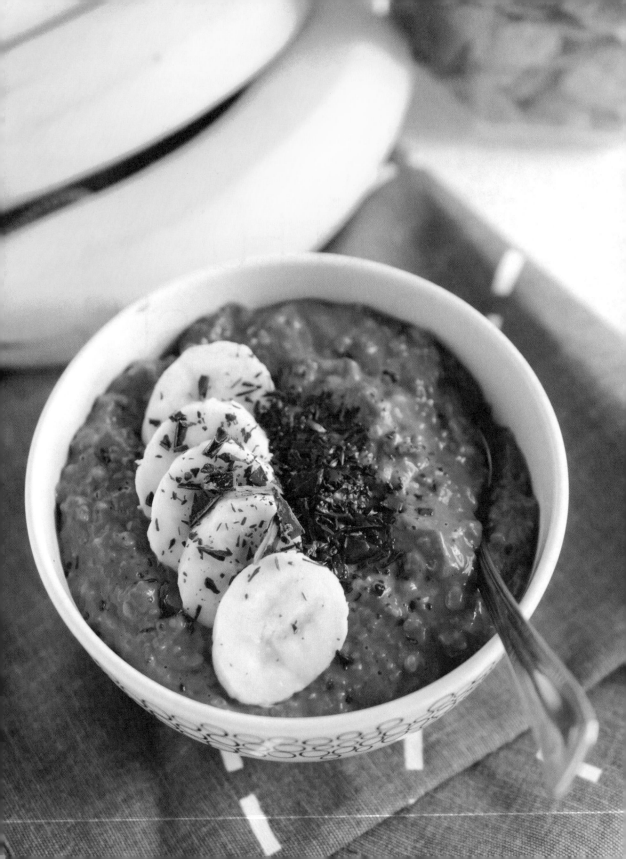

Cocoa Banana Oats

Serves 1

277 Calories

½ cup old fashioned rolled oats
1 tablespoon unsweetened dark cocoa powder
1 cup Silk unsweetened almond milk
1 scoop chocolate pea protein powder
½ banana, sliced

Optional:
½ ounce of dark cacao, shaved

1. Put the oats and cocoa into a large, microwave safe bowl. Pour ¾ cup of almond milk over the mixture and stir.
2. Microwave for 2 minutes, until thickened.
3. Whisk the remaining milk with the protein powder until dissolved.
4. Pour over the oatmeal and stir until all is incorporated.
5. Top with banana slices, and shaved cacao, if desired.

Banana Berry Bread

Serves 24

34 Calories per serving

3 mashed bananas
1 tablespoon coconut yogurt
1 teaspoon vanilla extract
½ cup stevia
1 dash salt
1 teaspoon baking powder
2 tablespoons Silk unsweetened almond milk
¾ cup buckwheat flour
1 cup blueberries

1. Preheat oven to 350°F.
2. Spray two mini-baking pans with nonstick cooking spray.
3. Place all ingredients in a medium-sized mixing bowl, except flour and blueberries, then mix until smooth.
4. Add flour and stir until just barely incorporated, then add blueberries.
5. Pour into greased pans and cook for about 20 minutes, or until golden brown.

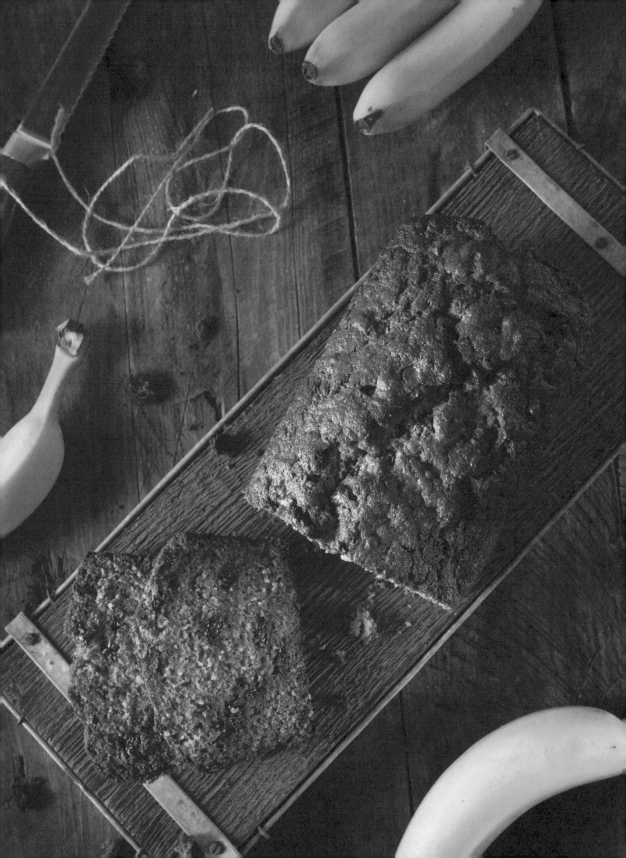

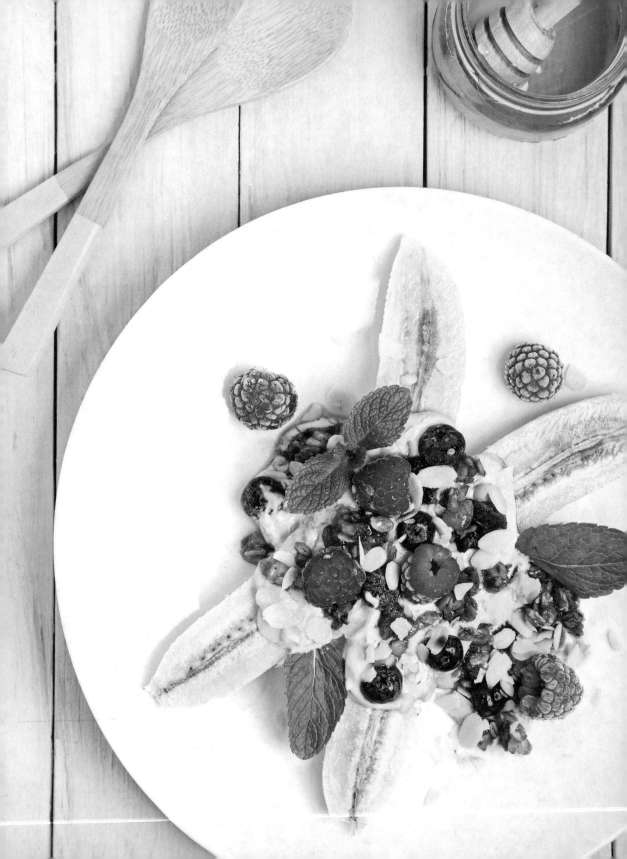

Beverly Banana Split

Serves 1

313 Calories

1 banana
½ cup coconut yogurt
½ cup blackberries
½ cup raspberries
¼ cup granola

Optional:
mint leaves, torn

1. Cut banana in half lengthwise and top with yogurt, blackberries, and raspberries.
2. Sprinkle granola on top.
3. If desired, add torn mint leaves.

Melrose Blueberry Muffins

Makes 12 Muffins

50 Calories per muffin

Nonstick cooking spray
1 cup buckwheat flour
1½ teaspoons baking soda
½ teaspoon salt
1 lemon, zested
½ cup Stevia
½ cup Silk unsweetened almond milk
3 tablespoons melted coconut oil
1 tablespoon apple cider vinegar
½ cup blueberries
Muffin cups

Optional:
1 scoop pea protein powder

1. Preheat the oven to 375°F.
2. Spray muffin tin with nonstick cooking spray.
3. In a medium bowl, combine flour, baking soda, salt, and lemon zest.
4. In a large bowl, combine sugar, milk, oil, and vinegar. Mix well.
5. Add the dry ingredients to the wet ingredients, stir until just combined.
6. Gently fold in the blueberries.
7. Place the muffin cups in the pan, and fill about two-thirds full.
8. Bake until tester comes out clean, about 22 minutes.

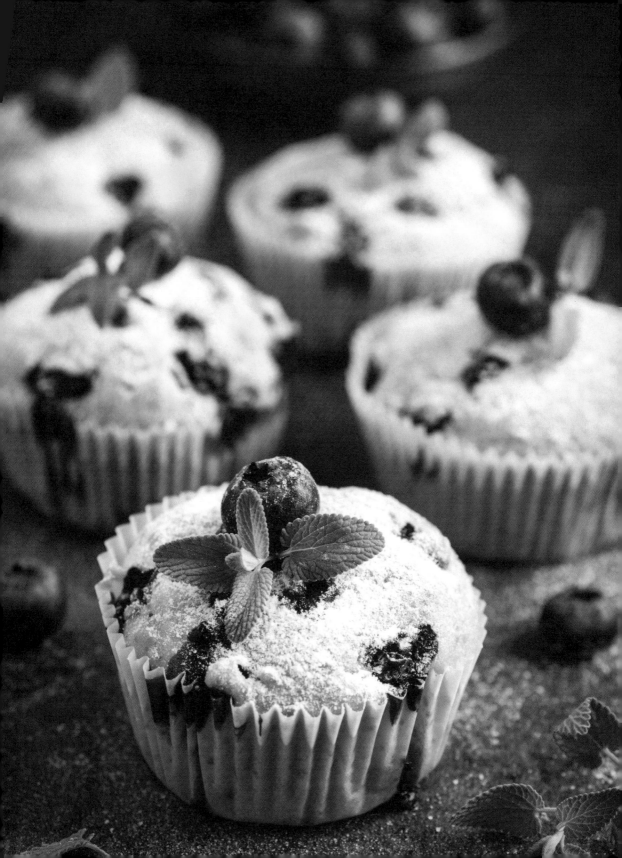

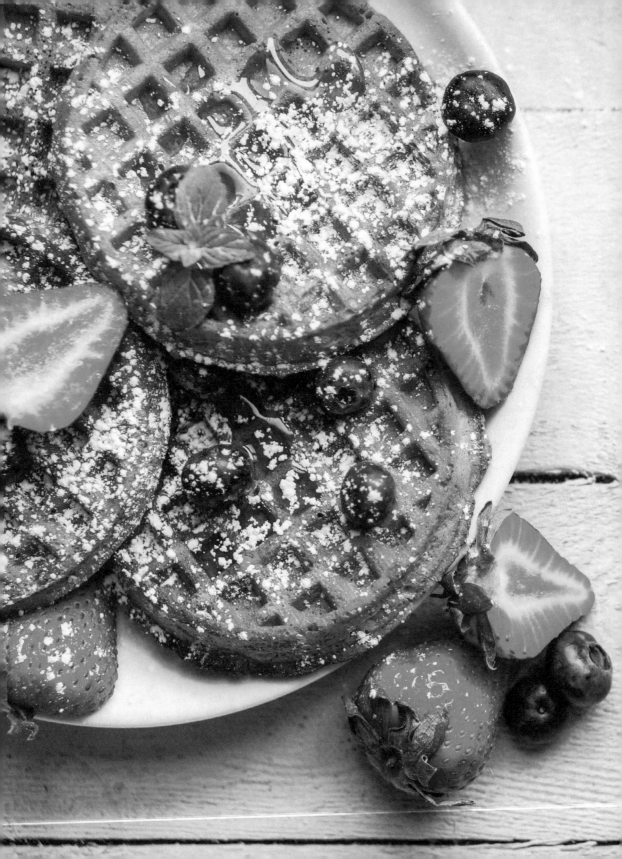

Sweet Potato Waffles

Makes 12 Waffles

109 Calories per waffle

1 cup mashed sweet potato
1 cup buckwheat flour
½ cup cornstarch
2 teaspoons baking powder
2 teaspoons cinnamon
2 Brazil nuts, finely chopped
½ teaspoon sea salt
4 tablespoons melted coconut oil
1½ cups Silk unsweetened almond milk
¼ teaspoon vanilla extract
1 tablespoon white vinegar
Nonstick cooking spray

Optional:
1 tablespoon agave
1 sliced banana
4 teaspoons stevia

1. Bake one large sweet potato at 375°F for about 1 hour, or until fork tender. Let cool and mash.
2. Preheat waffle iron.
3. In a large bowl, combine flour, cornstarch, baking powder, cinnamon, Brazil nuts, and salt.
4. In a medium bowl, stir oil, milk, vanilla extract, and vinegar. Add the wet ingredients into the dry ingredients and thoroughly combine.
5. Fold in the mashed sweet potato.
6. Spray the waffle iron with nonstick cooking spray before adding batter.
7. When waffles are cooked through, remove from iron and serve.
8. Optional: top with agave, bananas, or fruit tossed with stevia.
9. Freeze extra waffles, and toast when ready to enjoy.

California English Muffin

Serves 2

134 Calories per serving

1 English muffin (Ener-G, Udi's)
½ avocado
Lemon juice
Salt and pepper
Sliced tomato

1. Separate English muffin in half and toast.
2. Mash half of an avocado with lemon juice, salt, and pepper to taste.
3. Top both sides of the English muffin with avocado mixture.
4. Add a slice of tomato.

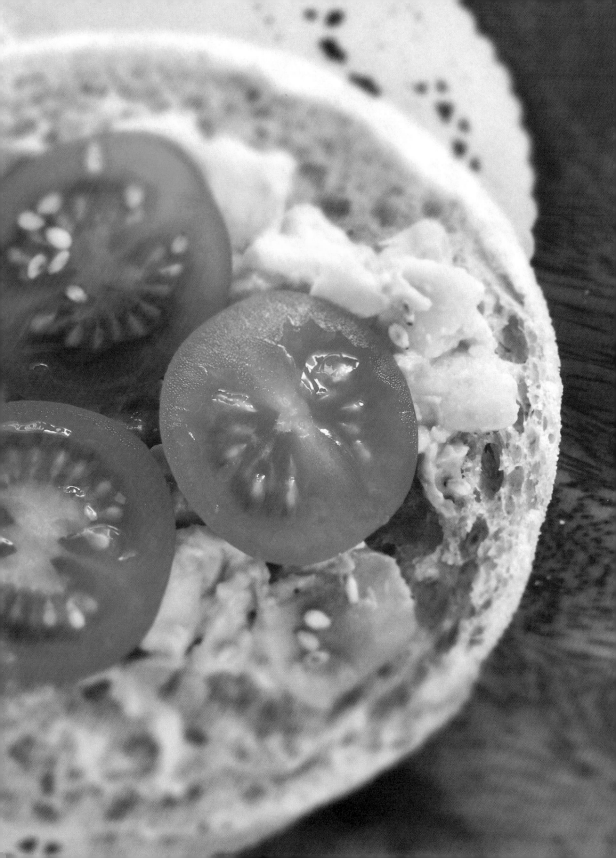

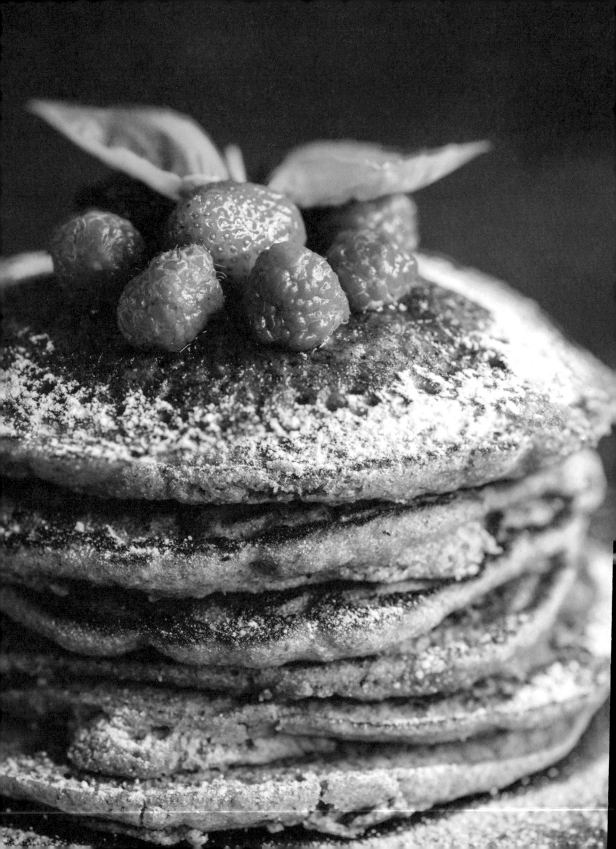

Promenade Protein Pancakes

Serves 2

160 Calories per serving

1 banana
½ cup rolled oats
½ cup Silk unsweetened almond milk
1 scoop vanilla pea protein powder
Nonstick cooking spray

Optional:
berries

1. Mash banana.
2. Add oats, almond milk, and protein powder.
3. Heat skillet on medium/low heat.
4. Spray with nonstick cooking spray.
5. Split batter on the skillet to make two pancakes.
6. Flip when golden brown, then cook through.
7. Top with berries, if desired.

Five Pea Protein Smoothies

Chocolate Peanut Butter Bliss

Serves 1

220 calories

1 banana
1 cup Silk unsweetened almond milk
2 tablespoons PB2 Powdered Peanut Butter
1 scoop chocolate pea protein powder
1 cup ice

1. Place all ingredients into a blender.
2. Blend until completely smooth.
3. Pour into a glass and enjoy!

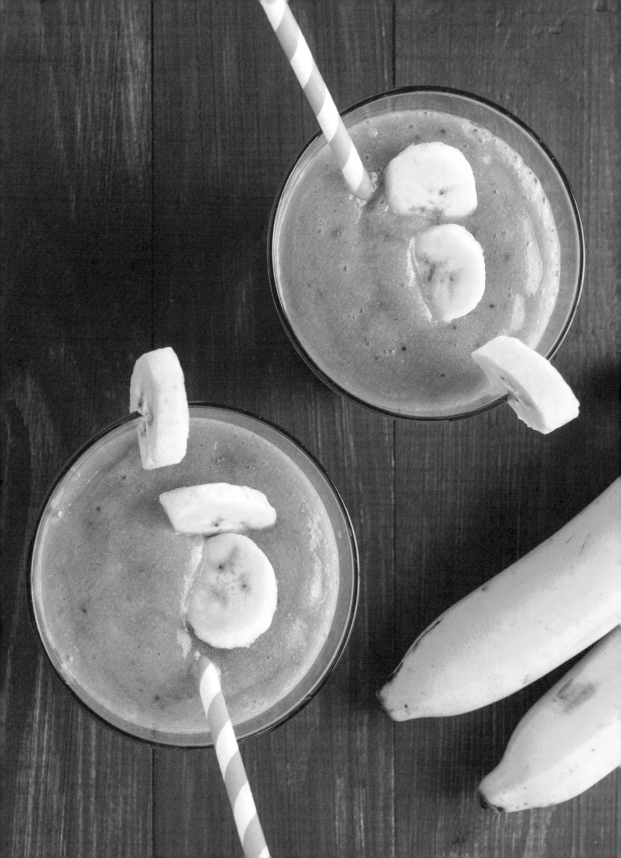

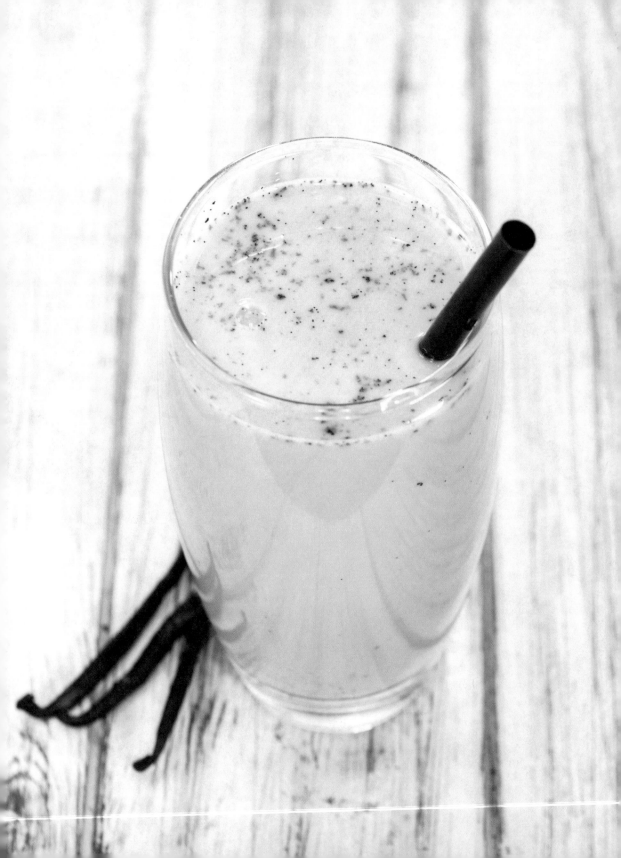

Vanilla Chai Spice

Serves 1

175 Calories

1 banana
1 Brazil nut
1 slice ginger
½ teaspoon cinnamon
Dash cardamom, ground cloves, and nutmeg
¼ teaspoon pure vanilla extract
1 cup Silk unsweetened almond milk
1 scoop vanilla protein powder

1. Place all ingredients into a blender.
2. Blend until completely smooth.
3. Pour into a glass and enjoy!

Blueberry Banana O's

Serves 1

120 Calories

½ cup Silk unsweetened almond milk
½ cup Honey Nut Cheerios™ cereal
½ banana

½ cup blueberries
1 cup ice

Garnishes:
banana slices and cereal

1. Combine all ingredients in a blender.
2. Puree until smooth.
3. Pour into a glass and enjoy!

Cafe Morning Mocha

Serves 1

246 Calories

1 banana
½ cup cold coffee
½ cup of Silk unsweetened almond milk

1 scoop chocolate pea protein powder
1 teaspoon mini dark chocolate chips
½ cup ice

1. Place all ingredients in a blender.
2. Blend until smooth.
3. Enjoy!

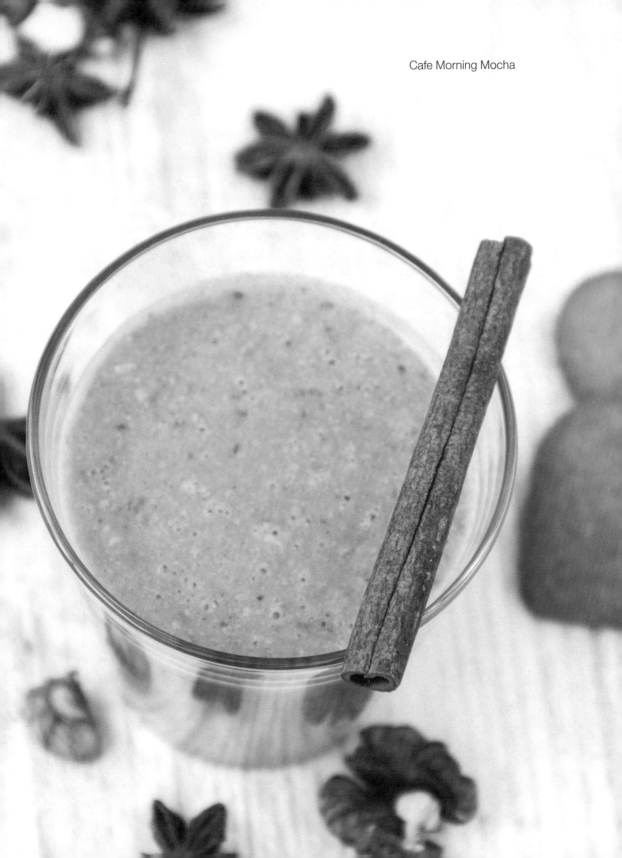

Cafe Morning Mocha

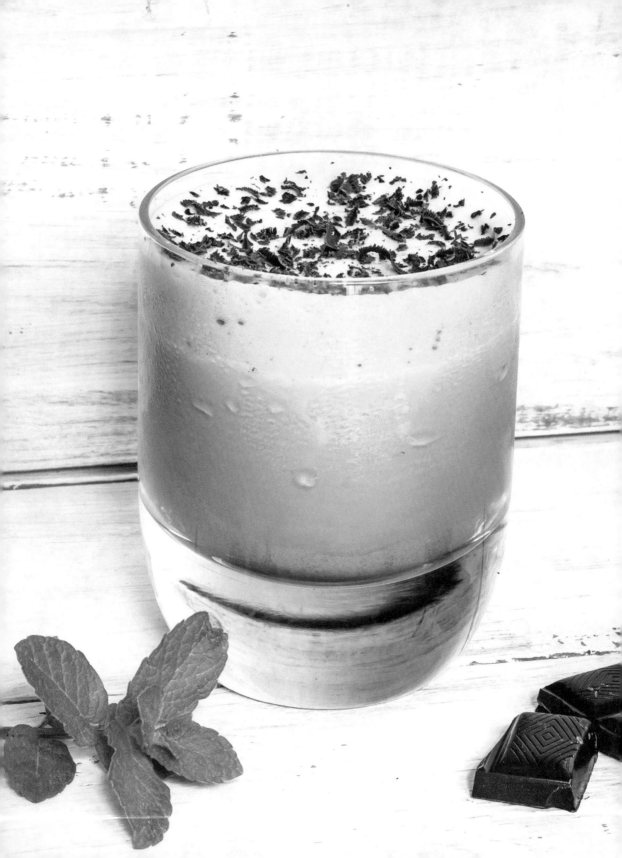

Skinny Mint Chip

Serves 1

140 Calories

1 banana
1 cup Silk unsweetened almond milk
1 scoop chocolate pea protein powder
1 tablespoon unsweetened cocoa powder
⅛ teaspoon peppermint extract
½ cup kale
½ cup ice

1. Add ingredients to a blender.
2. Blend until smooth.
3. Serve in a glass and enjoy!

9 Tiny and Full™ Entrée Recipes

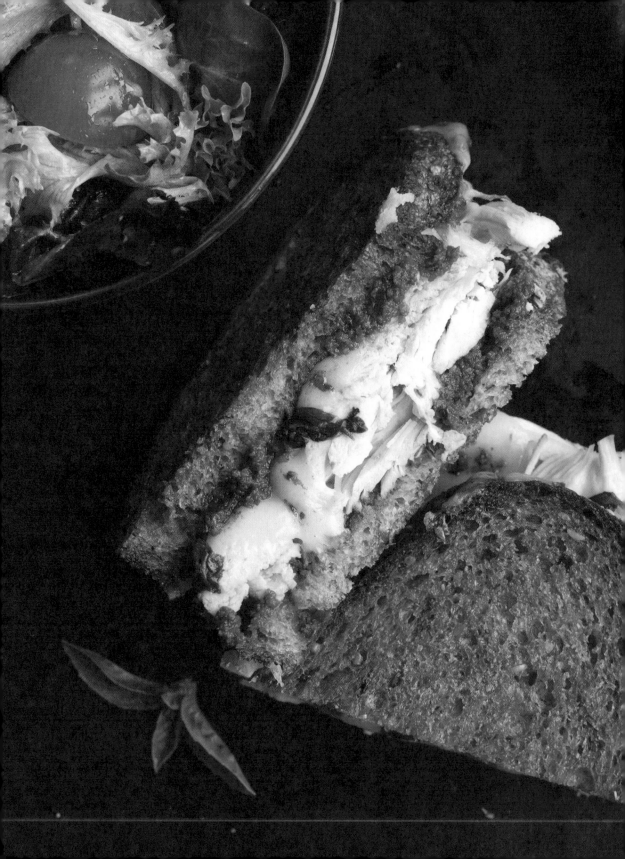

Lunch

Herb Chicken Salad Sandwich

Serves 1

275 Calories

1 slice bread (Udi's, Rudi's, Ezekiel 4:9)
2 tablespoons low fat plain Greek yogurt
1 tablespoon rosemary, finely chopped
Salt and pepper, to taste
2 dashes garlic powder
2 ounces shredded chicken breast
1 tablespoon celery, finely chopped
1 tablespoon red onion, finely chopped
1 lettuce leaf
1 tomato slice

1. Lightly toast bread and cut in half.
2. In a medium bowl, combine yogurt, rosemary, salt and pepper, and garlic powder. Mix well.
3. Add all remaining ingredients, and stir to coat.
4. Assemble sandwich with lettuce, tomato, and chicken salad.
5. Enjoy!

Spinach and Parmesan Portobellos

Serves 1

178 Calories

2 portobello mushrooms
1 teaspoon melted coconut oil
1 teaspoon garlic
1 cup spinach
1 tablespoon low fat Greek yogurt
3 tablespoons organic marinara sauce
2 tablespoons Parmesan cheese

1. Clean mushrooms and remove stems.

2. Brush mushrooms with oil on both sides.

3. Finely chop mushroom stems, and saute for 2-3 minutes in a large skillet.

4. Add garlic and allow to cook for another couple of minutes.

5. Add spinach to the pan, a handful at a time.

6. Once the spinach is wilted, remove from the heat, and stir in yogurt.

7. Preheat oven to 400°F.

8. Place oiled mushrooms on baking sheet, then spoon marinara sauce inside.

9. Spoon spinach mixture over marinara and top with Parmesan cheese.

10. Bake for 10-12 minutes, or until mushrooms are tender.

11. Broil for the last two minutes, or until cheese is melted and golden brown.

12. Let them rest for a couple of minutes, then serve warm!

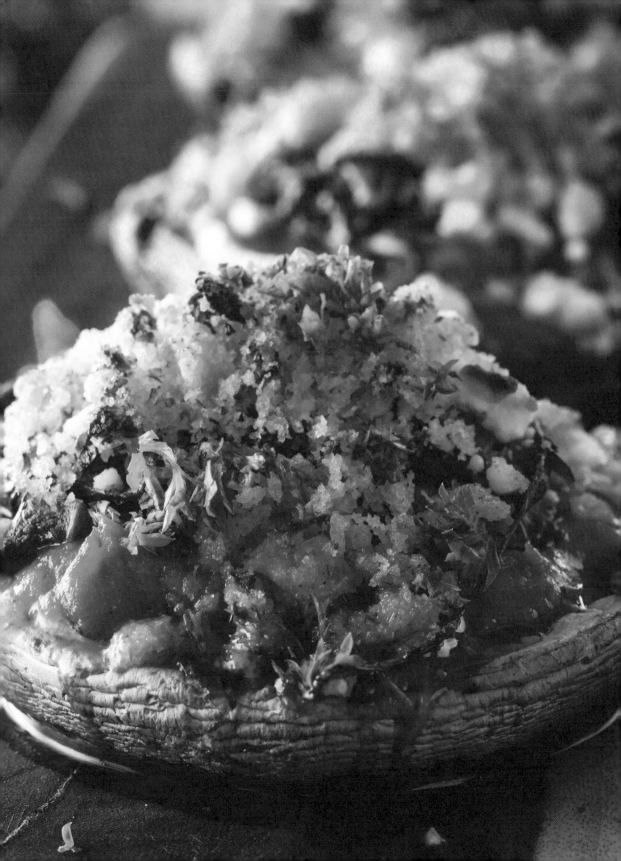

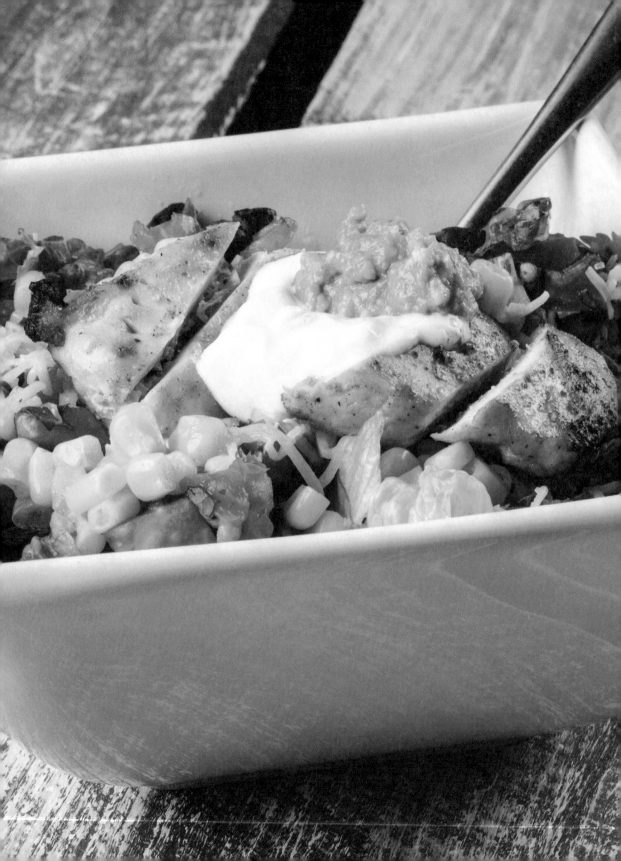

Santa Fe Chicken Elote Bowl

Serves 1

301 Calories

3 ounces boneless, skinless chicken breast
Salt and pepper
1 teaspoon coconut oil
1 tablespoon onion, diced
1 tablespoon bell pepper, diced
2 tablespoons corn, fresh or frozen
½ teaspoon cayenne pepper
1 clove garlic, minced
1 cup romaine lettuce, chopped
1 tablespoon avocado, mashed
1 tablespoon cilantro, chopped
Lime wedges

Optional:
low fat Greek yogurt

1. Cut chicken into bite-sized pieces, then season with salt and pepper.

2. In a large skillet, heat the oil over medium-high heat. Cook chicken until golden brown. Remove and set aside.

3. In the same skillet, increase the heat to high, and add the onion, bell pepper, corn, and cayenne pepper.

4. Stir occasionally, until vegetables are soft, then add garlic and decrease heat to low.

5. Plate chicken and vegetables on top of lettuce, then garnish with avocado, cilantro, and lime wedges. If desired, add one teaspoon of Greek yogurt to top.

6. Serve and enjoy!

Gooey Grilled Cheese

Serves 1

290 Calories

1 tablespoon coconut oil
2 slices bread (Udi's, Rudi's, Ezekiel 4:9)
½ cup shredded low fat cheddar cheese
Salt and pepper

1. Brush coconut oil on the outside of the slices of bread.
2. Assemble sandwich in hot pan, with the shredded cheddar cheese with salt and pepper in between bread with oiled sides on the outside.
3. Cook over medium-low heat until both sides are golden brown, about 3–5 minutes per side.
4. Cut in half and serve.

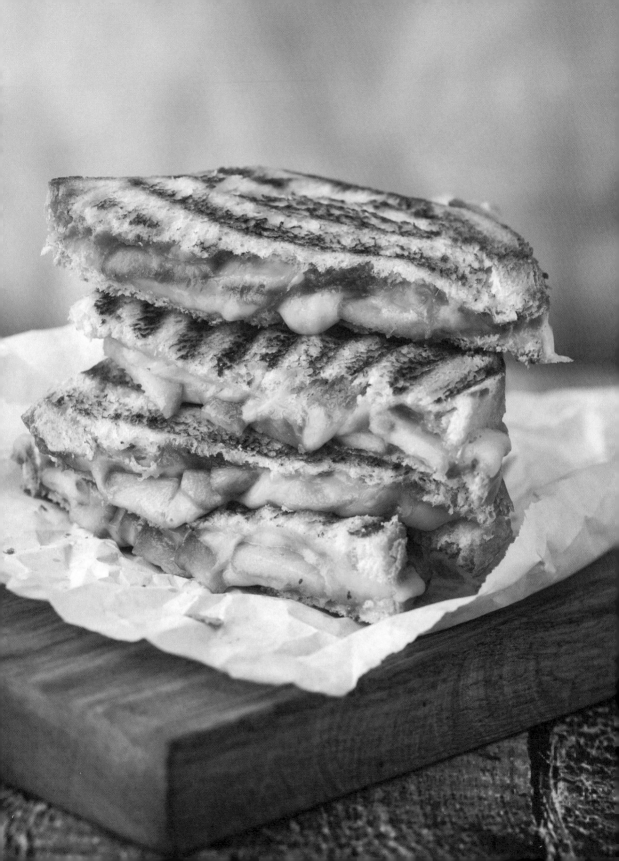

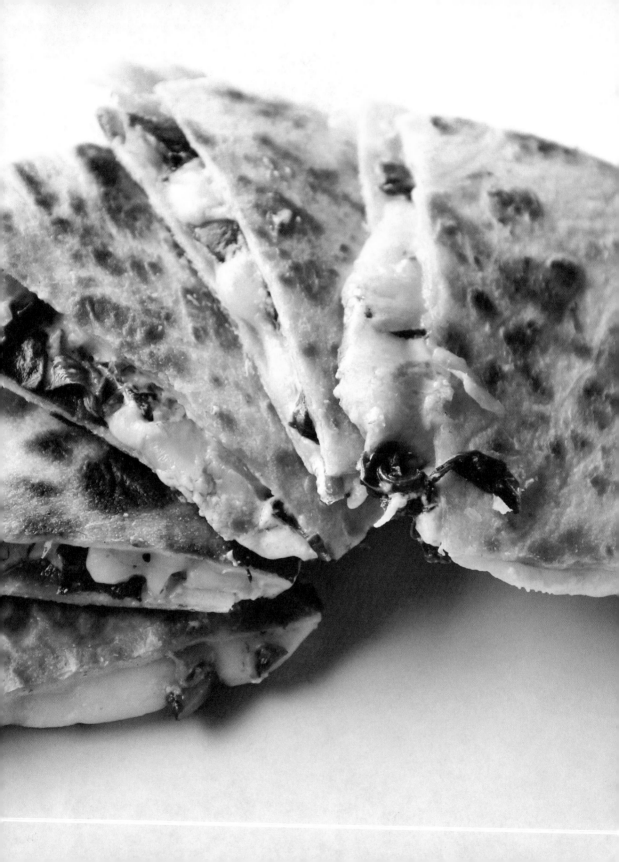

Creamy Spinach Quesadilla

Serves 1

256 Calories

¼ teaspoon coconut oil
1 ounce artichoke hearts, drained and chopped
¼ cup spinach
1 teaspoon low fat Greek yogurt
¼ cup nonfat mozzarella cheese, grated
1 tablespoon Parmesan cheese, grated
Salt and pepper, to taste
1 tortilla (Mission, Udi's, La Tortilla Factory)

1. Heat oil in a large pot over medium-high heat. Add artichokes and cook for one minute.

2. Reduce heat to medium, then add spinach and cook until wilted.

3. Add yogurt and both cheeses, and stir until cheese melts.

4. Season with salt and pepper to taste.

5. Remove from heat.

6. Meanwhile, heat tortilla until browned in dry, hot pan.

7. Assemble quesadilla, and cut into fourths.

8. Serve and enjoy!

Turkey Burger Sliders

Serves 2

167 Calories per slider

1 teaspoon coconut oil
1 tablespoon onion, diced
1 tablespoon green bell pepper, diced
¼ cup zucchini, grated
Salt and pepper, to taste
½ teaspoon garlic powder
1 teaspoon Worcestershire sauce
6 ounces ground turkey (93% lean)
4 romaine lettuce leaves
½ tomato, sliced

1. Combine oil, onion, green pepper, and zucchini in large skillet.
2. Sauté until vegetables are tender. Remove from heat and let cool.
3. In a large bowl, add salt, pepper, garlic powder, Worcestershire, and turkey.
4. Add cooled veggies and mix until evenly distributed
5. Form four small patties.
6. Add patties to hot grill and cook until golden brown.
7. Serve on lettuce leaves with a tomato slice.
8. Enjoy!

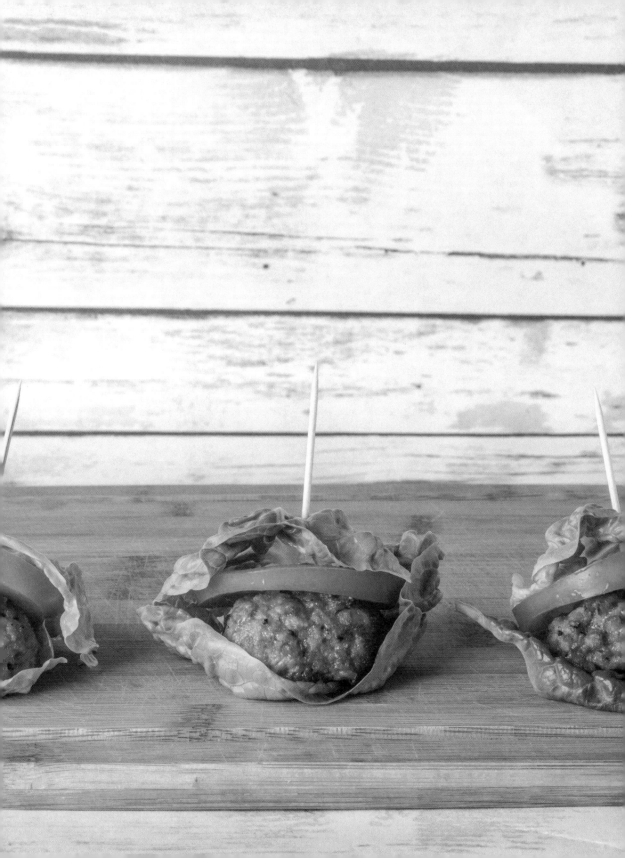

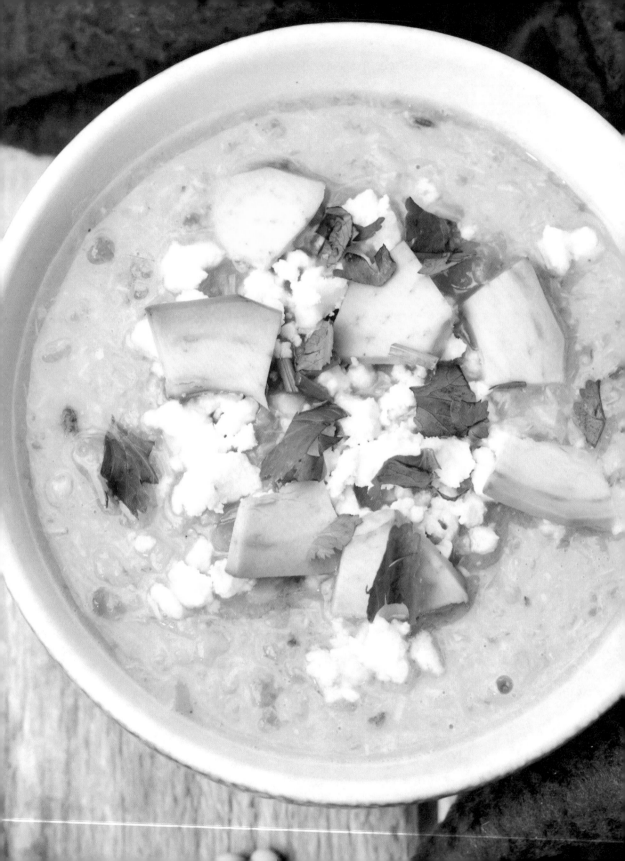

Creamy Avocado Spring Chicken Soup

Serves 2

224 Calories per serving

3 cups chicken broth
1 teaspoon Sriracha, or to taste
6 ounces boneless, skinless chicken breast
½ cup navy beans
1 clove garlic, minced
2 scallions, sliced
1 tablespoon low fat Greek yogurt
Salt and black pepper, to taste

Garnish:
diced avocado and chopped cilantro

1. Pour broth into large saucepan and heat to medium-high. Stir in Sriracha.
2. While broth heats, dice chicken into bite-size pieces.
3. When broth begins to boil, stir in chicken, navy beans, garlic, and chopped scallions.
4. Turn burner to low, and let simmer for 10 minutes.
5. Stir in yogurt and season with salt and pepper, to taste.
6. Ladle into bowls and garnish with avocado and cilantro. Enjoy!

Mediterranean Chicken Pita

Serves 2

332 Calories per serving

Juice of half a lemon
1 garlic clove, minced
1 teaspoon ground coriander
1 teaspoon cumin
Salt and pepper
6 ounces boneless, skinless chicken breast
2 tablespoons low fat Greek yogurt
¼ cucumber, grated
1 teaspoon mint, chopped
1 teaspoon coconut oil
2 pita breads (Udi's, Joseph's, Simply Balanced)
½ tomato, diced
1 cup spinach

1. Combine lemon juice, garlic, coriander, cumin, salt, and pepper—mix until smooth and use to marinate chicken.
2. Refrigerate chicken and allow to marinate for 30 minutes.
3. In a small bowl, stir together yogurt, cucumber, and chopped mint.
4. In a large skillet, heat oil over medium-high heat.
5. Add marinated chicken and cook for 8-10 minutes, stirring occasionally.
6. Heat pitas under a broiler or in a toaster oven.
7. Slice open pitas and stuff with chicken, tomatoes, and spinach, and top with yogurt dressing.
8. Serve and enjoy!

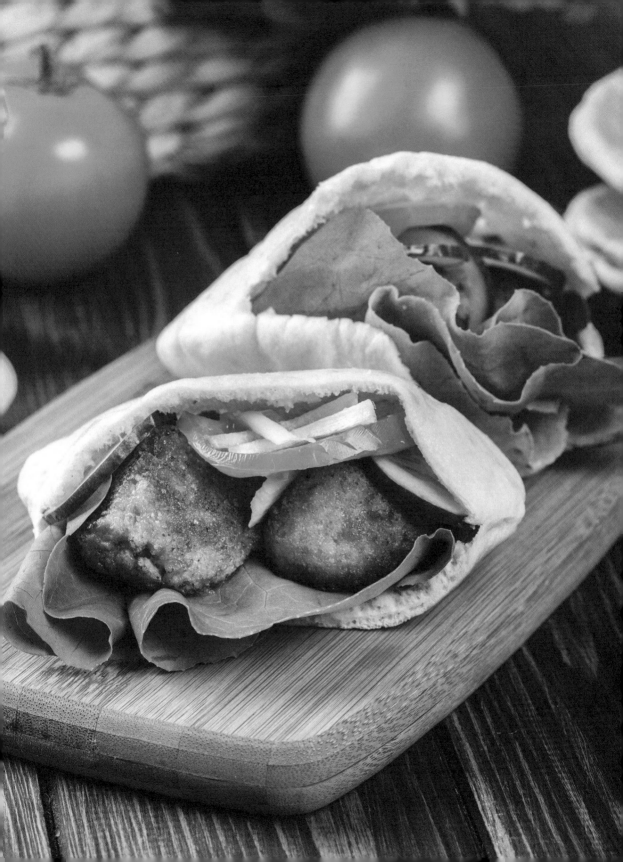

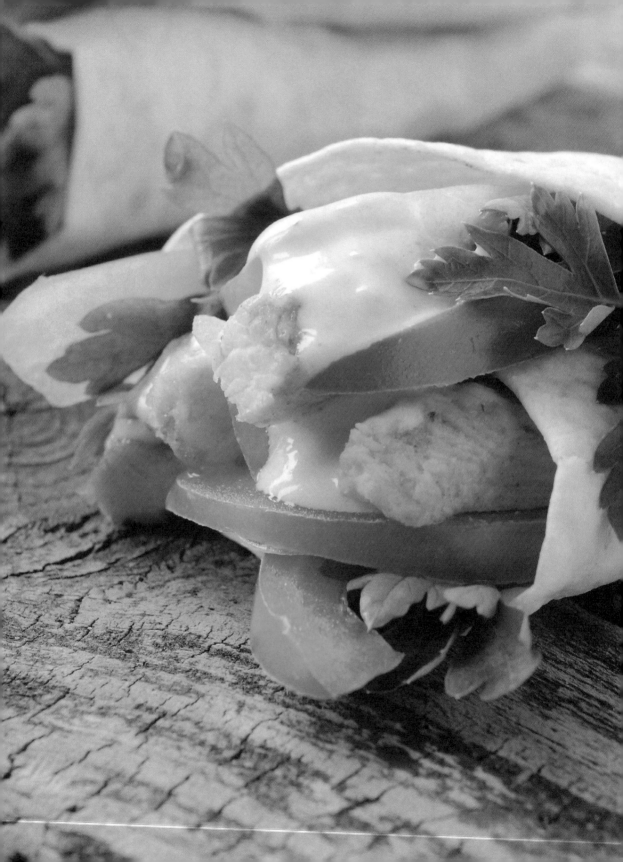

Brentwood BLT

Serves 1

295 Calories

1 slice extra lean turkey bacon
1 tortilla (Mission, Udi's, La Tortilla factory)
½ cup low fat Greek yogurt
3 slices deli turkey
½ cup shredded lettuce or cabbage
½ cup chopped or sliced tomatoes

1. In hot skillet, cook turkey bacon.
2. Heat tortilla.
3. Lay out tortilla and add yogurt, deli turkey, turkey bacon, lettuce, and tomatoes.
4. Wrap tightly and cut in half.
5. Enjoy!

Sweet and Spicy Asian Steak

Serves 2

219 calories per serving

6 ounces grass-fed flank steak
2 tablespoons low sodium soy sauce
½ teaspoon honey
½ teaspoon chili paste
1 teaspoon coconut oil

Suggested pairings:
brown rice and vegetables, cauliflower rice, or steamed broccoli

1. Slice the steak into bite-size pieces and place the chunks of beef into a medium size bowl.
2. Whisk soy sauce, honey, and chili paste. Pour over the beef and stir to coat.
3. Let the meat marinate for 20-30 minutes.
4. Heat up coconut oil in a medium sized pan.
5. Add meat and brown until desired doneness.
6. Serve on a plate with suggested pairings and enjoy!

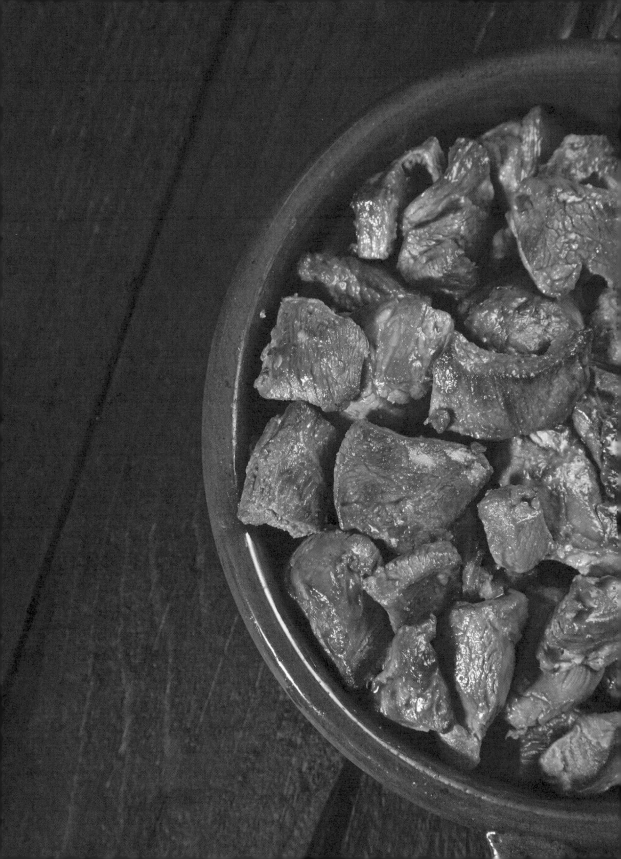

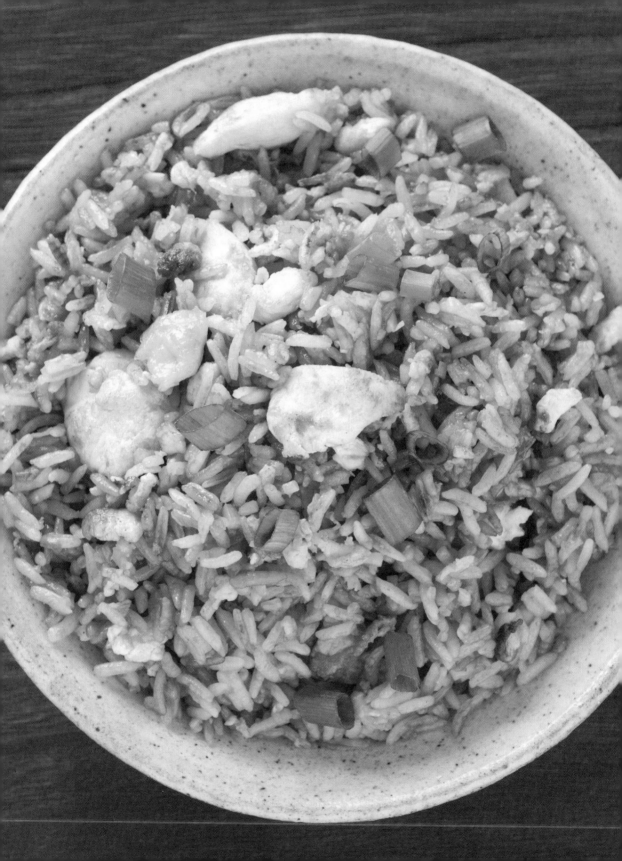

Guilt-Free Chicken Fried Rice

Serves 1

272 Calories

½ cup brown rice
2 teaspoons sesame oil
1 garlic clove, minced
¼ teaspoon red pepper flakes
3 ounces boneless, skinless chicken breast
½ small onion, diced
½ cup frozen peas and carrots
1 green onion, thinly sliced
1 ounce firm tofu, mashed or cubed
1 teaspoon low sodium soy sauce

1. Make the brown rice according to package directions.
2. In a wok or a large skillet, heat 1 teaspoon sesame oil over medium-high heat.
3. Add garlic and red pepper flakes, and stir constantly.
4. Increase the heat to high, and add the chicken.
5. Cook for 4 to 6 minutes, turning and moving the chicken constantly while cooking.
6. Scrape the chicken and garlic onto a plate and set aside.
7. Add the remaining 1 teaspoon of sesame oil to the pan. Once hot, add the onion, peas and carrots, and half of the green onion and stir-fry, constantly moving the mixture until the onion and carrots soften, 3 to 5 minutes.
8. Push the vegetables to the outer edges of the wok or skillet to make room in the center. Add tofu and let brown, about 2 minutes.
9. Reduce the heat to medium.
10. Add chicken, cooked brown rice, and soy sauce to the vegetable mixture and stir to combine.
11. Top with remaining green onions, and serve!

Hollywood Beet Salad

Serves 1

306 calories

2 ounces boneless, skinless chicken breast
Coarse salt and freshly ground pepper
1 teaspoon olive oil
2 cups chopped kale
1 teaspoon red wine vinegar
1 tablespoon fresh lemon juice
½ cup red beets, grated
1 ounce mild goat cheese

1. Season chicken with salt and pepper.
2. Heat oil in pan over medium heat.
3. Cook chicken on both sides until cooked through, 3 to 4 minutes per side. Slice.
4. Place kale and sliced chicken in a large bowl.
5. Drizzle with vinegar and lemon juice, then season with salt and pepper.
6. Top with beets and goat cheese, and toss.
7. Serve and enjoy!

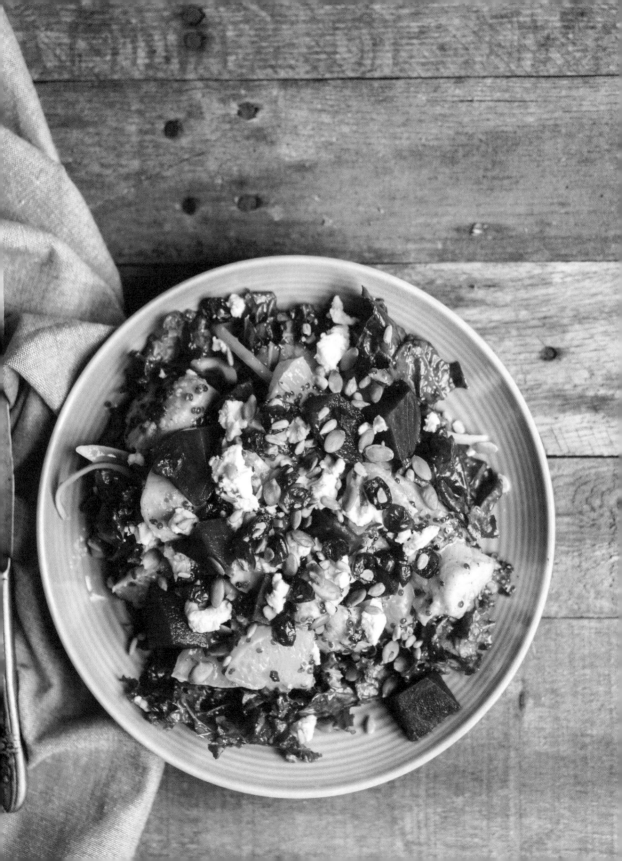

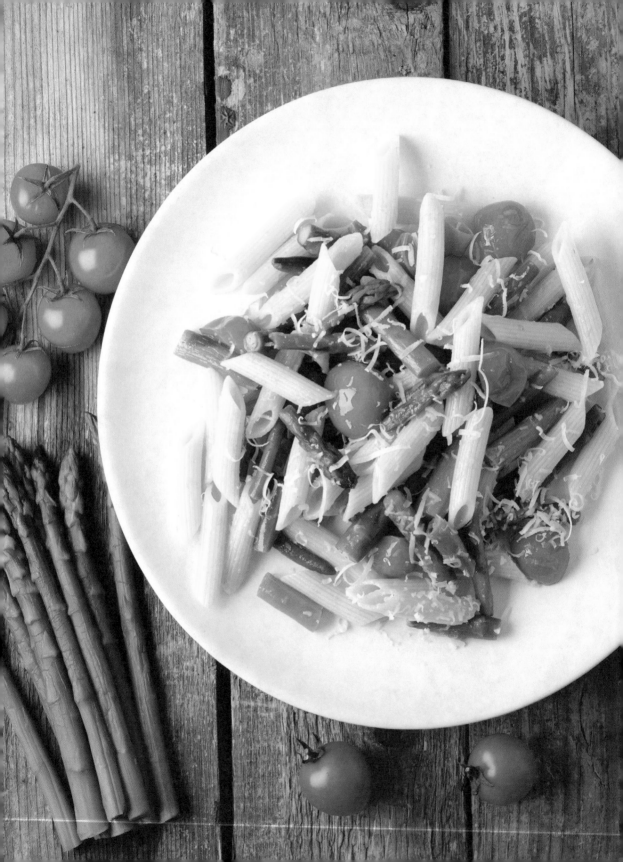

Capri Pasta

Serves 2

352 Calories per serving

2 cups pasta (Barilla, Ancient Harvest, etc.)
2 tablespoons olive oil
1 cup asparagus, chopped
1 cup cherry tomatoes, halved
1 tablespoon grated provolone

1. Cook pasta according to package directions.
2. In a large skillet over medium-high heat, add oil and chopped asparagus until soft.
3. Add cooked pasta and cherry tomatoes to the skillet.
4. Top with cheese and enjoy!

AB & J Sandwich

Serves 1

270 Calories

2 slices bread (Udi's, Rudi's, Ezekiel 4:9)
1 tablespoon unsalted almond butter
1 tablespoon sugar free jam, or pureed fruit

1. Toast bread.
2. Add almond butter to one slice and jam to the other slice.
3. Assemble sandwich and cut in half.
4. Enjoy!

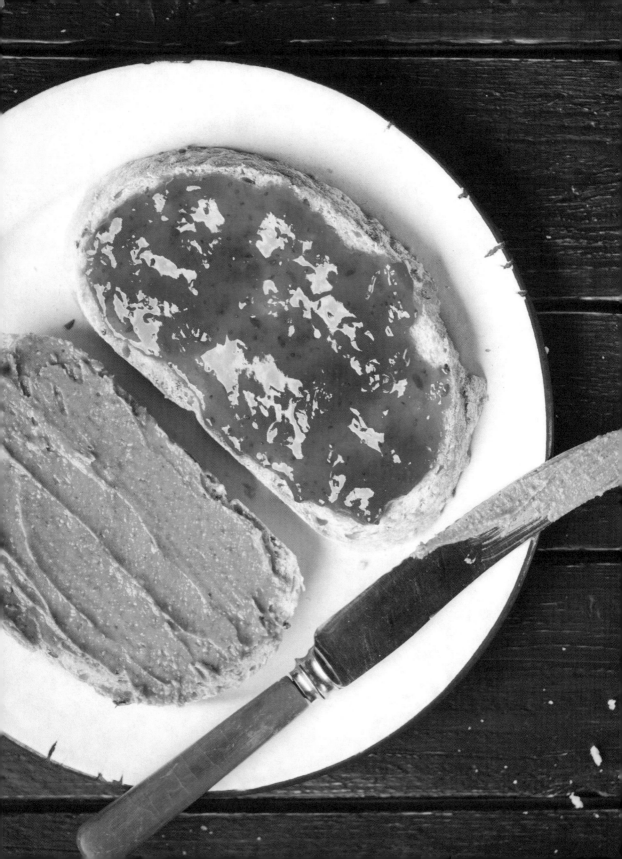

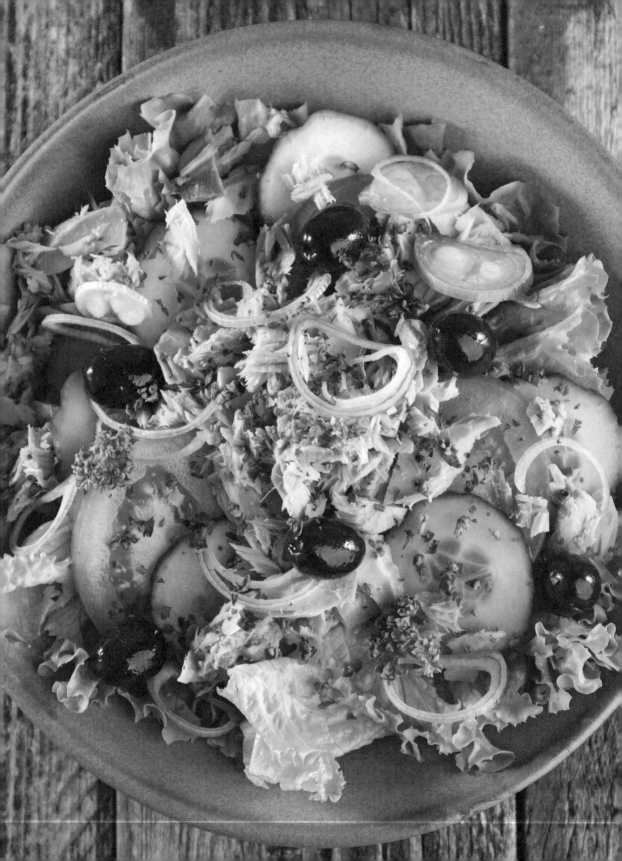

Pacific Tuna Salad

Serves 2

122 Calories per serving

6 ounce can tuna, drained
2 tablespoons low fat Greek yogurt
1 tablespoon sweet pickle relish
1 teaspoon Dijon mustard
1 stalk celery, chopped
¼ cup onion, chopped
¼ teaspoon ground black pepper
Juice of half a lemon
2 cups lettuce

1. Add all ingredients in a bowl and stir to combine.
2. Chill and serve on top of lettuce of your choice.

Kale Caesar

Serves 1

130 Calories

2 tablespoons lemon juice

1½ teaspoons Dijon mustard

4 anchovies, finely chopped

2 garlic cloves, finely chopped

¼ cup extra-virgin olive oil

Salt and pepper, to taste

1 tablespoon Parmesan cheese, grated

1 bunch kale, chopped

1. In a large bowl, whisk together lemon juice, mustard, anchovies and garlic.
2. Slowly whisk in oil until combined and thickened.
3. Whisk in salt, pepper, and grated cheese.
4. Add kale and toss until leaves are thoroughly coated.
5. Top with more cheese.

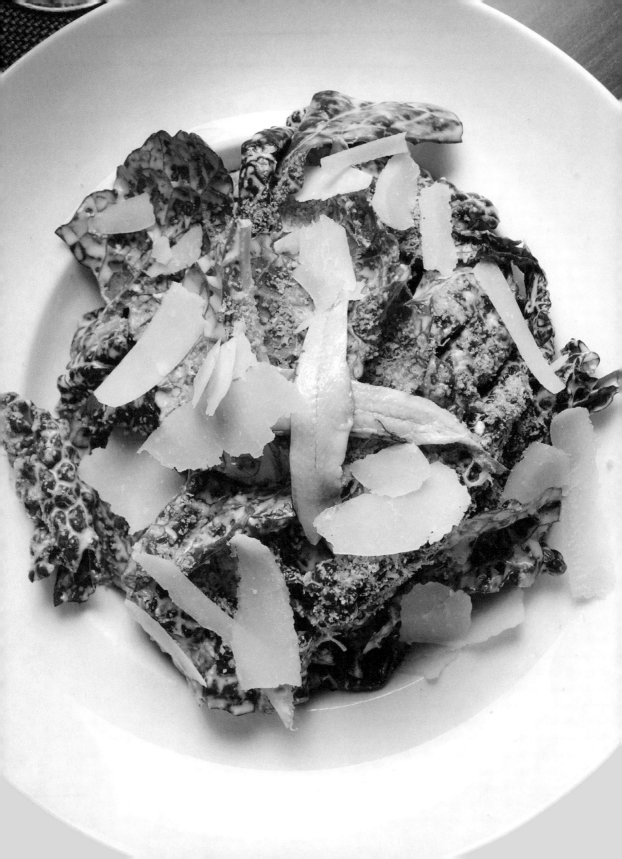

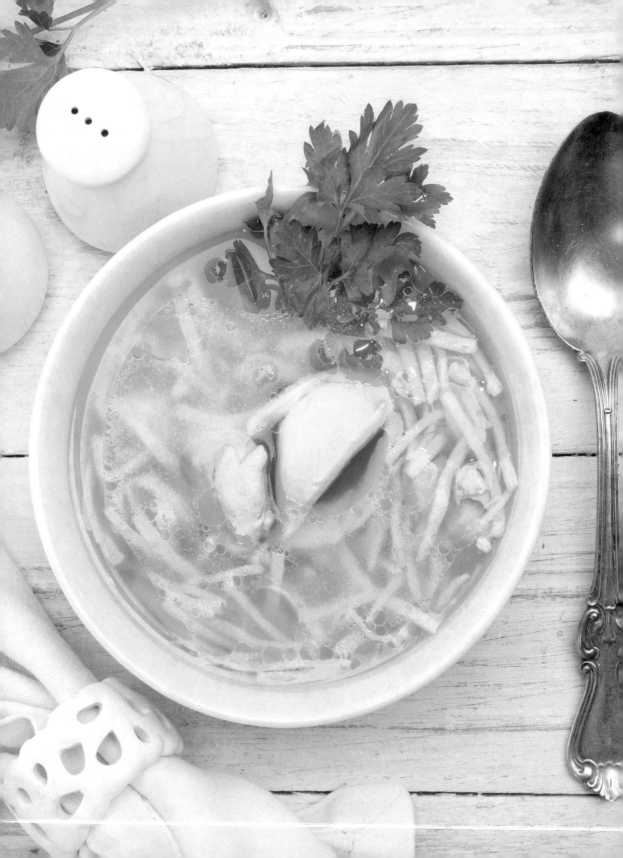

Chicken Zoodle Soup

Serves 2

215 Calories per serving

6 ounces boneless, skinless chicken breast, cubed
½ teaspoon poultry seasoning
1 teaspoon coconut oil
¼ onion, chopped
1 stalk celery, chopped
½ carrot, chopped
1 garlic clove, minced
2 cups reduced-sodium chicken broth
Salt and pepper, to taste
1 zucchini or yellow summer squash, spiralized
¼ cup fresh parsley, roughly chopped

1. In a large bowl, combine cubed chicken and poultry seasoning; toss to coat.

2. In a pot, heat oil over medium heat.

3. Add chicken and cook for 3 to 5 minutes, or until chicken is browned.

4. Remove chicken, and set aside.

5. In the same pot, sauté onion, celery, carrot, and garlic over medium heat about 5 minutes or just until tender, stirring occasionally.

6. Pour in chicken broth; bring to a boil.

7. Add salt and pepper to taste.

8. Add chicken and zucchini noodles.

9. Return to a boil; then reduce heat.

10. Cover and simmer for 5 minutes.

11. Garnish with parsley.

Three Minute Zucchini Pasta

Serves 1

301 Calories

Salt and pepper
3 ounces boneless, skinless chicken breast
1 large zucchini
1 teaspoon lemon zest
½ tablespoon extra-virgin olive oil
2 tablespoons Parmesan cheese

1. Salt and pepper chicken and cook through on hot skillet. Slice.
2. Spiralize zucchini into noodles.
3. Toss spiralized zucchini in lemon zest, olive oil, cheese, and salt and pepper.
4. Add sliced chicken.
5. Enjoy!

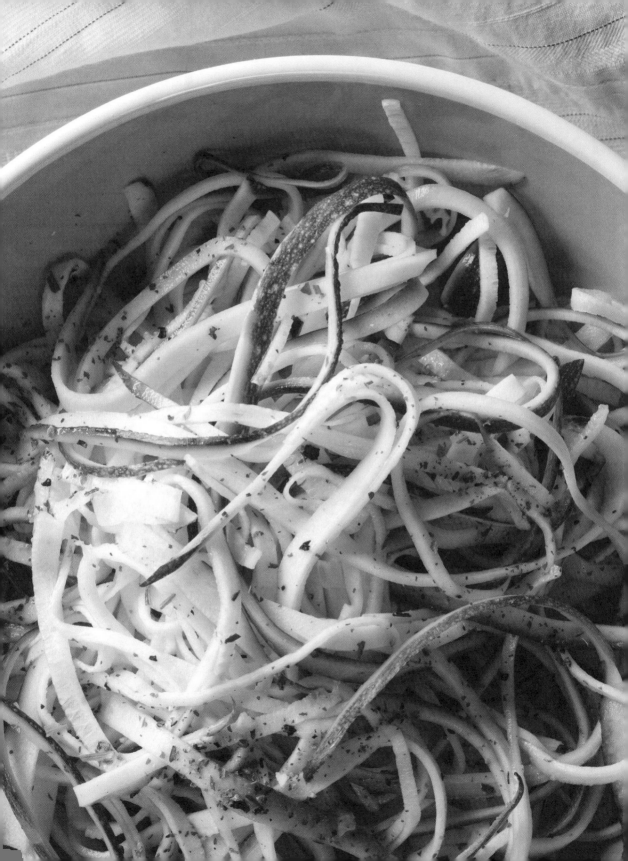

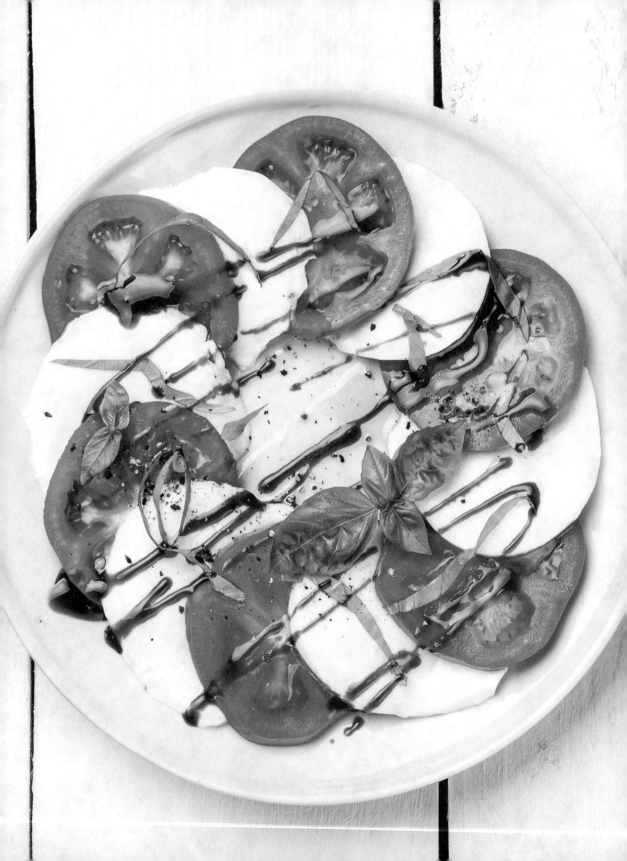

Dinner

Caprese Salad

Serves 1

230 Calories

4 ounces nonfat mozzarella cheese
1 tomato, sliced
Basil, torn
Salt and pepper
½ tablespoon olive oil
2 tablespoons balsamic vinegar

1. Slice mozzarella, and arrange on plate.
2. Top with tomato, basil, salt, and pepper.
3. Drizzle with olive oil and balsamic vinegar.
4. Serve and enjoy!

Revenge Body Soup

Serves 2

265 Calories per serving

6 ounces boneless, skinless chicken breast
1 teaspoon olive oil
1 celery, chopped
1 carrot, chopped
½ green pepper, chopped
1 garlic clove, minced
3 cups chicken broth
1 can diced tomatoes
½ teaspoon basil
¼ teaspoon oregano
¼ teaspoon rosemary
Pepper, to taste
¼ cup lentils
¼ cup fava beans

1. Cut chicken into cubes, and cook in large saucepan until fully cooked.
2. Remove chicken and set aside.
3. Heat olive oil and add celery, carrot, pepper, and garlic; cook until tender.
4. Stir in chicken broth, tomatoes, basil, oregano, rosemary, black pepper, lentils, and fava beans.
5. Bring to a boil, then reduce heat.
6. Cover and simmer for 20 minutes.
7. Add cooked chicken.
8. Cover and cook for 10 more minutes.
9. Ladle into bowls and enjoy!

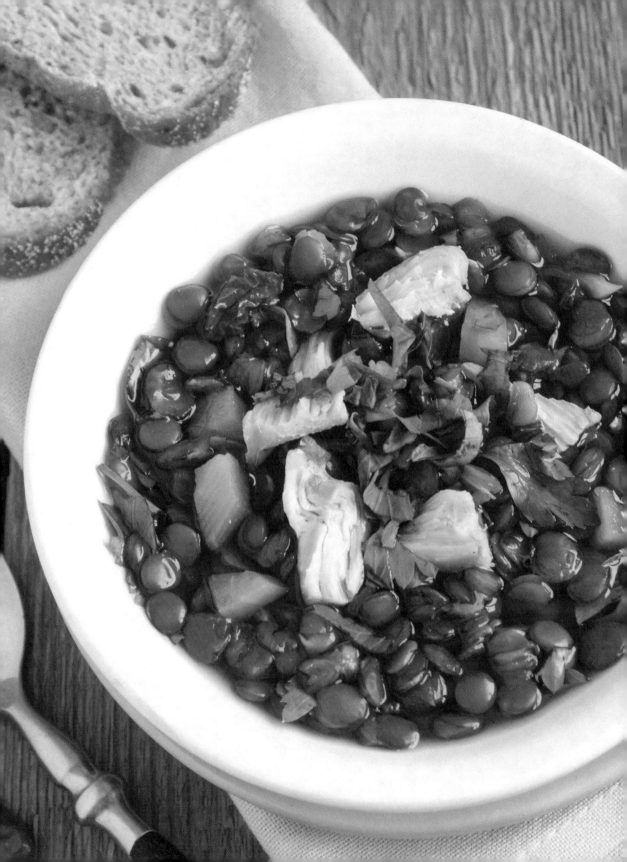

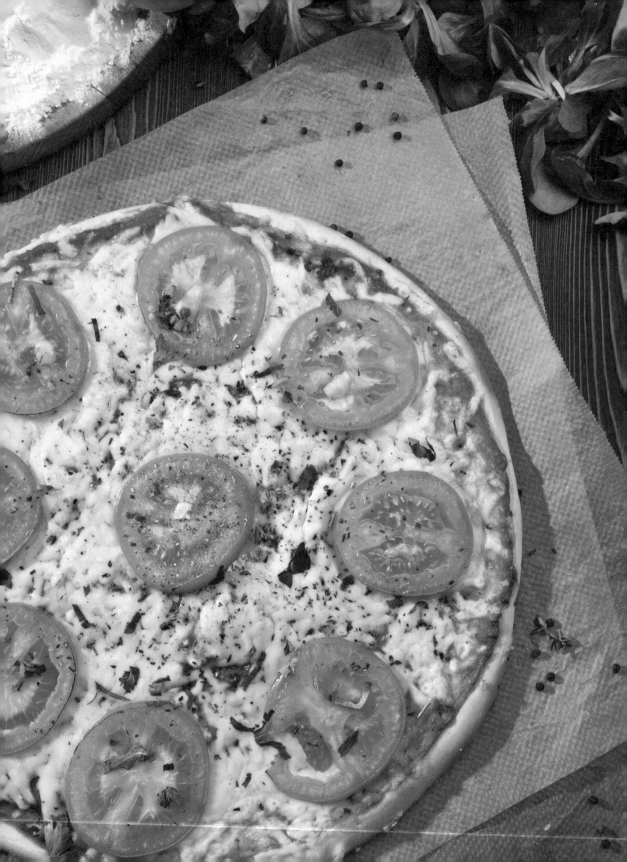

Margherita Tortilla Pizza

Serves 1

256 Calories

1 large tortilla (Mission, Udi's, La Tortilla Factory)
⅓ cup organic marinara sauce
½ cup nonfat mozzarella cheese
1 plum tomato, thinly sliced
½ cup fresh basil, thinly sliced

1. Preheat oven to 400°F.
2. Lay tortilla on baking sheet and spread thin layer of marinara sauce on top.
3. Sprinkle with cheese.
4. Arrange tomato slices on top.
5. Bake for 10 minutes or until cheese melts and crust is golden brown.
6. Sprinkle pizza evenly with sliced basil.
7. Cut slices and enjoy!

Venice Beach Street Tacos

Serves 1

245 Calories

3 ounces grass-fed flank steak
½ lime, juiced
1 tablespoon cilantro
Salt and pepper
2 corn tortillas
¼ white onion, chopped
Lime wedges, for serving

1. Marinate steak in lime juice, cilantro, and salt and pepper for at least 1 hour.
2. Heat up grill or pan.
3. Cook steak for 4–6 minutes each side for medium. Remove steak and let rest.
4. Heat up corn tortillas.
5. Slice steak into small pieces.
6. Assemble tacos with sliced steak topped with onion and cilantro.
7. Serve with lime wedge.
8. Enjoy!

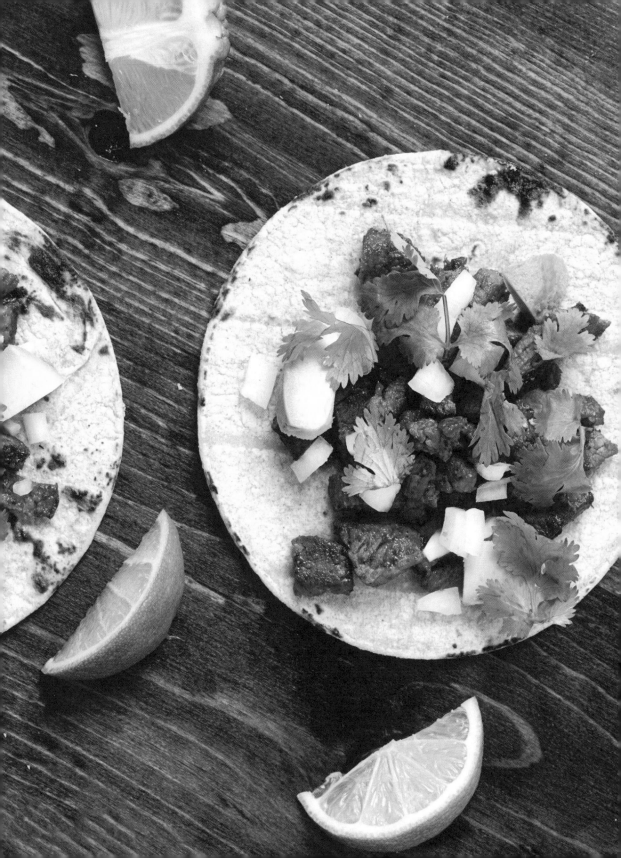

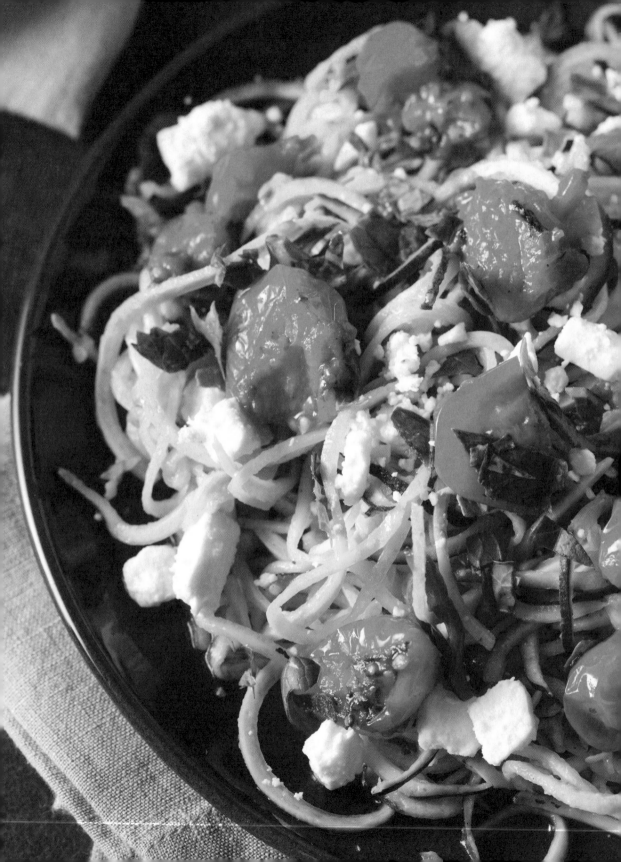

Tomato Feta Pasta Primavera

Serves 2

167 Calories per serving

2 large zucchini
1 tablespoon olive oil
1 cup cherry tomatoes
1 large clove of garlic, minced
2 tablespoon chopped basil
Salt and pepper, to taste
4 tablespoons reduced fat feta cheese

1. Using a spiralizer, create the zucchini noodles and set aside.
2. Heat saucepan over medium heat and add oil to saute tomatoes and garlic.
3. Reduce heat, then add basil and zucchini noodles; season with salt and pepper.
4. Toss in pan for 2–3 minutes.
5. Serve topped with feta cheese.

Tiny and Full™ Entrée Recipes

Zucchini Rad Thai

Serves 2

164 Calories per serving

2 large yellow squash
2 ounces firm tofu, mashed
2 tablespoons lime juice
1 tablespoon low sodium soy sauce
1 tablespoon chili sauce
½ tablespoon coconut oil
1 garlic clove, minced
1 shallot, minced
1 tablespoon cilantro
1 tablespoon roasted unsalted peanuts, finely chopped
Lime wedges

1. Spiralize yellow squash into noodles and set aside.
2. Whisk tofu, lime juice, soy sauce, and chili sauce in a bowl until smooth.
3. Heat a large skillet over medium heat, and add oil, garlic, and shallot. Cook for about 1-2 minutes, stirring frequently, until the shallot softens.
4. Add the sauce and reduce for 2-3 minutes or until sauce has slightly thickened.
5. Once the sauce is thick, add in the squash noodles and cilantro and stir to combine thoroughly.
6. Cook for about 2 minutes, then add chopped peanuts.
7. Cook for 30 seconds, tossing to fully combine.
8. Plate onto dishes and garnish with cilantro leaves.
9. Serve with lime wedges.

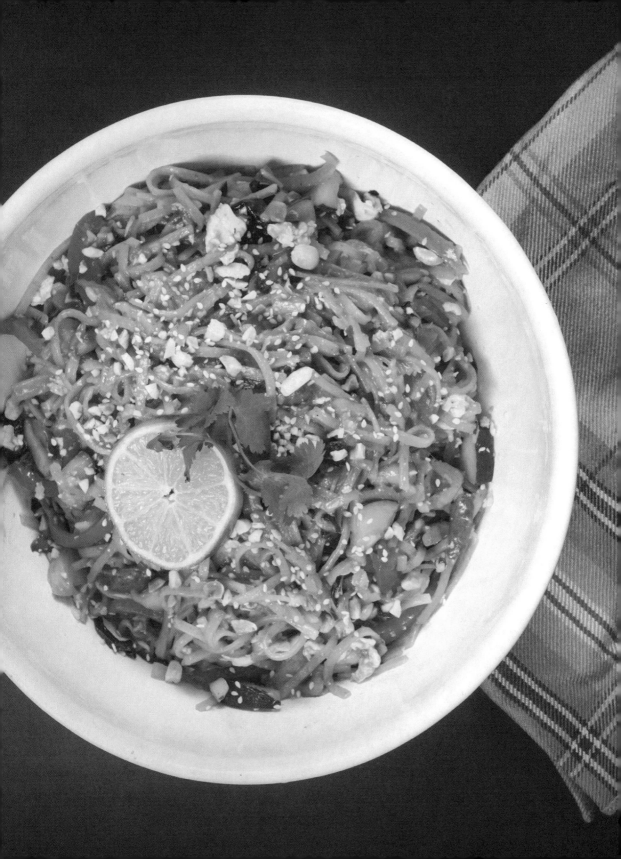

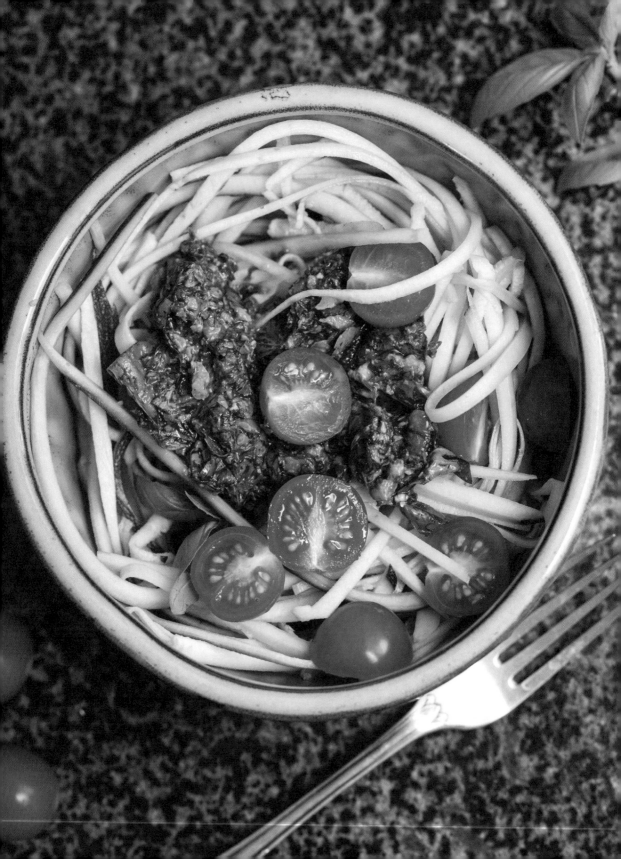

Zucchini Basil Fresca

Serves 2

242 Calories per serving

2 large zucchini
1 cup basil
2 garlic cloves
1 Brazil nut
1 tablespoon extra-virgin olive oil
2 tablespoons fresh lemon juice
¼ cup Parmesan cheese, freshly grated
Salt and pepper, to taste
1 cup cherry tomatoes

1. Spiralize the zucchini into noodles.
2. Combine the basil, garlic, and Brazil nut in a food processor and pulse until coarsely chopped.
3. Slowly add the olive oil in a constant stream while the food processor is on.
4. Stop the machine and scrape down the sides of the food processor with a rubber spatula.
5. Add the lemon juice and Parmesan cheese. Pulse until blended.
6. Season with salt and pepper.
7. Heat the zucchini noodles in a pan over medium heat for 2-5 minutes.
8. Plate the zucchini and add pesto and the cherry tomatoes.
9. Enjoy!

Spaghetti Squash Lasagna

Serves 4

349 Calories per serving

1 large spaghetti squash
Salt and pepper, to taste
2 cups organic marinara sauce
1 cup part-skim ricotta
8 teaspoons Parmesan cheese
6 ounces nonfat shredded mozzarella
4 cups spinach
Basil, to garnish

1. Cut spaghetti squash in half lengthwise, and scoop out the seeds with a spoon.
2. Place on a baking sheet, cut side up, and sprinkle with salt and pepper.
3. Bake at 350°F for about an hour or until the inside is tender. Remove from oven and let cool.
4. Using a fork, remove squash meat out of skin.
5. Increase oven temperature to 375°F.
6. In a baking dish, layer marinara sauce, spaghetti squash, ricotta, Parmesan cheese, and spinach—spreading each layer smooth.
7. Repeat steps until dish is almost full, making the top layer mozzarella cheese.
8. Cover with foil and bake for 15–20 minutes, or until the cheese is melted and the edges begin to bubble.
9. Uncover and cook an additional 5 minutes.
10. Garnish with basil.
11. Serve and enjoy!

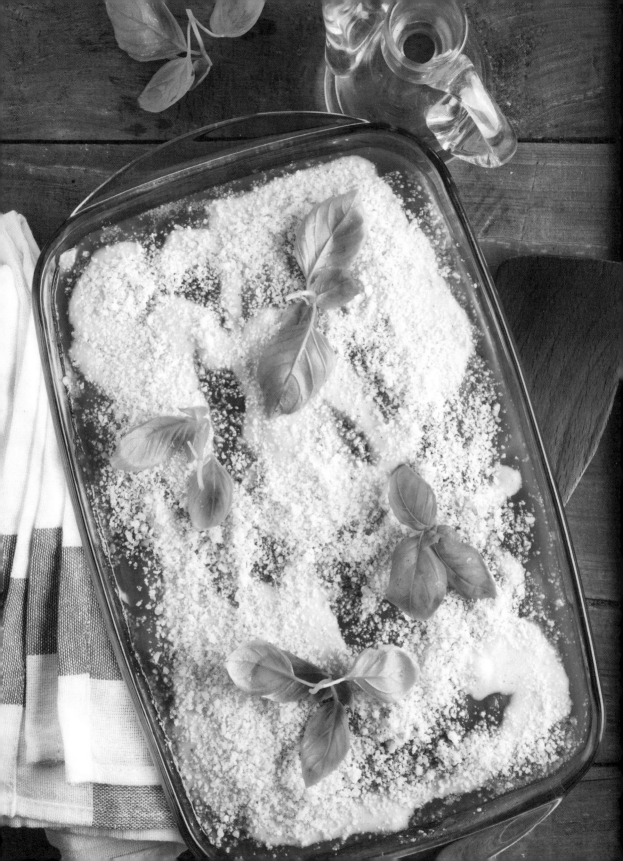

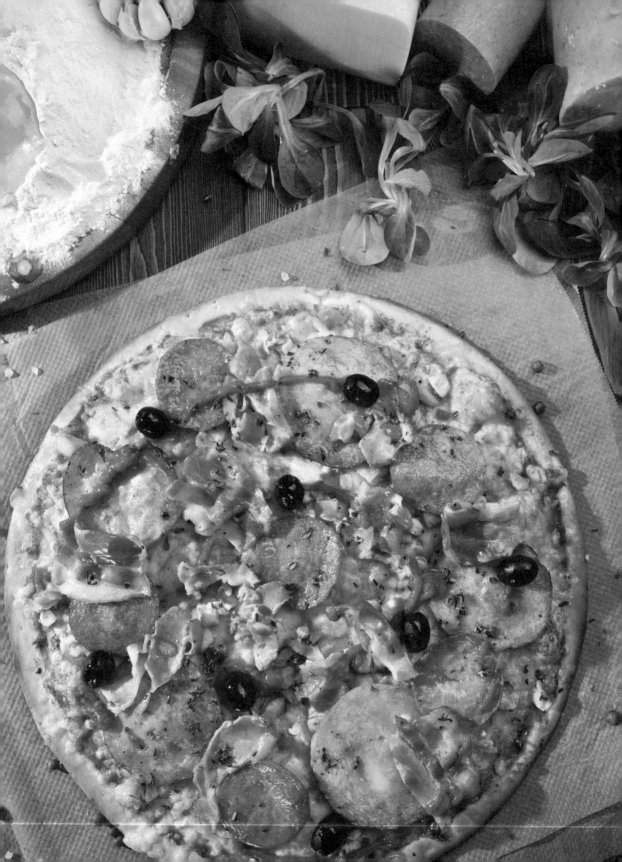

Downtown Pita Pizza

Serves 1

321 Calories

1 pita bread (Udi's, Joseph's, Simply Balanced, Ezekiel 4:9)
1 tablespoon organic marinara sauce
1 ounce nonfat mozzarella cheese
2 slices extra lean turkey deli meat
5 pepperonis
1 teaspoon black olives, sliced
Fresh basil, thinly sliced
Red pepper flakes

1. Preheat oven to 400°F.
2. Place pita bread on baking sheet and spread a thin layer of organic marinara sauce on top.
3. Add mozzarella cheese, deli meat, pepperonis, and olives.
4. Bake for 15–20 minutes until cheese is melted.
5. Garnish with basil and red pepper flakes. Enjoy!

Malibu Tortilla Pizza

Serves 1

205 Calories

1 teaspoon coconut oil

¼ yellow bell pepper, finely sliced

⅓ small eggplant, finely sliced

¼ onion, finely sliced

1 garlic clove, minced

Salt and pepper, to taste

1 tortilla (Mission, Udi's, or La Tortilla Factory)

1 tablespoon organic marinara sauce

2 tablespoons nonfat mozzarella, grated

1 teaspoon basil, thinly sliced

1. Preheat oven to 375° F.
2. In a medium saucepan, heat oil and add pepper, eggplant, onion, garlic, salt, and pepper and cook until just softened, about 6 to 8 minutes.
3. Lay tortillas on a baking sheet.
4. Spread a thin layer of marinara sauce and top with vegetables and cheese.
5. Bake for 8 to 10 minutes, or until cheese is melted.
6. Garnish with basil and enjoy!

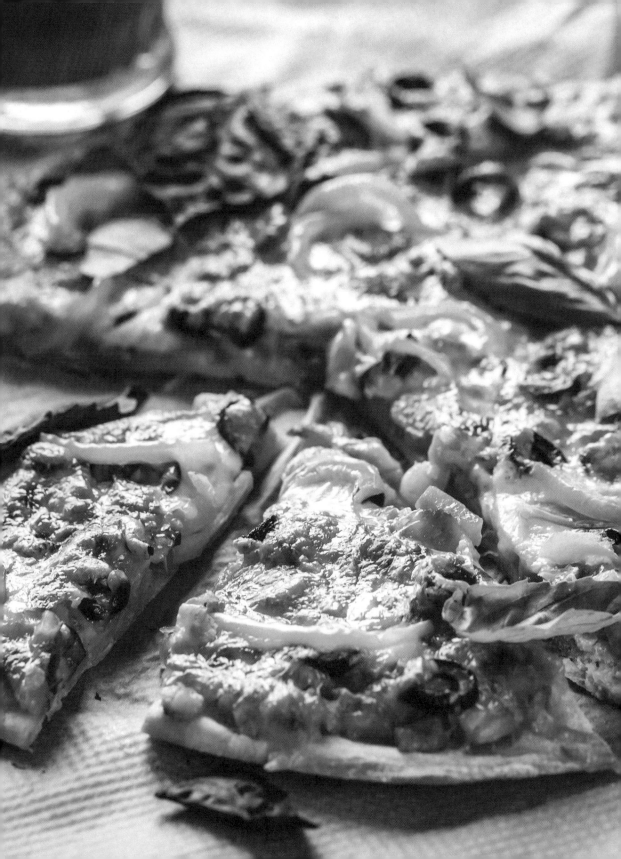

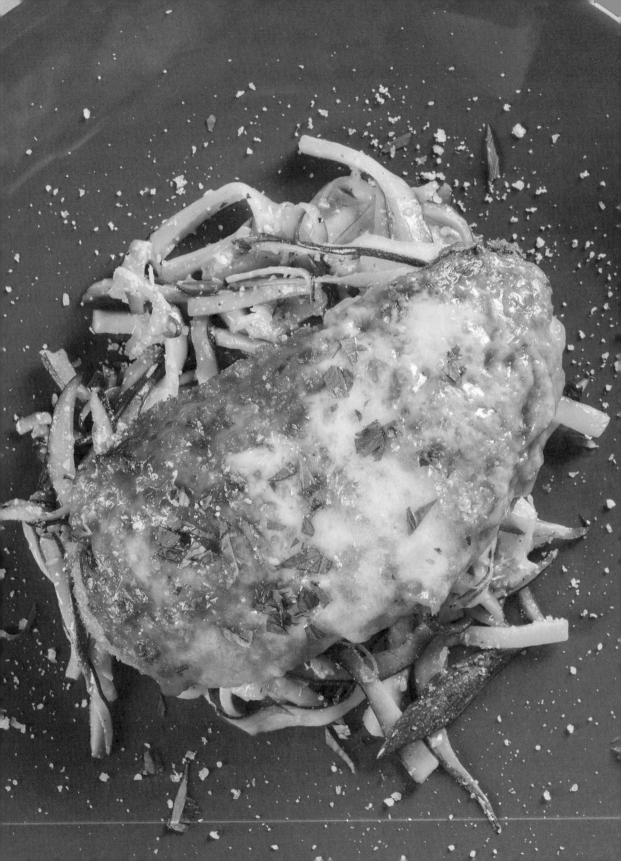

Chicken Parmesan

Serves 1

216 Calories

1 tablespoon Parmesan cheese
1 teaspoon dried Italian herbs
Salt and pepper, to taste
2 tablespoons Silk unsweetened almond milk
1 teaspoon olive oil
3 oz boneless, skinless chicken breast
½ cup organic marinara sauce
1 slice nonfat mozzarella cheese

Optional:
1 zucchini

1. Preheat the oven to 425°F.
2. Toss the Parmesan cheese with the Italian herbs, salt, and pepper in a shallow plate.
3. In another shallow dish, mix almond milk with pepper.
4. Heat the oil in a skillet over medium heat.
5. Dredge chicken in almond milk, then coat with Italian herbs and Parmesan cheese mixture.
6. Add the chicken to the hot skillet and fry for 3–4 minutes on each side or until golden brown.
7. Pour organic marinara sauce into a baking dish.
8. Add chicken breasts to baking dish and top with a slice of cheese.
9. Transfer the baking dish to the oven and bake for 5–10 minutes or until the chicken is fully cooked and the cheese is melted.
10. Use a spiralizer to create zucchini noodles, if desired.
11. Serve chicken and sauce over the raw zucchini noodles.
12. Enjoy!

Glazed Grilled Halibut

Serves 1

168 Calories

½ teaspoon light brown sugar
1 teaspoon chili powder
¼ teaspoon ground cumin
¼ ounce dried seaweed
⅛ teaspoon salt
⅛ teaspoon freshly ground black pepper
3 ounces halibut filet
½ teaspoon olive oil

Suggested pairings:
grilled asparagus, eggplant, green beans, or Brussels sprouts

1. Coat your grill with nonstick cooking spray, and preheat for medium heat.
2. While the grill is heating, combine the brown sugar, chili powder, cumin, dried seaweed, salt, and pepper.
3. Brush filet with oil, then rub on spice mixture.
4. Grill the fish until charred, 4 to 5 minutes.
5. Flip and cook another 5 to 6 minutes for medium doneness.
6. Remove and serve immediately.

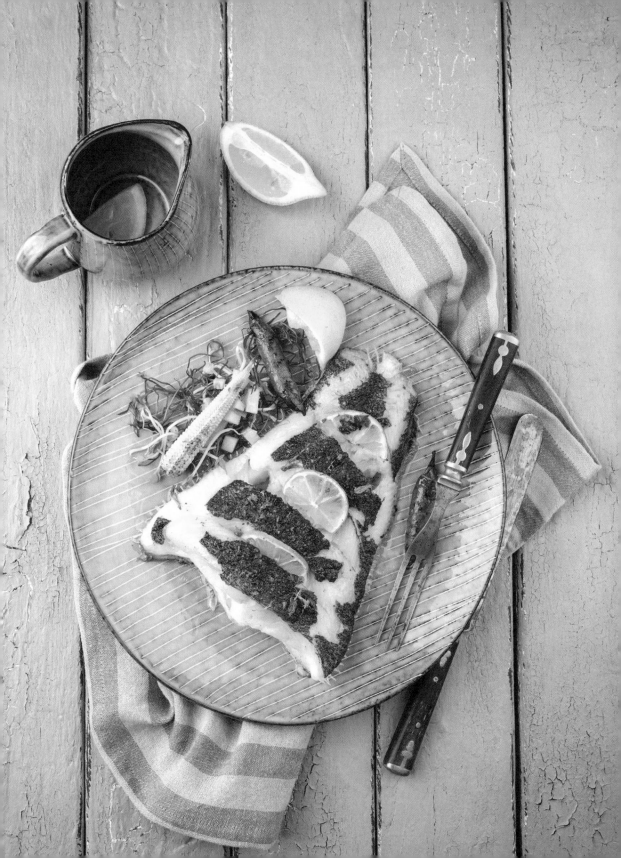

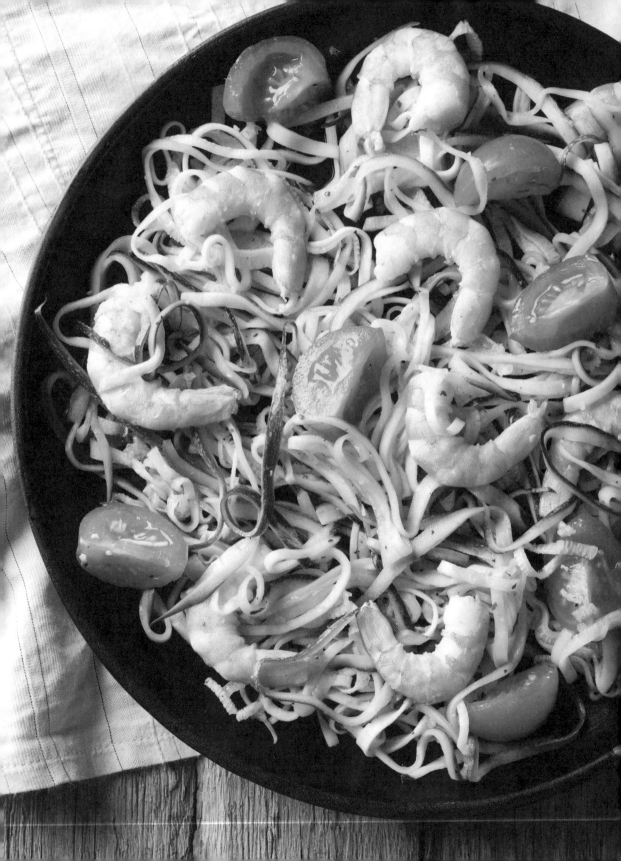

Zoodle Linguine with Garlic Shrimp

Serves 2

202 Calories per serving

2 zucchini
1 tablespoon olive oil
3 garlic cloves, minced
½ cup onion, diced
Red pepper flakes
Salt and pepper
10 large shrimp
½ cup white wine
1 cup Roma tomatoes, wedged
3 tablespoons parsley, chopped

1. Spiralize zucchini into noodles.
2. Heat up large skillet with oil and add garlic, onion, red pepper flakes, and salt and pepper to taste. Cook until onion is soft.
3. Season shrimp with salt and pepper and add to pan.
4. When shrimp turn pink, add white wine and tomatoes to simmer for 7–10 minutes.
5. Toss in zucchini and coat well.
6. Top with parsley.
7. Serve and enjoy!

90210 Chicken Nuggets

Serves 2

225 Calories per serving

6 ounces boneless, skinless chicken breast
¼ cup almond flour
½ teaspoon paprika
½ teaspoon garlic powder
¼ teaspoon cumin
¼ teaspoon cayenne pepper
¼ teaspoon black pepper
Pinch of salt
¼ cup Silk unsweetened almond milk
Nonstick cooking spray

1. Preheat oven to 375° F.
2. Slice chicken into strips.
3. Mix flour, paprika, garlic, cumin, cayenne, pepper, and salt.
4. Dredge each piece of chicken in almond milk and then coat with flour spice mixture.
5. Place on a baking sheet sprayed with nonstick cooking spray.
6. Bake for 20–25 minutes, until golden.
7. Serve!

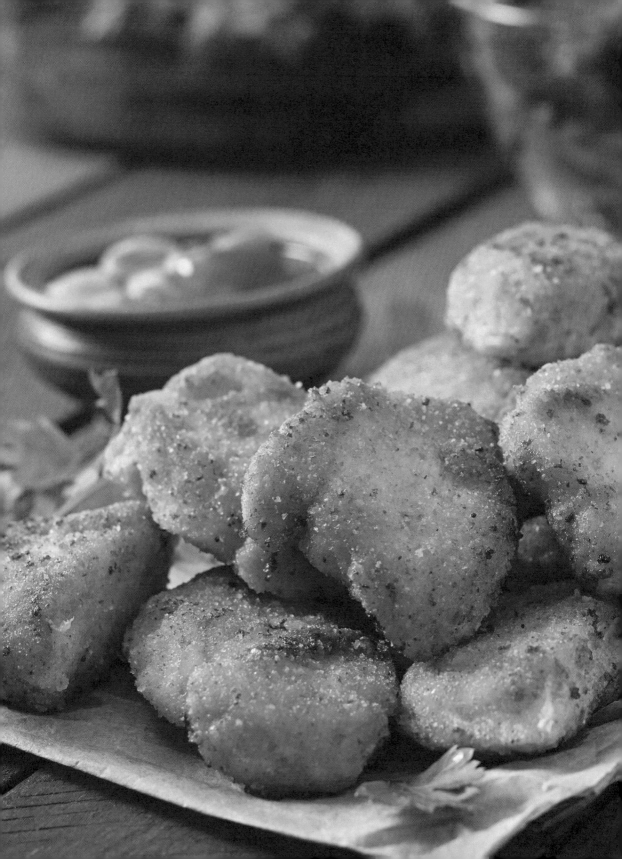

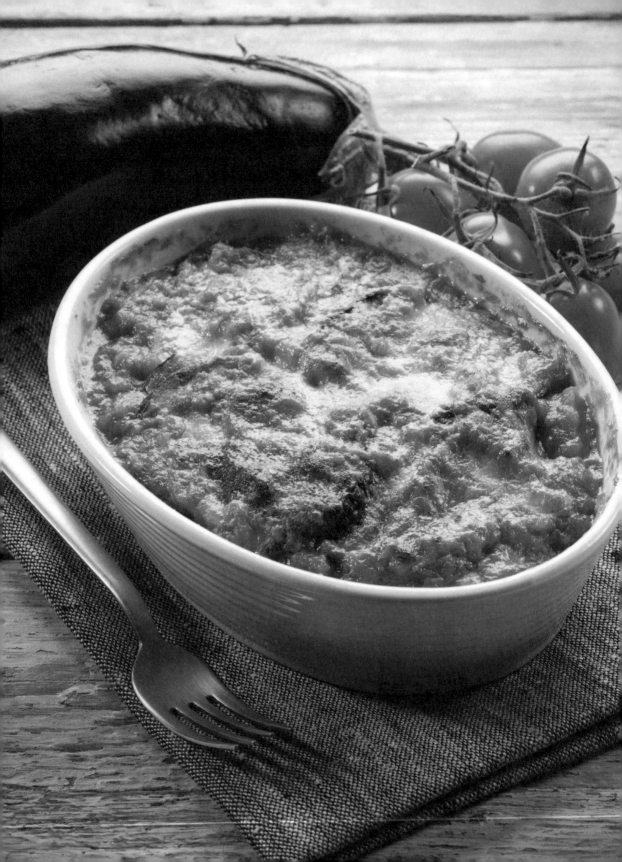

Roasted Eggplant Parmesan

Serves 4

302 Calories per serving

½ cup Parmesan cheese
1 tablespoon garlic powder
Salt and pepper
1 large eggplant, sliced into ¼ inch rounds
½ cup chickpea flour
½ cup Silk unsweetened almond milk
Nonstick cooking spray
1 cup organic marinara sauce
1 cup nonfat mozzarella cheese

1. Preheat oven to 450°F.

2. Mix Parmesan cheese, garlic powder, salt, and pepper in a shallow bowl.

3. Dredge eggplant slices in chickpea flour, then almond milk, then coat with Parmesan cheese mixture.

4. Place on baking sheet coated with cooking spray.

5. Bake for 15–20 min, turning halfway, until browned and crispy.

6. Layer eggplant and sauce in a baking dish.

7. Top with cheese and bake until melted.

Spaghetti Squash N' Cheese

Serves 2

165 Calories per serving

1 spaghetti squash
1 teaspoon coconut oil
1 tablespoon coconut flour
1 cup Silk unsweetened almond milk
Salt and pepper
½ cup nonfat mozzarella cheese
Parmesan cheese, to garnish

1. Preheat the oven to 375°F.
2. Cut the squash in half lengthwise; remove seeds.
3. Place squash on a baking sheet and bake until fork tender, about 1 hour.
4. Separate the strands of squash with a fork and place in a medium bowl.
5. Heat oil in a large saucepan over medium heat.
6. Stir in flour.
7. Reduce heat to low and add milk.
8. Once flour is incorporated, raise heat to medium-high until it comes to a boil and becomes smooth and thick.
9. Season with salt and pepper.
10. Remove from heat, add cheese, and mix well until cheese is melted.
11. Add cooked spaghetti squash.
12. Plate with Parmesan on top.
13. Serve and enjoy!

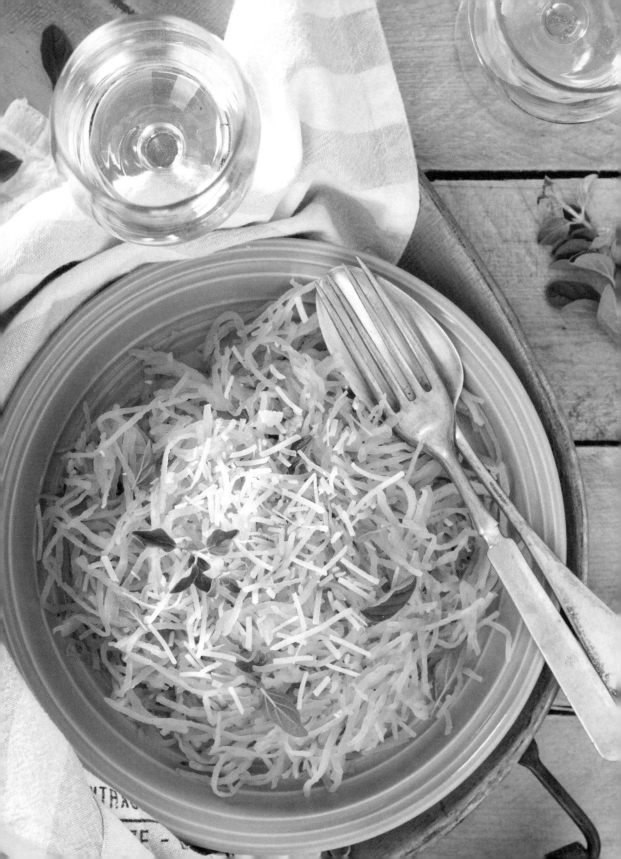

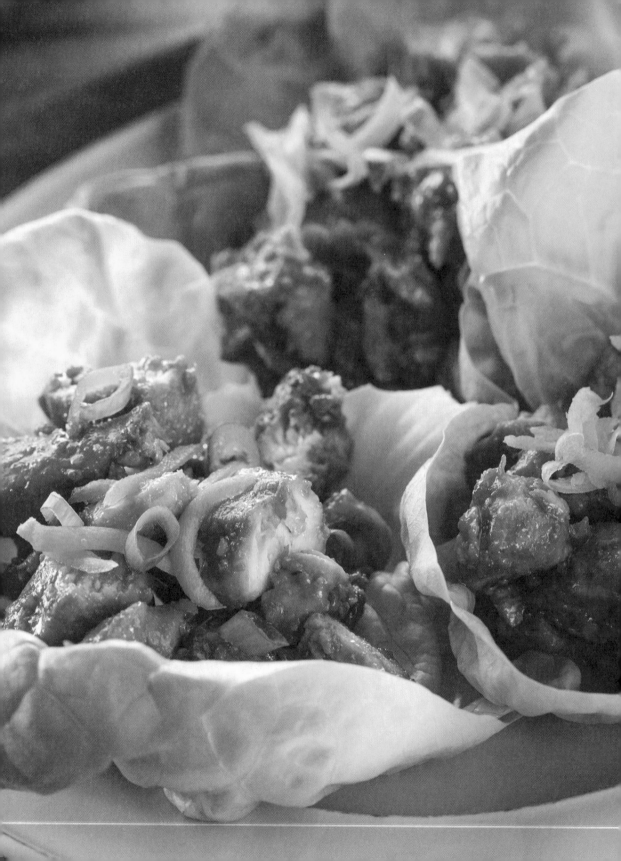

Asian Turkey Lettuce Cups

Serves 2

194 Calories per serving

1 tablespoon carrots, grated
2 tablespoons rice wine vinegar
1 tablespoon reduced sodium soy sauce
1 teaspoon sesame oil
Pepper, to taste
6 ounces ground lean turkey
¼ cup water chestnuts, chopped fine
1 garlic clove, minced
4 butter Bibb lettuce leaves
1 tablespoon scallions, diced

1. Quick pickle the grated carrots in 1 tablespoon of rice wine vinegar; let rest.

2. Combine soy sauce, ½ teaspoon sesame oil, remaining rice wine vinegar, and pepper in a bowl.

3. Add turkey and water chestnuts, stir to combine.

4. Let marinate for 15 minutes.

5. Heat remaining sesame oil in a wok or skillet over high heat. Add garlic; cook until fragrant, about 30 seconds.

6. Add turkey mixture; stir-fry until browned, breaking the turkey apart as it cooks, about 4–5 minutes.

7. To serve, spoon ¼ cup of the turkey into each lettuce leaf.

8. Garnish with scallions and more carrots.

Spaghetti and Meatballs

Serves 2

289 Calories per serving

Nonstick cooking spray
6 ounces ground turkey, 93% lean
1 garlic clove, minced
½ teaspoon Italian seasoning
Salt and pepper, to taste
2 zucchini, or 1 spaghetti squash
1 cup organic marinara sauce
½ tablespoon olive oil
¼ cup Parmesan cheese, grated

Optional:
½ cup cherry tomatoes

1. Preheat oven to 350°F and coat baking sheet with nonstick cooking spray.

2. In a large bowl, combine turkey, garlic, Italian seasoning, salt, and pepper to taste. Gently mix and form six meatballs about one inch in diameter. Place meatballs on baking sheet to bake for 20 minutes.

3. While the meatballs are baking, spiralize the zucchini or scoop out spaghetti squash.

4. Pour marinara sauce into a small saucepan and heat over medium-low heat for 5–10 minutes.

5. Heat olive oil in a nonstick skillet and sauté squash for 3–5 minutes, stirring frequently. Season with salt and pepper to taste.

6. Divide squash between two plates and top with 3 meatballs each. Spoon marinara sauce over the meatballs, sprinkle with Parmesan cheese, and enjoy!

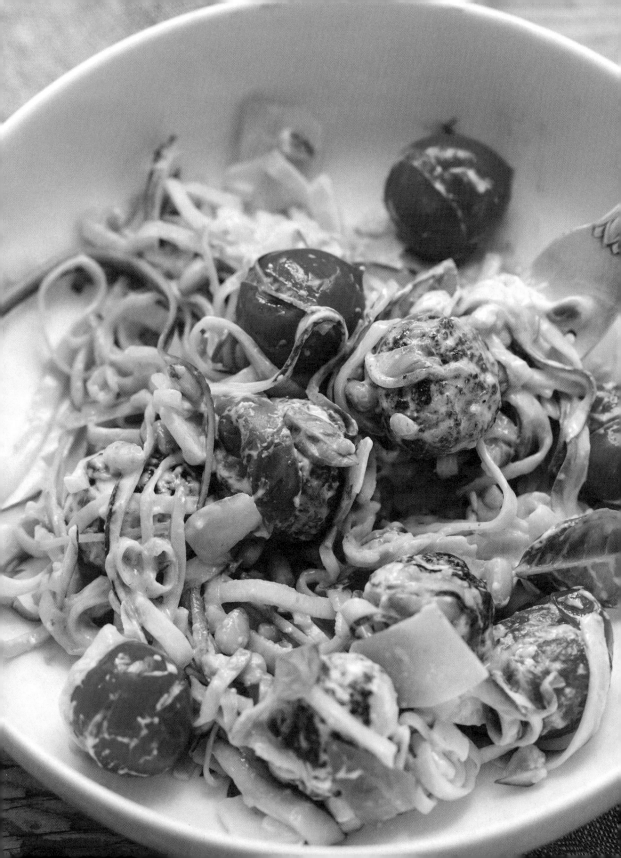

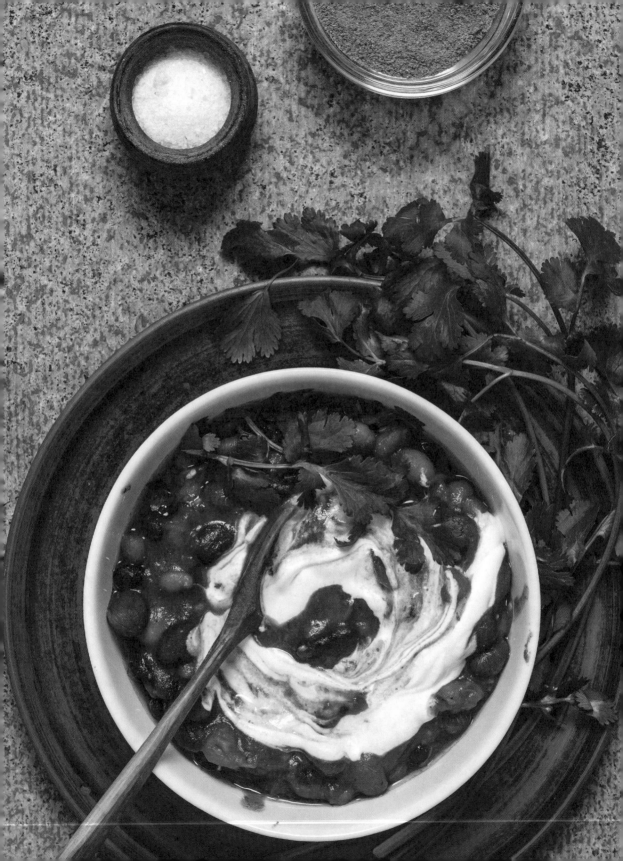

Chipotle Chili

Serves 2

163 Calories per serving

1 tablespoon chipotle chili purée (instructions below)
1 teaspoon olive oil
½ onion, diced
1 garlic clove, minced
½ cup black beans
½ cup fava beans

½ cup navy beans
½ cup crushed tomatoes
½ teaspoon ground cumin
1 zucchini, grated
1 tablespoon cilantro, chopped
1 teaspoon rice wine vinegar
Salt and pepper

Optional:
Low fat Greek yogurt

1. Prepare chipotle purée: Blend a 7-ounce can of chipotle chilies, including the adobo sauce, in a blender or food processor until smooth. Store remainder of sauce in an airtight container in the refrigerator up to 1 week, or freeze for several months.

2. In a 3- to 4-quart pan over medium-high heat, add the olive oil, and cook the onion and garlic, stirring often, until onion softens and starts to brown, 6 to 8 minutes.

3. Add beans, tomatoes and their juice, cumin, and 1–2 cups water; bring to a boil, then reduce heat and simmer, stirring occasionally, to blend flavors, about 15 minutes.

4. Stir in zucchini, cilantro, chipotle purée, and rice vinegar. Add salt and pepper to taste.

5. Spoon chili into two bowls and top each with 1 tablespoon low fat Greek yogurt, if desired.

Garlic and Parmesan Noodles

Serves 2

184 Calories per serving

1 tablespoon butter

3 garlic cloves, minced

2 zucchini, spiralized

1 teaspoon extra-virgin olive oil

1 teaspoon Italian seasoning

Red pepper flakes, to taste

2 tablespoons Parmesan cheese

1. Heat butter in saucepan, and add garlic and zucchini; cook until garlic is fragrant.
2. Stir in EVOO and seasonings.
3. Remove from heat, and top with cheese.

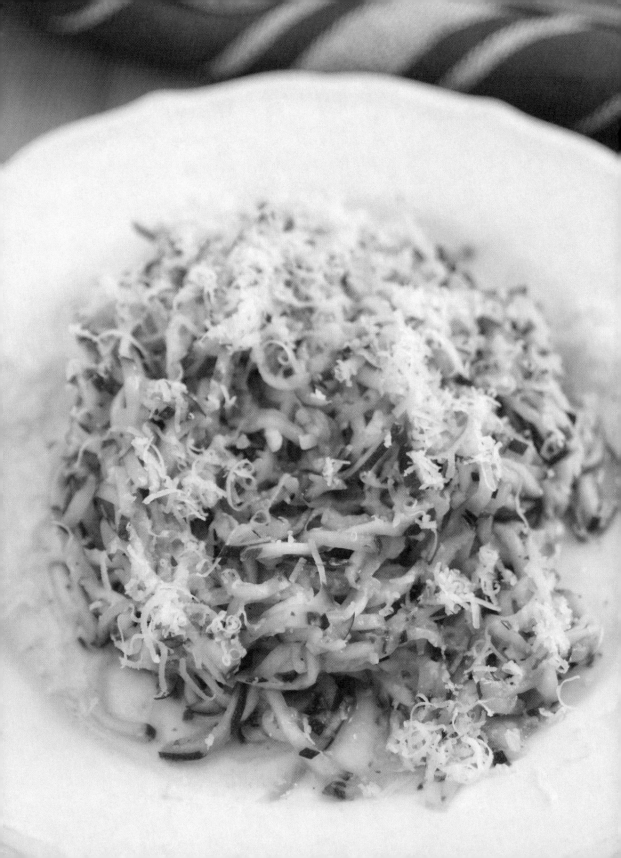

10 Tiny and Full™ Snack Recipes

There's nothing better than a great snack before a big meeting at work or right after a workout. I am so excited to introduce to you new Tiny and Full snacks. Use these anytime you need something in between your next meal. They are great to share with friends and family. Don't forget to look at the calorie counts and adjust portions or reduce treats to make sure you don't go over your daily calorie goal.

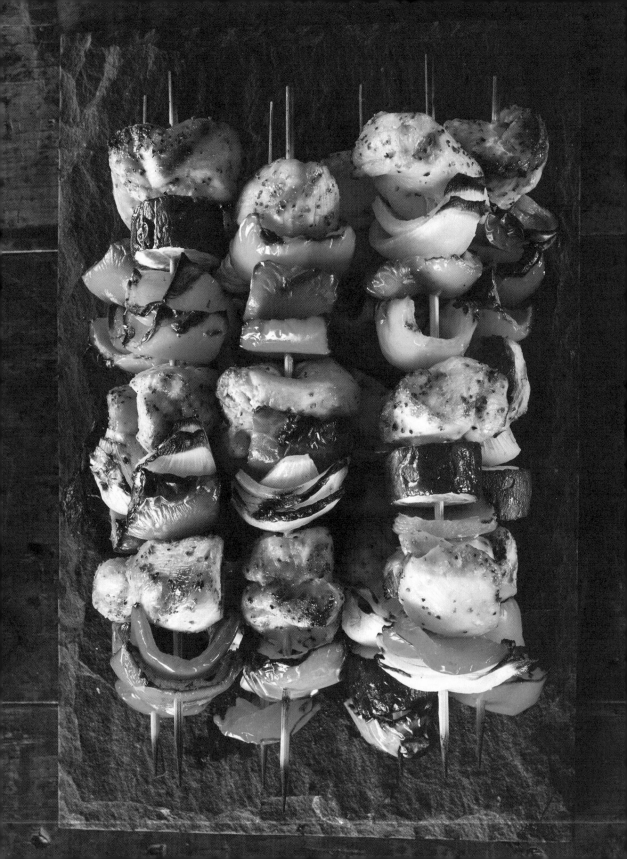

Grilled Chicken and Summer Vegetable Skewers

Serves 2

127 Calories per serving

1 tablespoon lemon juice
1 tablespoon olive oil
1 teaspoon rosemary, chopped
Salt and pepper
1 garlic clove, finely chopped
6 ounces boneless, skinless chicken breast, cubed
1 red bell pepper, cut into 1-inch pieces
1 zucchini or yellow summer squash, cut into 1-inch pieces
1 onion, cut into wedges

1. In a medium bowl, mix lemon juice, olive oil, rosemary, salt, pepper, and garlic clove.

2. Add chicken, stirring to coat with marinade.

3. Cover and refrigerate for 1–6 hours.

4. Heat coals or gas grill for direct heat.

5. Remove chicken and reserve marinade.

6. Thread chicken, bell pepper, zucchini, and onion alternately on skewers.

7. Brush vegetables with marinade.

8. Grill kabobs over medium heat 10 to 15 minutes, turning and brushing frequently with marinade, until chicken is cooked through.

9. Share and enjoy!

The Grove Grilled Nachos

Serves 2

134 Calories per serving

1 zucchini, sliced
Olive oil
Salt and pepper, to taste
1 tablespoon fat free cheddar cheese, grated
½ cup black beans, rinsed and drained
1 small tomato, chopped
½ avocado, chopped
1 green onion, chopped
1 tablespoon cilantro, chopped
1 lime

1. Place the sliced zucchini chips into a large bowl and toss with olive oil, salt, and pepper.
2. Place zucchini on a grill pan or directly on a hot grill over medium heat. Grill for 4 to 5 minutes or until zucchini is tender.
3. Sprinkle cheese directly over zucchini chips and cook until cheese is melted, about 1 minute.
4. Remove zucchini from grill and arrange on a platter.
5. Top with black beans, tomato, avocado, green onion, cilantro, and a squeeze of fresh lime.
6. Serve and enjoy!

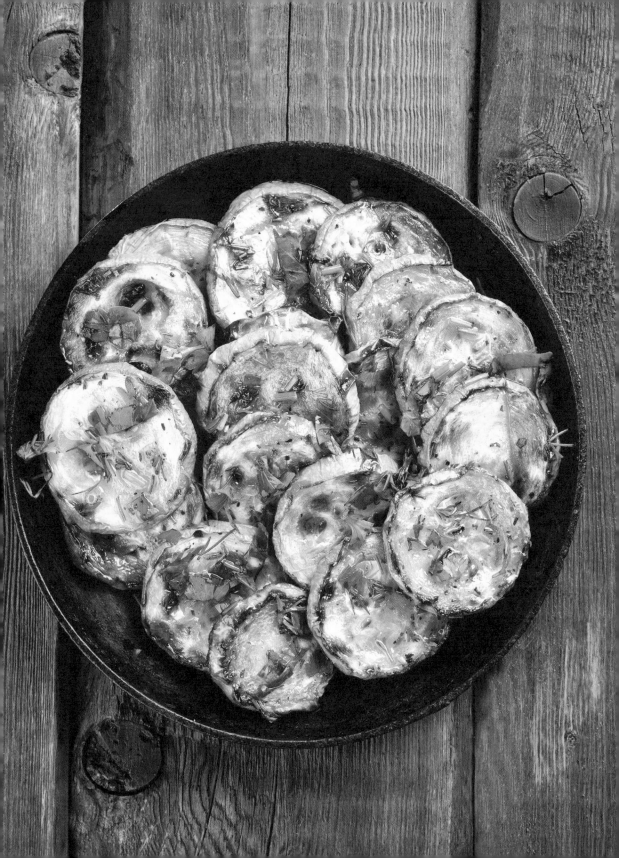

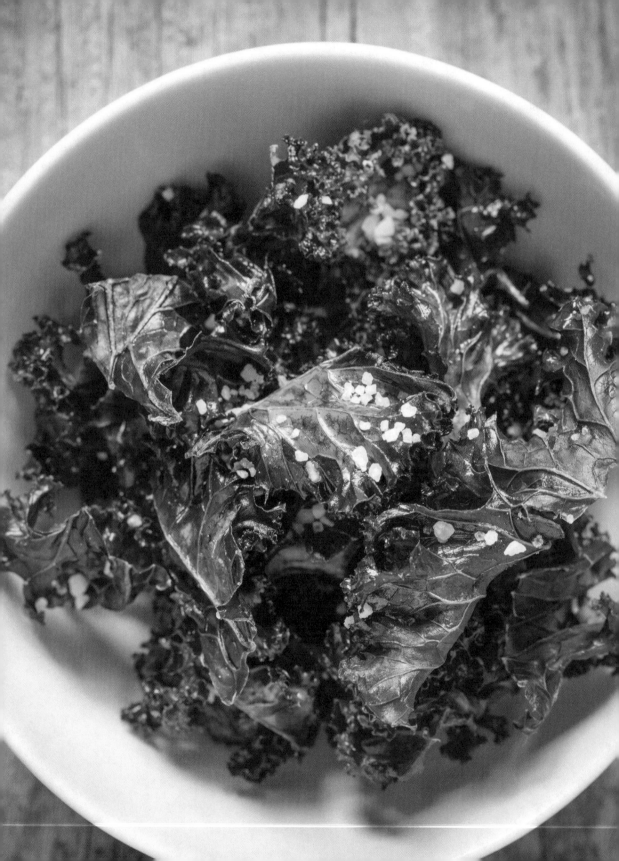

Santa Monica Kale Chips

Serves 4

93 Calories per serving

4 cups torn kale leaves
2 tablespoons extra-virgin olive oil
Salt
1 lemon, zested

1. Heat oven to 350°F.
2. Toss kale with olive oil and salt, and coat evenly.
3. Arrange seasoned kale on two rimmed baking sheets.
4. Bake until crisp, about 12 to 15 minutes.
5. Toss with lemon zest, then enjoy!

Cauliflower Mashed Potatoes

Serves 2

100 Calories per serving

1 head cauliflower
½ cup Silk unsweetened almond milk
1 teaspoon coconut oil
2 tablespoons light sour cream
¼ teaspoon garlic salt
Freshly ground black pepper
Chives, thinly chopped

Optional:
1 tablespoon Earth Balance Organic Coconut Spread

1. Steam cauliflower for 12–15 minutes or until very tender.
2. Drain and dry cauliflower, and transfer to a large bowl.
3. Add the milk, oil, sour cream, salt, and pepper, then mash until smooth.
4. Top with chives and a pat of the coconut spread, if desired.
5. Enjoy!

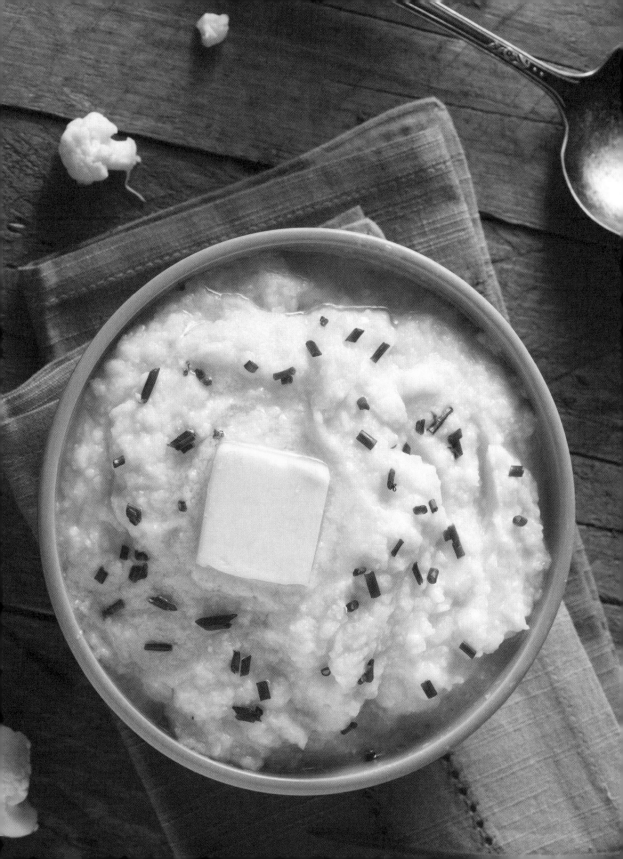

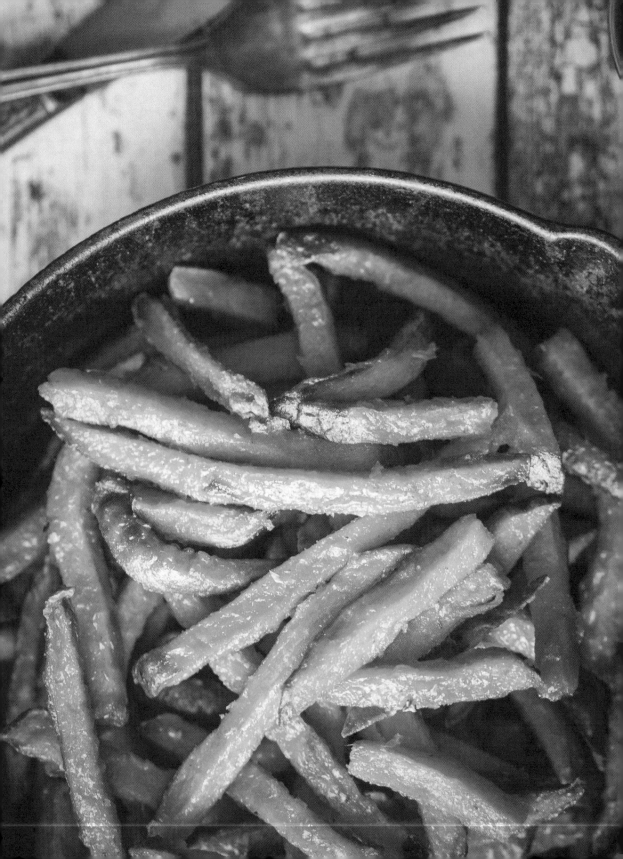

Sweet Potato Fries

Serves 2

210 Calories per serving

Nonstick cooking spray
2 medium sweet potatoes
½ teaspoon salt
½ teaspoon chili powder
½ teaspoon paprika
¼ teaspoon ground black pepper

1. Preheat oven to 425°F.
2. Lightly coat a baking sheet with nonstick cooking spray.
3. Cut potatoes lengthwise into thin strips or wedges.
4. Arrange potatoes in a single layer in pan.
5. Sprinkle seasonings over potatoes.
6. Bake for 20 minutes or until brown and tender.
7. Serve and enjoy!

Sweet and Salty Popcorn

Serves 2

185 Calories per serving

1 tablespoon coconut oil
¼ cup popcorn kernels
1 ounce dark chocolate
½ teaspoon sea salt

1. Pour oil into a large, deep pan and heat to medium, then add three test kernels and cover.
2. When the kernels pop, remove the lid and add remaining kernels.
3. Cover the pot, hold the lid down, and give it a few shakes.
4. Cook the popcorn, shaking the pot occasionally, until the popping sound stops, about 4–5 minutes.
5. While the corn is popping, melt the dark chocolate in the microwave.
6. Once the corn stops popping, immediately remove and spread out on a baking sheet.
7. Drizzle the popcorn with the melted chocolate, and sprinkle with the sea salt. Toss to coat.
8. Allow the chocolate to cool and set before eating, about 20 minutes.
9. Enjoy!

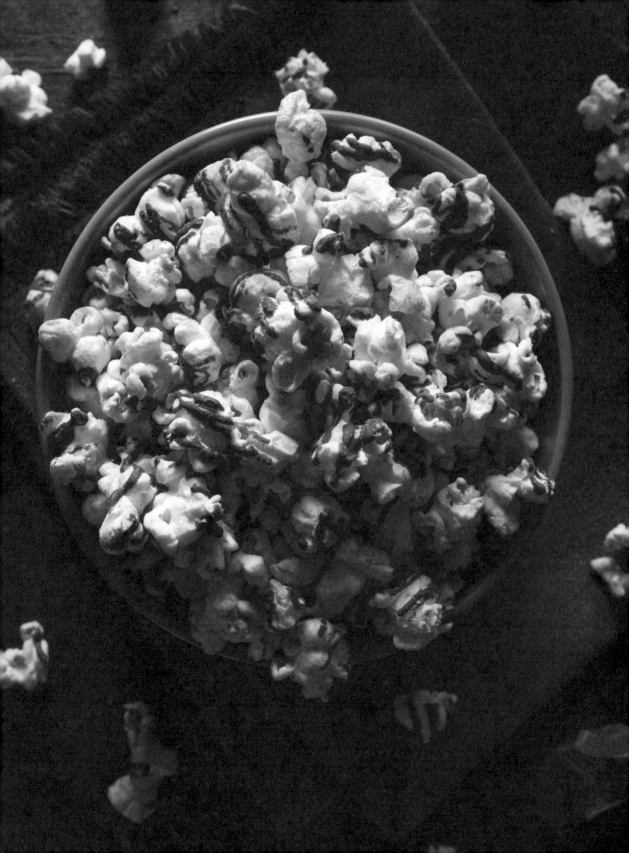

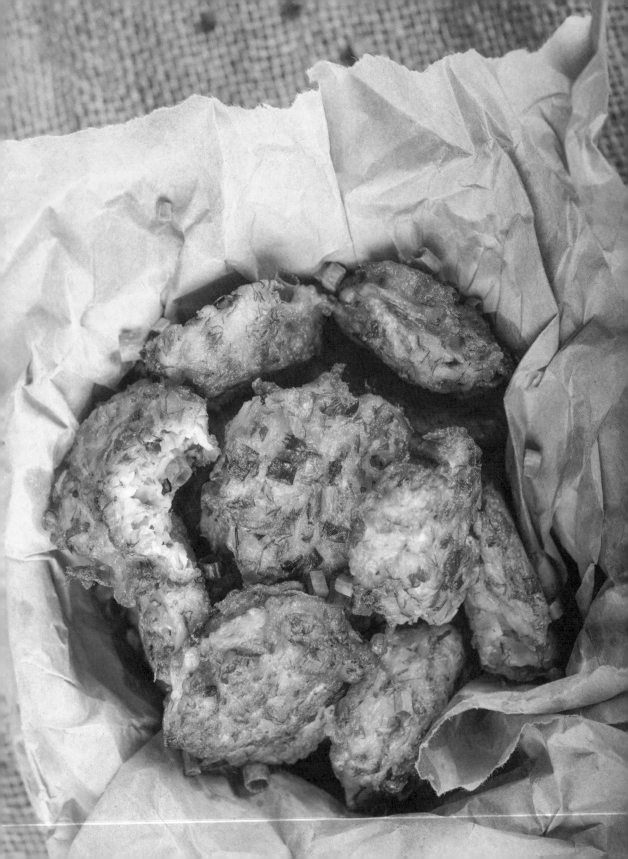

Tater Tots

Serves 2

116 Calories per serving

1 potato
1 zucchini, shredded
½ teaspoon salt
1 teaspoon olive oil

Optional:
organic ketchup

1. Boil potato for 20–30 minutes, until just barely fork tender.

2. Drain water and let cool.

3. Preheat oven to 425°F.

4. Grate potato and zucchini into a bowl.

5. Squeeze out the liquid using a clean dish towel or paper towels.

6. Season with salt.

7. Line a large baking sheet with parchment paper, then make small balls out of the mixture, about 1 tablespoon for each.

8. Place the baking sheet in the freezer for about 10 minutes to firm mixture.

9. Brush the top of each tater tot with olive oil.

10. Bake until browned and crispy, about 30 minutes, flipping halfway through.

11. Serve with organic ketchup, if desired.

Buffalo Cauliflower

Serves 4

113 Calories per serving

1 large head cauliflower
½ cup cornstarch
Sea salt and garlic powder, to taste
½ cup water
1 tablespoon Earth Balance butter, melted
½ cup Frank's Red Hot Buffalo hot sauce, or desired brand

1. Preheat oven to 425°F.
2. Chop cauliflower head into even pieces.
3. Mix cornstarch, sea salt, garlic powder, and water together in a large bowl.
4. Toss cauliflower in mixture, coated evenly.
5. Place cauliflower on a baking sheet and roast in the oven for 15-20 minutes.
6. In a separate bowl, melt the butter, then stir together with hot sauce.
7. Remove cauliflower from oven and coat all pieces in hot sauce.
8. Place cauliflower back in the oven and roast for an additional 20-25 minutes.
9. Serve and enjoy!

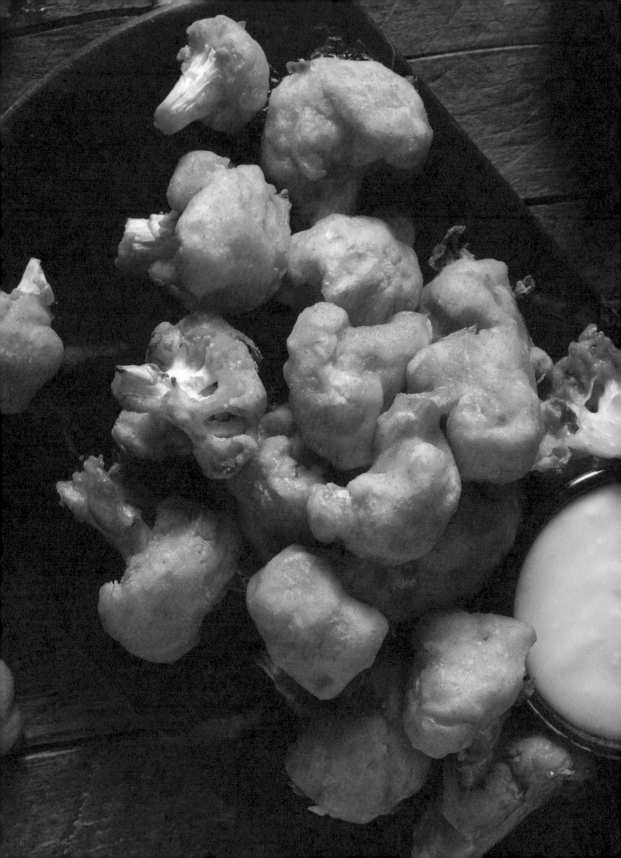

11

Tiny and Full™ Dessert Recipes

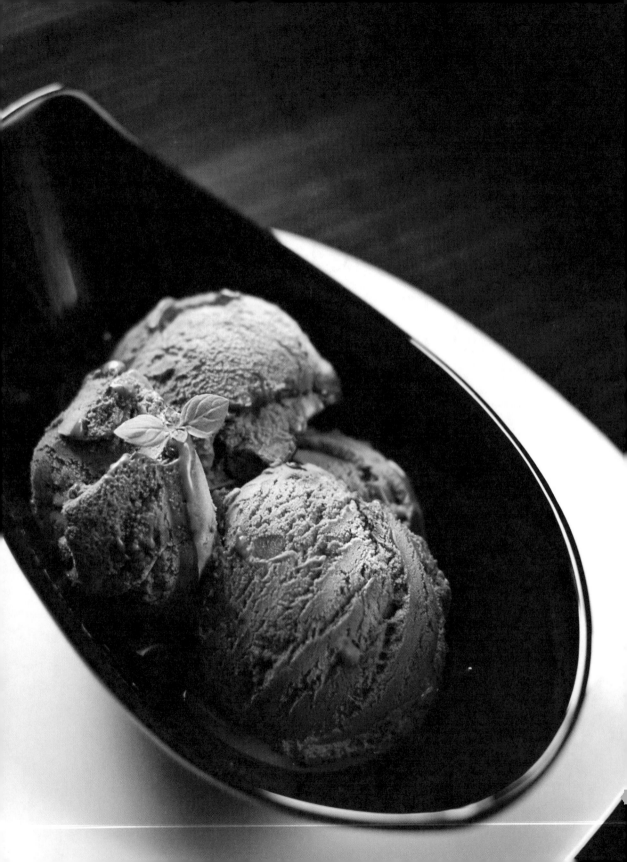

Three Ingredient Chocolate Ice Cream

Serves 1

143 Calories per serving

1 frozen banana, diced
2–3 tablespoons Silk unsweetened almond milk
2–3 tablespoons cocoa powder

Optional:
1 tablespoon mini dark chocolate chips

1. Place all ingredients into blender and mix until thick and smooth, about one minute.
2. Scoop into bowl and let freeze for 15 minutes.
3. Garnish with chocolate chips, if desired.
4. Serve and enjoy!

Banana Berry Ice Cream

Serves 2

96 Calories per serving

1½ medium bananas, peeled, sliced, and frozen until solid
⅓ cup chopped frozen strawberries
2 tablespoons cream

1. Place frozen bananas in a blender.
2. Mix until they are the consistency of soft serve ice cream.
3. Add strawberries and cream and blend until smooth.
4. Transfer mixture to a freezer container and freeze until solid.
5. Serve when completely frozen and enjoy!

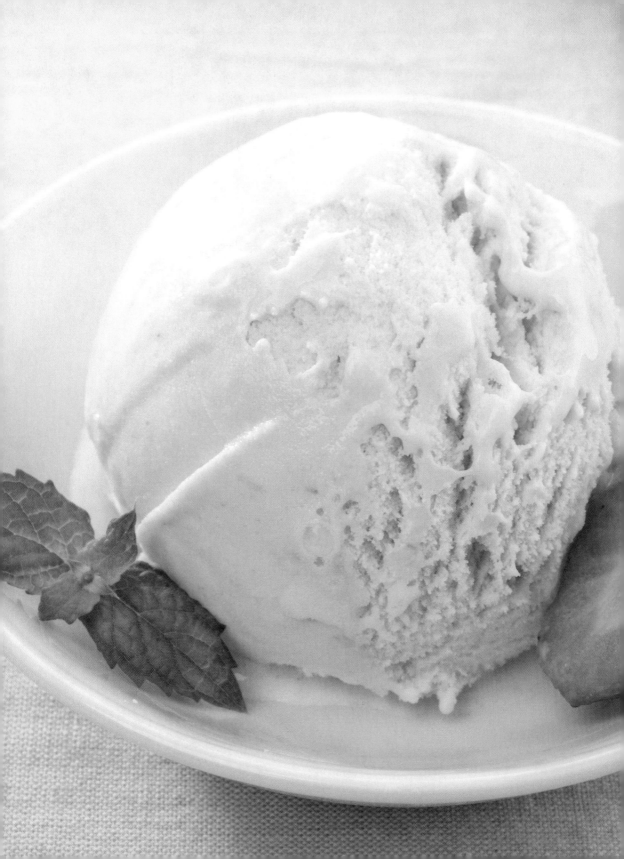

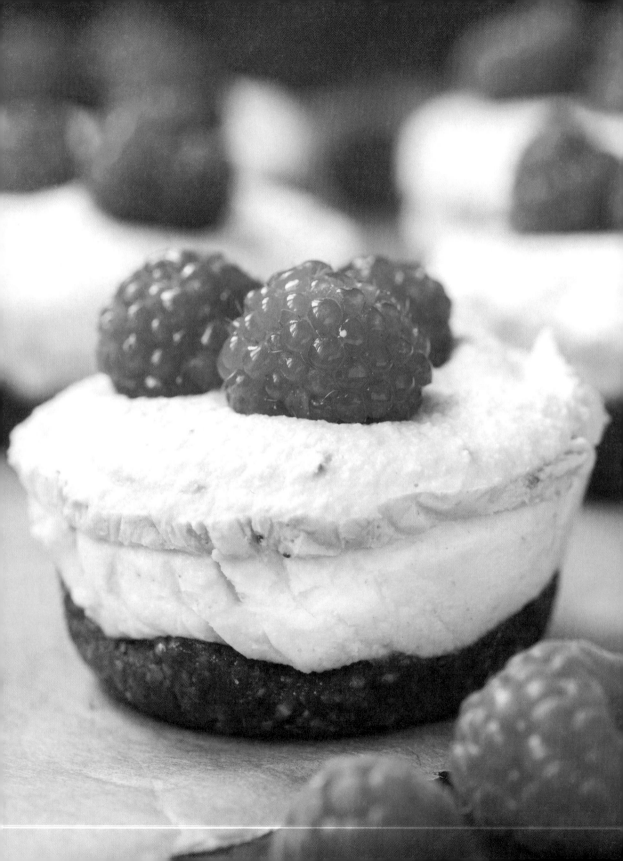

Rodeo Drive Cheesecake Cups

Makes 12 Cups

201 Calories per serving

Nonstick cooking spray
2 tablespoons coconut flour
2 dates
1 tablespoon coconut oil
2 tablespoons Silk unsweetened almond milk
14 ounces fat-free cream cheese, room temperature
½ cup stevia
2 teaspoons cornstarch
1 teaspoon vanilla extract
6 ounces raspberries, mashed

1. Preheat the oven to 300°F, and lightly coat muffin pan with nonstick cooking spray.

2. To prepare the crust, add coconut flour and dates to food processor or blender, and pulse until even.

3. Add mixture to a bowl, and mix in the oil and milk.

4. Press the mixture into the prepared muffin pan.

5. Bake for 8 minutes, then cool completely.

6. To prepare the filling, beat cream cheese and stevia in a large bowl until smooth, then add cornstarch and vanilla extract.

7. Gently fold in the raspberries.

8. Spread the filling on top of the cooled crust. Bake at 300°F for 25-30 minutes, or until the center only jiggles slightly.

9. Cool completely to room temperature, then chill for at least 3 hours before serving.

10. Garnish with fresh berries, if desired.

Belly Burning Donuts

Makes 20 Donuts

78 Calories per serving

For Donut Dough:
½ cup Silk unsweetened almond milk
½ teaspoon apple cider vinegar
½ teaspoon pure vanilla extract
¼ cup unsweetened applesauce
4 tablespoons Earth Balance butter
½ cup almond flour
½ cup vanilla pea protein powder
½ cup stevia
1½ teaspoons baking powder
¼ teaspoon salt
¼ teaspoon nutmeg
¼ teaspoon cinnamon

For Icing:
1 tablespoon stevia
3 tablespoons arrowroot
1 tablespoon Silk unsweetened almond milk
1 teaspoon maple extract

Optional:
Vegan sprinkles

1. Preheat oven to 350°F.
2. Place wet ingredients in a small pot on the stovetop on low.
3. Whisk ingredients on stove to blend well.
4. Mix the dry ingredients together in a large bowl.
5. Add the wet to the dry, and mix until just incorporated.
6. Do not overmix—the batter should be very sticky.
7. Scoop the batter into the greased doughnut pans.
8. Bake for 12 minutes.
9. Whisk icing ingredients until fully incorporated.
10. Let doughnuts cool on a wire rack, then add icing and decorate!

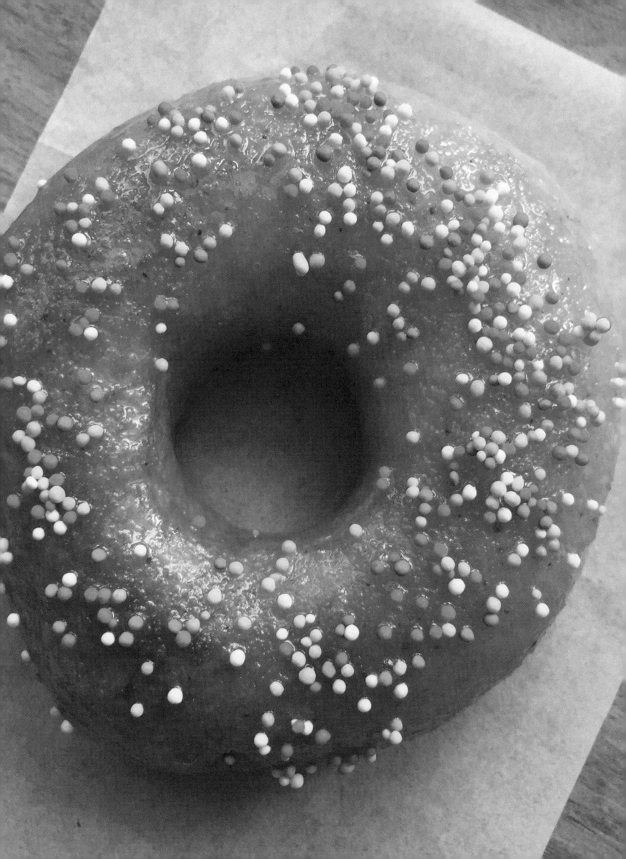

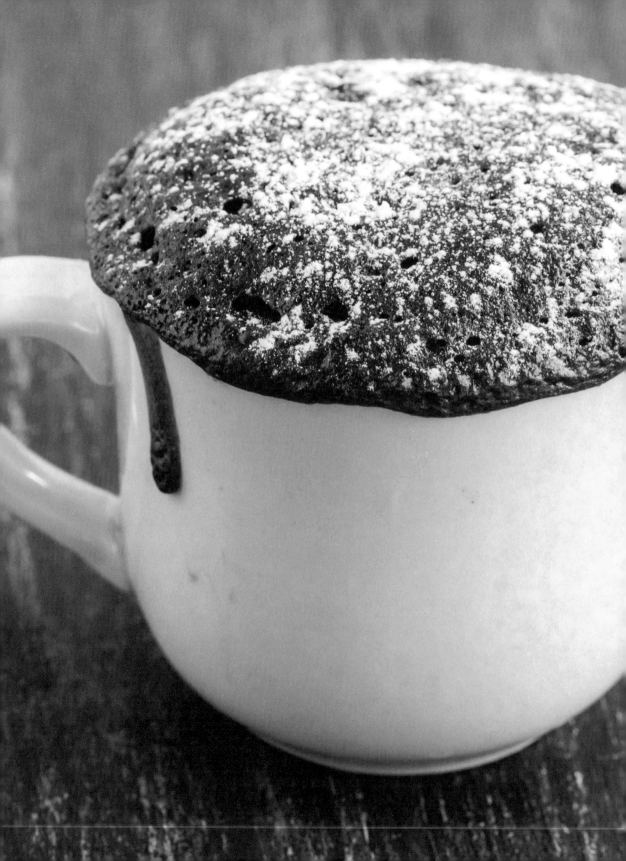

One Minute Mug Cake

Serves 1

100 Calories per serving

Nonstick cooking spray
2 tablespoons almond flour
1½ tablespoons stevia
2 teaspoons cocoa powder
¼ teaspoon baking powder
Pinch of salt
2 tablespoons Silk unsweetened almond milk
1 teaspoon coconut oil
1 drop vanilla extract

1. Spray a mug with cooking spray.

2. In the mug, combine the flour, sweetener, cocoa powder, baking powder, and salt.

3. Stir in the milk, oil, and vanilla until smooth.

4. Bake in the microwave on high for 30–60 seconds.

Protein Butter Cups

Makes Fourteen Cups

17 calories per serving

Chocolate Layer:
¼ cup Silk unsweetened almond milk
¼ cup plain lowfat Greek yogurt
¼ cup unsweetened cocoa powder
2 tablespoons chocolate pea protein powder
Pinch salt
1 tablespoon stevia

Peanut Butter Layer:
¼ cup PB2 powdered peanut butter
¼ cup water
Pinch salt
½ tablespoon stevia

1. In two separate small bowls, combine ingredients for chocolate and peanut butter layers, then stir each until smooth.
2. Line muffin pan with cups, and spray with cooking spray.
3. Pour 1 teaspoon of the chocolate mixture into each liner.
4. Follow with 1 teaspoon of the peanut butter mixture on top of the chocolate layer.
5. Finish off by pouring 1 teaspoon of the chocolate mixture on top of the peanut butter layer.
6. Freeze for 1–2 hours, or until they are firm enough to remove from the muffin cups.
7. Enjoy!

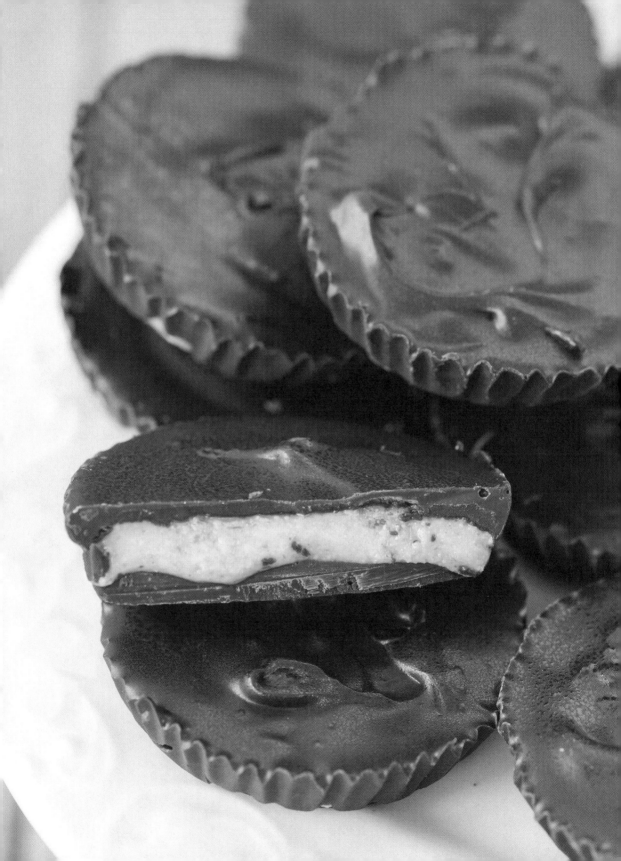

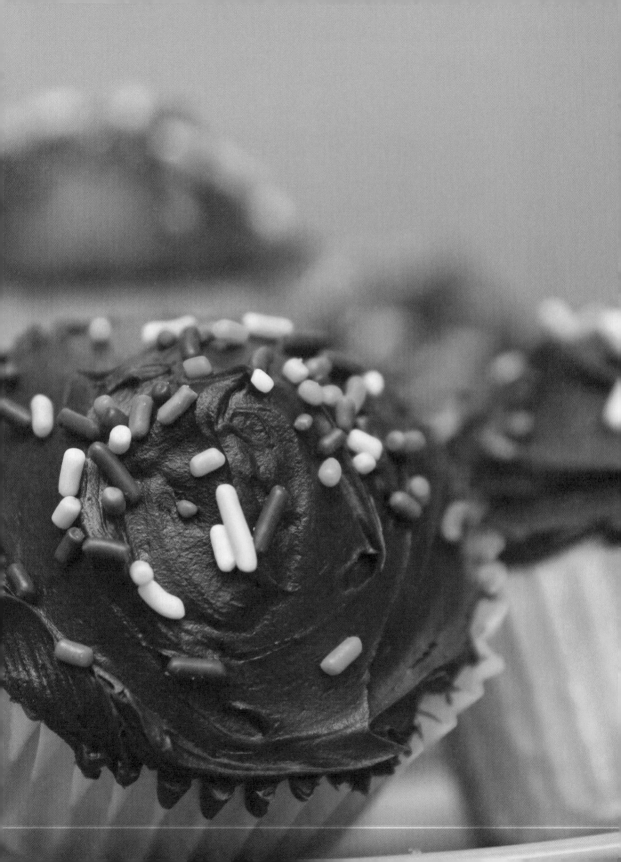

Chocolate Frosted Vanilla Cupcakes

Makes Twelve Cupcakes

55 Calories per serving

1¼ cups buckwheat flour
¾ cup coconut flour
¾ cup stevia
1 teaspoon baking soda
½ teaspoon salt
1 cup Silk unsweetened almond milk
1 tablespoon vanilla extract
⅓ cup unsweetened applesauce
1 teaspoon apple cider vinegar

For the Frosting:
2 tablespoons unsweetened cocoa
   powder
2 tablespoons Silk unsweetened almond
   milk
1 tablespoon chia seeds

Optional:
Vegan sprinkles

1. Preheat oven to 350°F.

2. Line a 12 cup muffin pan with cupcake liners.

3. In a large bowl, combine the flours, stevia, baking soda, and salt.

4. Add in the almond milk, vanilla extract, applesauce, and vinegar until the batter is uniform and no pockets of flour remain.

5. Evenly distribute the batter into the cupcake liners.

6. Bake for about 25 minutes, or until a tester comes out clean.

7. For the frosting, whisk ingredients until smooth, then chill while cupcakes cool.

8. Spread the frosting over the cooled cupcakes and decorate with vegan sprinkles.

Chocolate Avocado Cookie

Makes Ten Cookies

67 Calories per serving

¾ cup avocado

½ cup stevia

2 tablespoons coconut oil

1 tablespoon coconut milk

½ cup unsweetened cocoa powder

½ teaspoon baking soda

1 teaspoon of salt

2 ounces dark chocolate chunks

1. Preheat oven to 350°F.

2. Blend avocado and stevia until smooth.

3. Add coconut oil and milk.

4. Mix in the cocoa powder, baking soda, and salt, then add chocolate chunks.

5. Place dollops of cookie dough in a baking sheet lined with parchment paper.

6. Flatten dough slightly with the back of a spoon.

7. Bake for 8–10 minutes.

8. Let cool, then store in an airtight container in the fridge.

9. Enjoy!

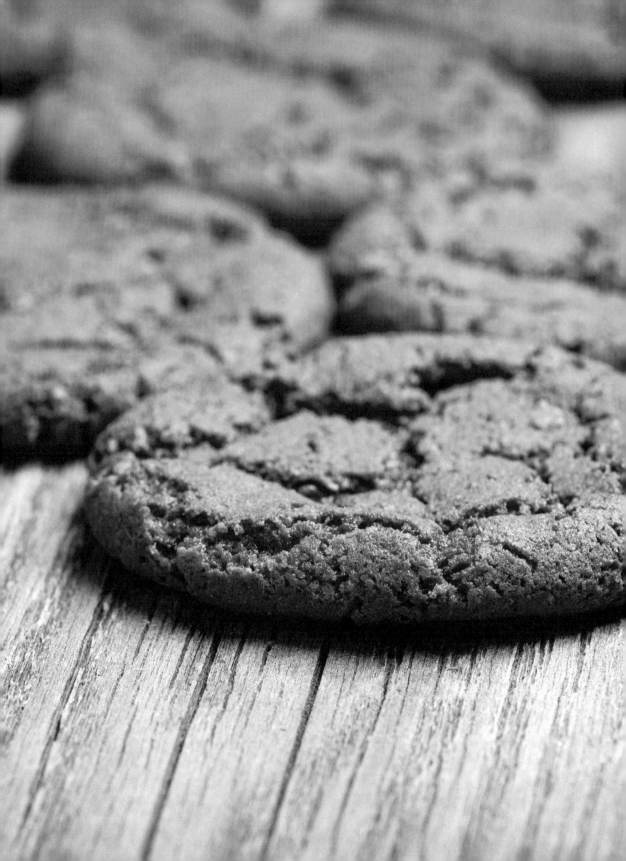

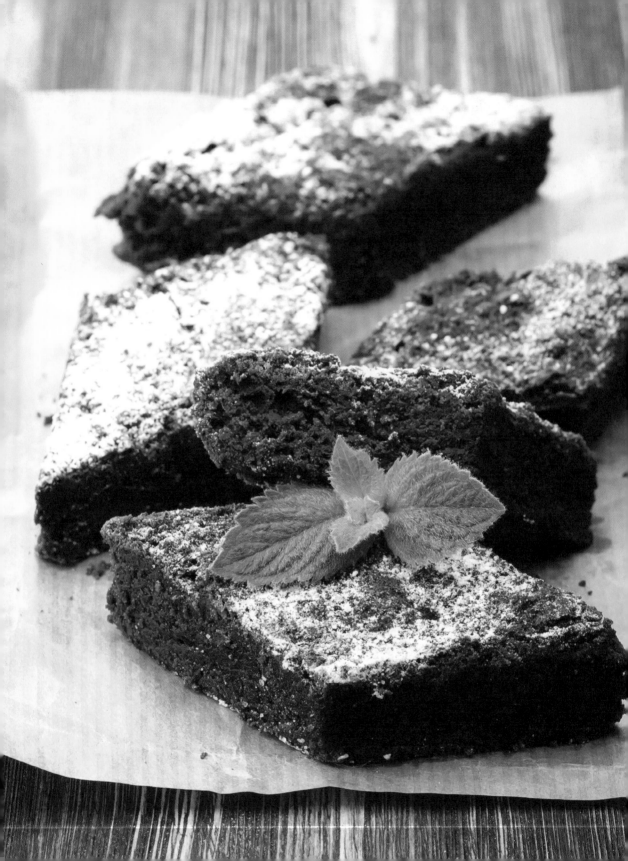

37 Calorie Brownie

Makes Nine Brownies

37 Calories per serving

¾ cup nonfat Greek yogurt
¼ cup coconut milk
½ cup cocoa powder
½ cup old fashioned rolled oats
½ cup stevia
1 egg
1 teaspoon vanilla extract
1 teaspoon baking powder
1 pinch salt

1. Preheat the oven to 400°F. Grease a square 8x8 baking dish.
2. Combine all ingredients into a food processor or a blender, and blend until smooth.
3. Pour into the prepared dish and bake for about 15 minutes.
4. Allow to cool completely before cutting into 9 large squares.
5. Enjoy!

Blackberry Oatmeal Bars

Makes Sixteen Bars

97 Calories per serving

1 cup rolled oats

¾ cup almond flour

⅓ cup light brown sugar

¼ teaspoon ground ginger

¼ teaspoon kosher salt

6 tablespoons Earth Balance butter,
   melted

2 cups blackberries, cut in half

1 teaspoon cornstarch

1 tablespoon freshly squeezed lemon
   juice

1 tablespoon stevia

1. Place a rack in the center of your oven and heat to 375°F.
2. Line an 8x8 baking pan with parchment paper so that the paper hangs over two sides for handles.
3. In a medium bowl, combine the oats, flour, brown sugar, ginger, and salt.
4. Pour in the melted butter and stir until it forms clumps and the dry ingredients are evenly moistened.
5. Press mixture into an even layer in the bottom of the prepared pan, and reserve a half cup.
6. Scatter half of the blackberries over the crumble in pan. Sprinkle the cornstarch evenly over the top, then sprinkle on the lemon juice, and ½ tablespoon of the stevia.
7. Add another layer of the remaining berries, then the remaining ½ tablespoon stevia.
8. Sprinkle the reserved mixture evenly over the top.
9. Bake for 35 to 40 minutes, until the fruit is bubbly and the crumb topping smells toasty and looks golden brown.
10. Place the pan on a wire rack to cool, then remove bars from pan.
11. Slice and enjoy!

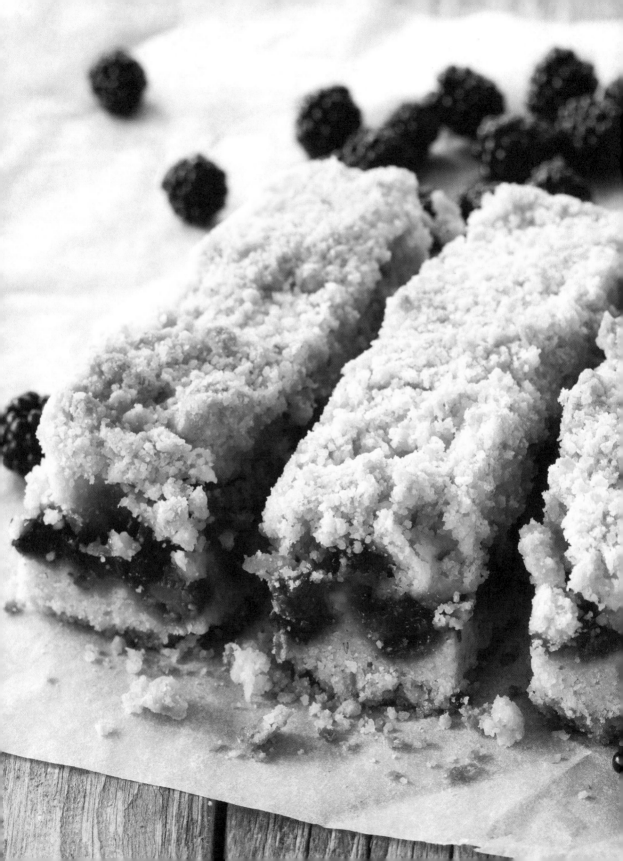

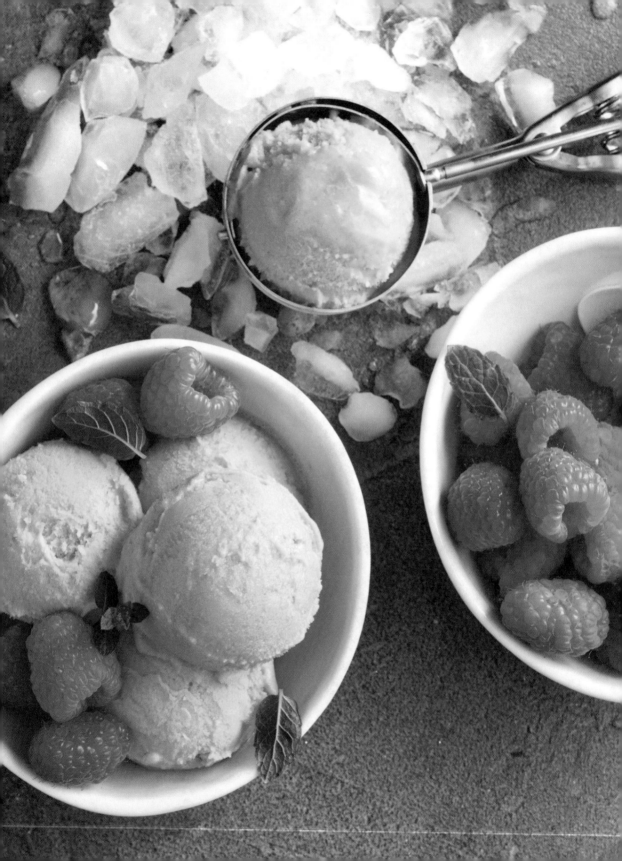

Lemon Raspberry Belly Burning Sherbet

Serves 5

101 Calories per serving

1 cup plain Greek yogurt
12 ounces frozen raspberries
⅓ cup fresh lemon juice
⅓ cup ice
2 teaspoons fresh lemon zest
3 tablespoons honey

1. Add Greek yogurt, raspberries, lemon juice, ice, lemon zest, and honey to a blender.
2. Blend until smooth.
3. Serve immediately or freeze for 1–2 hours.
4. Enjoy!

Wonderful Watermelon Cake

Serves 12–16

80 Calories per serving

4 cans full fat coconut milk
1 teaspoon vanilla extract
2 tablespoons raw honey
2 large seedless watermelons

1. Make sure to place the can of coconut milk in the refrigerator for at least 6 hours (overnight). This will cause the cream to separate from the milk. The cream will be at the top of the can.

2. Open the can of coconut milk and scrape out the cream into a medium-sized bowl.

3. Add the vanilla and raw honey to the mixture. Whip the cream with a hand mixer on medium speed and work your way up to high speed until the cream is fluffy, about 5 minutes (it will not be as fluffy as dairy-whipped cream). Place the bowl of whipped cream in the fridge until ready to use.

4. Remove the top and bottom from the watermelons and remove the rinds from the middle section. You should be left with cake-shaped pieces of watermelon. You can cut one watermelon smaller than the other to make a two-tiered cake.

5. Pat the outside of the watermelon dry with paper towels (this is important because it will help the coconut whipped cream adhere better).

6. Spread the coconut whipped cream around the watermelon cake.

7. Serve or store in the refrigerator until ready to serve.

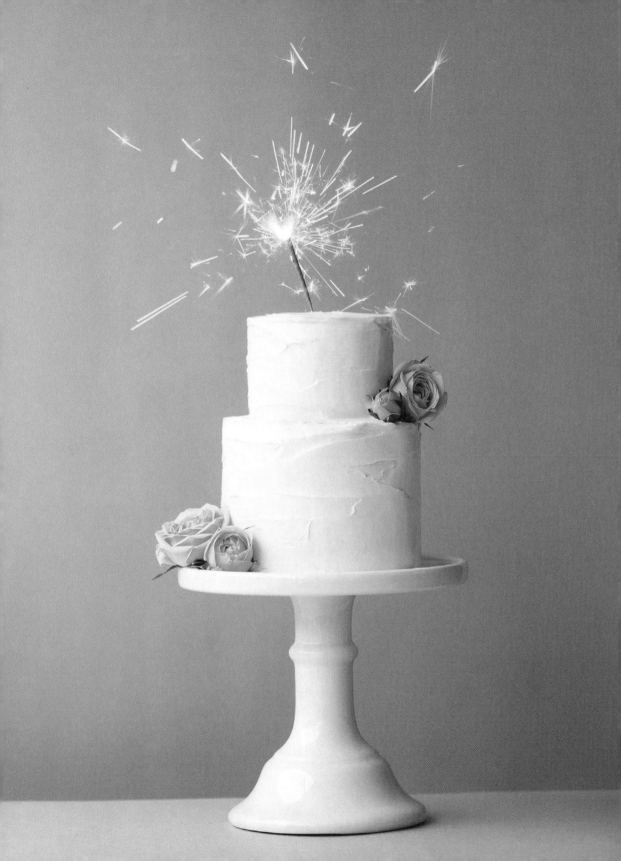

12 Tiny and Full™ Adult Beverages Recipes

n this new edition, I've included Adult Beverages because so many of you requested some low-calorie Tiny and Full approved drinks. And I know sometimes the only way to celebrate is with a drink. If you are indulging in one of these delicious drink recipes you should probably skip the "treat" you are having to make sure you don't overindulge in calories. Take note of calorie counts and sip away on these refreshing drink recipes.

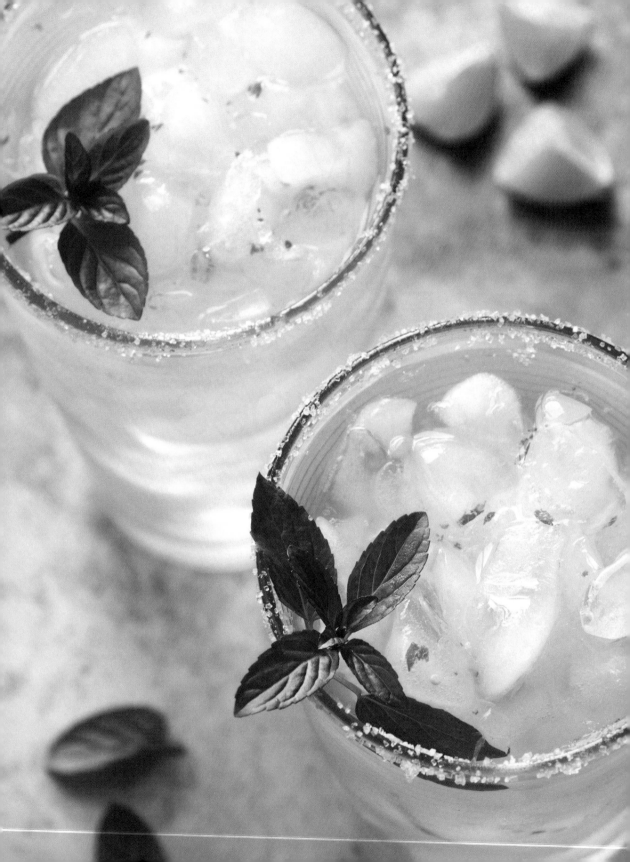

Minty Mojito

Serves 1

96 Calories

Simple Syrup
4-6 packets stevia
1 cup water
5-8 fresh mint leaves

2 oz simple syrup with stevia
1 ounce white rum
5 fresh mint leaves
Juice of ½ a lime
Chilled sparkling water
Ice

Garnish:
Mint and lime wedge

1. To make simple syrup, bring water to a boil in a small pot and add stevia.

2. Stir to dissolve, then remove from heat.

3. Add mint leaves, then cover to steep about 30 minutes.

4. Let simple syrup cool.

5. In a 12 ounce glass, pour 2 ounces simple syrup, 1 ounce rum, a few fresh mint leaves, and juice of half a lime, then muddle.

6. Fill glass with sparkling water and ice, then stir.

7. Garnish with fresh mint and a lime wedge.

8. Cheers!

Sweet Strawberry Raspberry Daiquiri

Serves 1

165 Calories

1 ounce rum
1 packet Stevia
1 cup frozen strawberries
¼ cup raspberries
½ cup water
¾ cup ice cubes
A squeeze of fresh lime

1. Add all ingredients to blender.
2. Blend until smooth.
3. Enjoy!

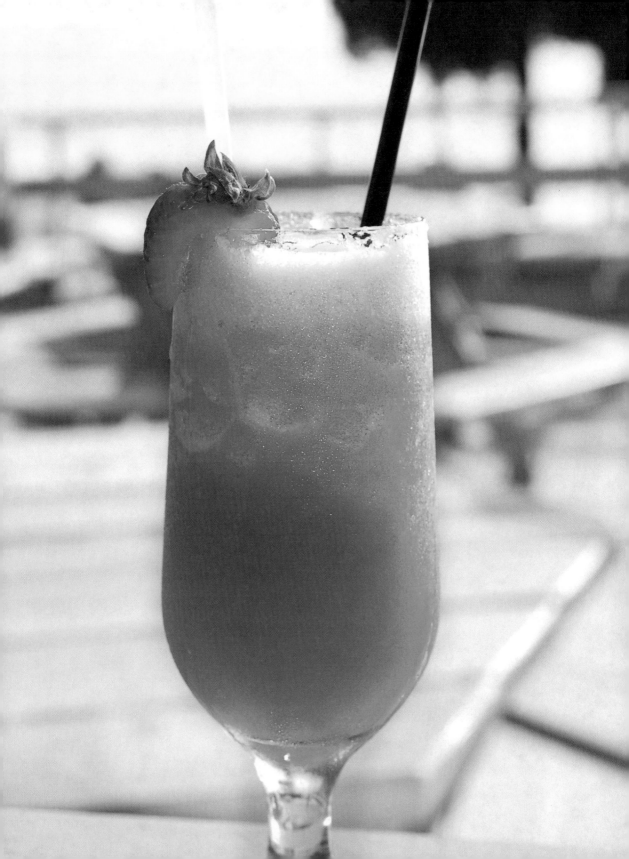

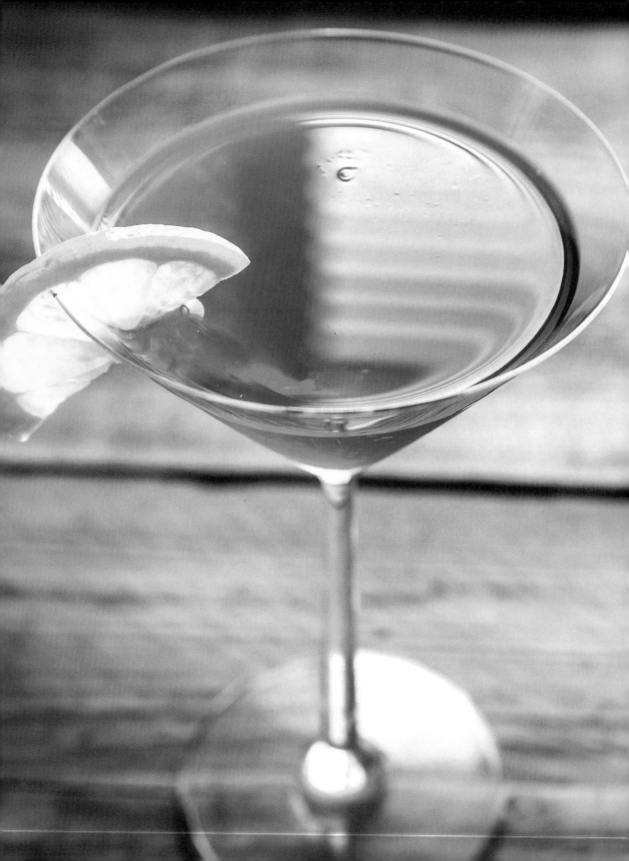

Pomegranate Cosmo

Serves 1

112 Calories

Zest from ½ lemon
Zest from ½ orange
1 packet stevia
½ ounce unsweetened pomegranate juice
1½ ounces vodka

Garnish:
1 lemon slice

1. In a cocktail shaker, muddle the lemon and orange zest with the stevia.
2. Add the pomegranate juice and vodka.
3. Fill the shaker halfway with ice, then shake vigorously.
4. Strain into a chilled glass.
5. Garnish with the lemon slice.

Raspberry Champagne Float

Serves 1

78 Calories

4 ounces champagne

Garnish:
raspberries and mint

1. Pour chilled champagne into a glass.
2. Top with a few raspberries and mint.
3. Cheers and enjoy!

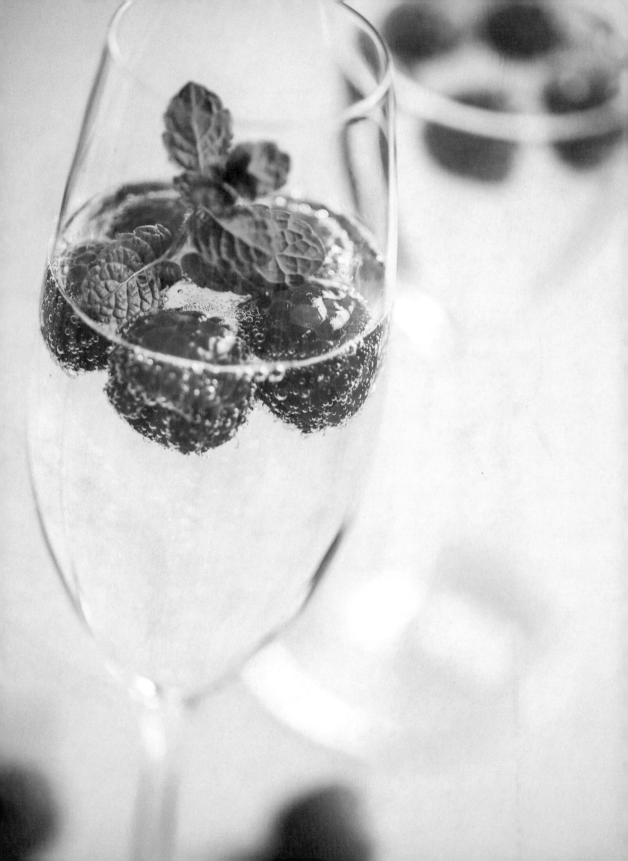

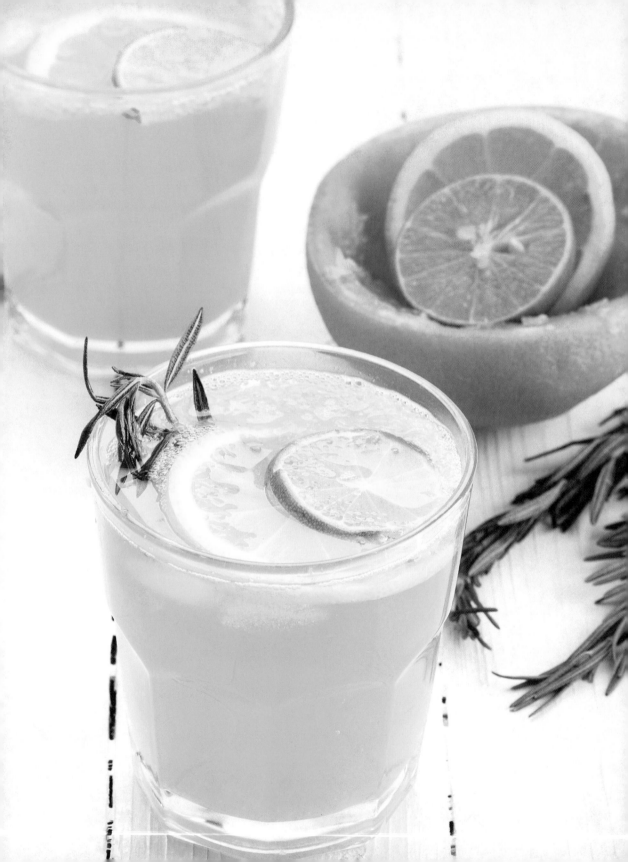

Grapefruit Margarita

Serves 1

96 Calories

Grapefruit slice, for garnish
Coarse sea salt, for rim
1 cup crushed ice
⅓ cup freshly squeezed red grapefruit juice
1 ounce silver tequila

1. Rub rim of glass with grapefruit slice and crust with salt.
2. Fill glass with crushed ice.
3. Combine juice and silver tequila in shaker.
4. Pour over glass.
5. Enjoy!

Tiny Sparkling Margarita

Serves 1

76 calories

3 ounces lime flavored Perrier
1 ounce tequila
1 ounce fresh squeezed lime juice
Salt, for rim
Lime slice, for garnish

1. Shake Perrier, tequila, and lime juice.
2. Pour into a chilled glass rimmed with salt.
3. Garnish with lime slice.

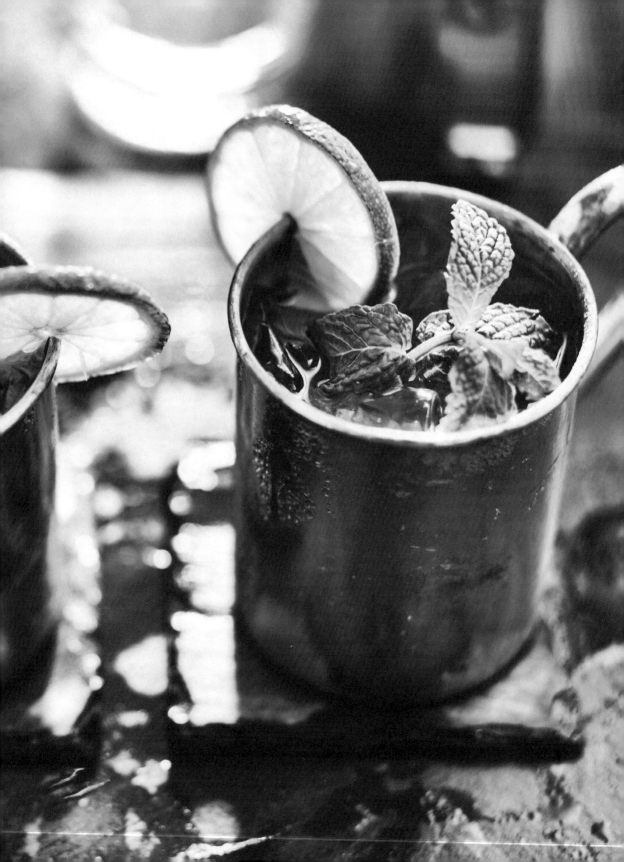

Slim & Sexy Moscow Mule

Serves 2

132 Calories per serving

2 ounces vodka

1 ounce lime juice

12 ounces ginger beer, or ginger ale

1 cup ice

Garnish:

lime slice and mint

1. Shake vodka and lime together.

2. Split ginger beer between two glasses, then pour over vodka with lime juice.

3. Add ice and garnish.

4. Enjoy!

Sparkling Citrus Berry Sangria

Serves 8

160 Calories per serving

1 cup vodka
Oranges, blueberries, peaches, raspberries
1 bottle sparkling white wine or Brut Champagne
1 bottle sparkling water

1. Combine vodka and fruit in a carafe and refrigerate at least 4 hours, or overnight.
2. When ready to serve, add the sparkling wine and sparkling water and gently stir.
3. Cheers!

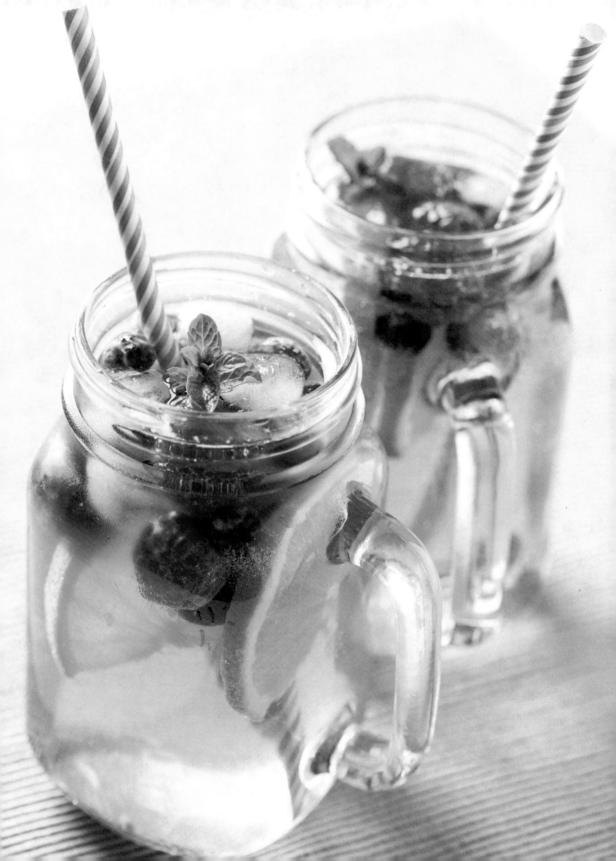

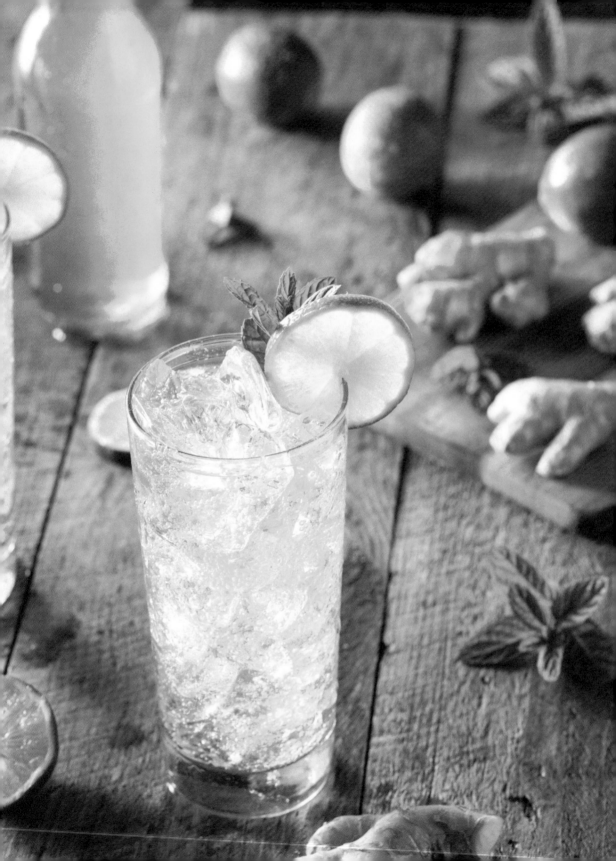

Be My Corona and Lime

Serves 1

100 Calories

1½ ounces lime juice
Ginger, grated
1 lime, zested
1 bottle of Corona Light Beer

Garnish:
lime slice and mint

Optional:
ice

1. Combine lime juice, grated ginger, and lime zest in a glass.
2. Add beer and stir gently.
3. Garnish with a lime wheel and mint.
4. Salud!

Vodka con Agua Mineral

Serves 1

66 Calories

Ice
1 ounce vodka
Perrier or sparkling water
Lime slices

1. Add ice and vodka to glass.
2. Fill glass with bubbly.
3. Garnish with lime slices.

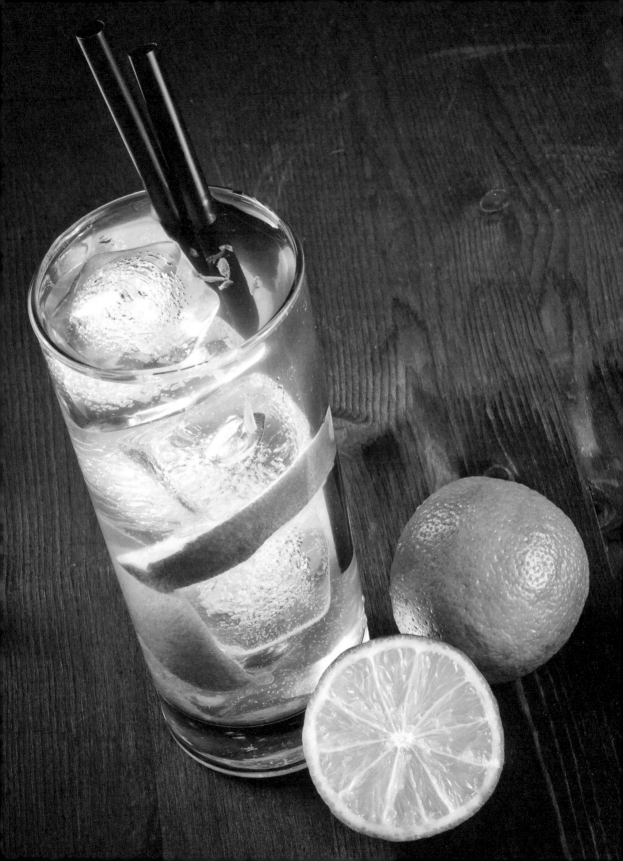

Conclusion

You've reached the end of the book! I want to take this moment to thank you for reading and I hope you now know that you deserve to be Tiny, but don't have to suffer getting there.

If you have yet to start your 12-week challenge to kick off your new Tiny and Full™ lifestyle, I encourage you to turn to the meal planners in Chapter 4 and get started today.

If you're reading this and you have completed your 12-week challenge, congratulations! I want to invite you to share this message with your friends and family as well as share your success with me personally. Please visit TinyandFull.com as well as tag me on social media (@TinyandFull, #TinyandFull). Share your stories of success, your favorite meals, and be inspired by all of the others following this lifestyle. I can't wait to find out how you did and how you will continue on this journey!

No matter what stage you are at, I encourage you to be an ambassador for Tiny and Full so we can change the world together! Let's do this!

Real Results

Learn how to get real results from real people

Jen

Lost 46 Pounds

Before starting Tiny and Full, Jen struggled with her portion control because she found that the foods she typically ate NEVER filled her up. With Tiny and Full, Jen ate meals that were BIG in size but also LOW in calories such as Cocoa Banana Oats, Chicken Salad Sandwich, Margherita Tortilla Pizza, and even Chocolate Ice Cream.

Now that Jen has lost the weight, she can finally walk down the aisle in her dream wedding dress. Jen has now created a life of empowerment where no matter what obstacle life throws at her, she is ready to conquer it all. What's next? Jen plans to start a family with her new husband and now after losing 46 pounds, she no longer fears having a high-risk pregnancy.

"Before Tiny and Full, I felt like I didn't get the respect I'd deserved because of my size. Now after losing 46 lbs., I have a new sense of empowerment because people treat me differently and I believe I can do anything I want now."

Real Tips

Create a workout schedule that FITS in your schedule. Whether it be in the morning or at night, finding the right time for you is key when starting a new lifestyle. Jorge's at-home workouts can be done at home with no gym or equipment required, and that saved me!

Set goals. I learned the importance of this very early on. Jorge suggested that in addition to our big goals such as buying my dream wedding dress, we must set small weekly goals so that you never lose focus.

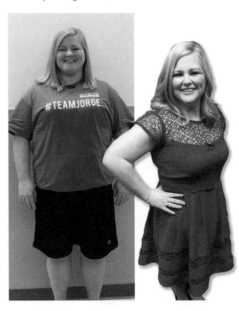

Alisha

Lost 65 Pounds

After 7 years of yo-yo dieting, Alisha has finally found the plan that has helped her shed 65 stubborn pounds. The same girl that used to be out of breath trying to catch the subway is now running up the stairs to catch the subway every morning with no huffing or puffing. Alisha's physical transformation inspired a mental transformation as well. No longer does Alisha feel insecure or depressed about herself; she now feels empowered and confident. Today, Alisha is no longer afraid to walk into a room, she now makes an entrance. Alisha's plans are to go after her dreams of becoming a Hollywood actress and making Jorge her official trainer when she hits it big.

"The food plan really helped me reset my body. I was able to turn off my hunger because the foods I ate were so big in size but also low in calories, allowing me to really control my appetite and literally eat off the pounds. Today, I am so grateful for the body that I have and I have a new sense of empowerment. I now believe I can do anything and I can finally show the world who Alisha really is, because every time I look in the mirror I'm just so proud of what I've accomplished and the person I've become."

Real Tips

Pack emergency snacks. Working as a receptionist, I always get hungry throughout the day. I learned to choose the right snacks to help me feel full on fewer calories. My typical snack bags included: strawberries, blueberries, bananas, chia seeds, carrots, and popcorn.

Find your after picture. One motivation tip Jorge gave me that really helped me stay on track was finding a picture of a girl that I wanted to look like. I put this picture as my screen saver on my phone so that anytime I felt like I was reversing back to my old ways I was reminded of the goals I have set for myself.

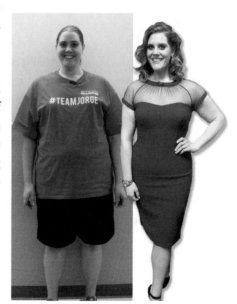

Kaitlyn

Lost 44 Pounds

Tiny and Full helped educate Kaitlyn on the power of plant-based foods and how they can help slim her down without her feeling starved or unsatisfied. Kaitlyn focused on incorporating more fruits and veggies into her diet and started moving more during the day. She started small by just doing a lap around the office every hour and is now on her way to run that marathon she's always dreamed about doing.

Now Kaitlyn looks and feels better than ever. She is a go-getter at work and now has the confidence to be a go-getter wherever she is. She's ready to run a marathon and to take that trip to Europe she's always wanted because she has the energy and willpower to accomplish anything she wants now!

"Before this diet I was at my highest size ever, a 16 . . . But now I've lost 44 pounds and I've never felt better in a size 8 dress! Everyone has been so supportive. I've had people reach out on Facebook! It's extremely rewarding to have everyone see the person on the inside showcased on the outside."

Real Tips

Automation, automation, automation! I ate the same thing for breakfast, lunch, and dinner all week. It sounds boring, but it works! And it makes meal prep super easy!

Think BIG. Tiny and Full has really allowed me to think differently when it comes to food now. Before I was very robotic and didn't necessarily think of what I was putting into my body 24/7. Now when I pick out what food I want to eat I think: Will this fill me up? Is this healthy? How many calories is this? Learning how to eat MORE food for fewer calories was truly the reason I was able to do this program without being hungry.

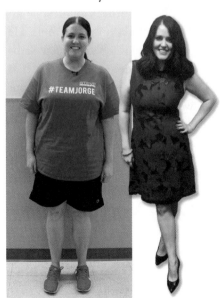

Suresh

Lost 55 Pounds

Suresh, like many of us, has had success losing weight in the past, but has always gained it back because of hunger and lack of variety. With Tiny and Full, Suresh learned how to incorporate plant-based pea protein into his morning breakfast routine to help detox the body from unhealthy toxins and waste AND, most importantly, turn off hunger for FOUR hours. In addition, Suresh stuck to the Tiny and Full meal planners to bring variety, flavor, and appetite control into his diet.

Now that Suresh has lost the 55 pounds he is feeling confident and determined to keep the weight off. He has even quit smoking in order to help him on his path to a healthier lifestyle.

"When I walk into a store to buy clothes I used to walk away depressed because I could only buy clothes in the Big and Tall section, but now I can go in and choose the clothes that I've always wanted to wear. This plan has given me the confidence and skills to be healthy for the rest of my life."

Real Tips

Get enough sleep. This was a challenge for me because I work a lot and help out with my family. I never put sleep as a priority, but once I learned about the benefits sleep has for weight loss, I focused on getting more z's. It actually made a difference and helped me break through my plateau. I was shocked!

Find your go-to meals. Jorge taught me that having a healthy lifestyle all comes down to keeping it simple. He encouraged me to choose a few sample days from the meal planners that I liked and to repeat them throughout the week. This way I was eating the meals I wanted to, but still sticking to the Tiny and Full routine.

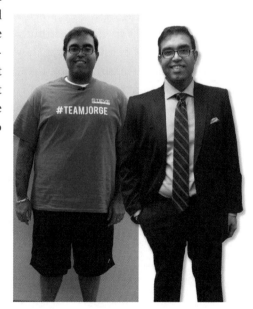

Emily

Lost 45 Pounds

Before Tiny and Full, Emily had a tendency to skip meals throughout the day and overeat at night. She decided to give the plan a try so that she could look amazing on her wedding day. Emily worked on automating her breakfast and lunch so that she DID eat throughout the day and wouldn't sabotage herself by binge eating at night. Prepping her meals the night before and sticking to the daily meal planners helped her control the amount of food she put in her body without overeating.

Today, Emily is the confident woman she always knew she could be. Her goals before starting the Tiny and Full included looking "drop-dead gorgeous" in her wedding dress. It's safe to say, "Mission accomplished!" She is going to make a GORGEOUS bride!

"I finally feel like the person who I feel on the inside is the same person who is being portrayed on the outside. Tiny and Full has taken my life outside of this box that I was living in for so long and helped blossom into the person I've always wanted to become. This plan has 100 percent changed my life."

Real Tips

Move more. I work at a typical desk job so I sit all day. Jorge encouraged me to set an alarm on my phone to go off every hour to remind me to get do a lap around the office or use the restroom. This little change in my work routine really helped my energy stay high and burn an extra 300 calories throughout the day.

Take selfies. When Jorge first told me to take a selfie every week I was a bit skeptical. But I will tell you a selfie shows what the scale doesn't. It's a great monitoring tool and it really helps you stay on track and hold yourself accountable. I look back at old selfies I took and look at the selfies I take now and am so proud of all the accomplishments I've made.

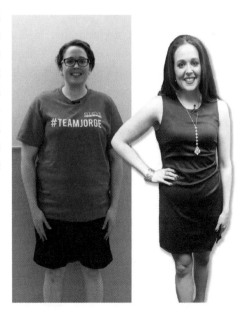

Danielle

Lost 45 Pounds

Being a mother of four and managing a successful blog (City Girl Gone Mom), Danielle had put her diet on the back burner after having her fourth child. However, after nursing was established and routines started to come into play, she finally had the desire to lose those leftover pregnancy pounds. Being a person who loves organization and lists, Danielle really utilized the Tiny and Full food lists and meal planners so that she always knew what to eat to stay on track.

Today, Danielle is 45 pounds lighter and now has the energy to keep up with her husband and their four children and the confidence and drive to take her blog to the next level.

"Being an Italian mom, I love to cook, especially for my family. I didn't know that the recipes within this book could be so sustainable and delicious not only for me, but for my entire family. Tiny and Full helped me lose 45 pounds, but it also helped my whole family get healthy again."

Real Tips

Make it a family affair. When I started this diet I decided that the whole family was going to get healthy . . . including my kids. I made meals like Zucchini Lasagna and Spaghetti Squash that I loved, but more importantly, so did my family. It was so great to see my kids eating plant-based foods instead of the usual chicken nuggets or pizza. By having my family's support and encouragement it really helped me stay focused and on track.

Retail therapy. I decided that I was going to buy a dress that I loved 3 sizes smaller than I normally am and I hung it in my closet in a place where I would see it every day. This outfit not only was motivating, it helped me stay on track and focused. Every day, I would wake up and see it hanging in my closet and it would remind me of my goals and how each day I could make a choice that would either bring me closer or farther away from wearing it. This was a great strategy, not to mention a great excuse for buying a new outfit. Highly recommend.

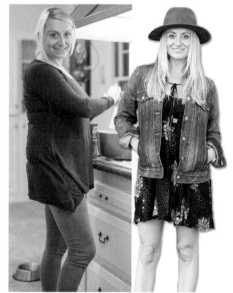

Cristina

Lost 70 Pounds

Growing up in a Mexican family Cristina was taught that food was to be enjoyed, not restricted. Unfortunately Cristina gained weight after years of eating the high-calorie processed foods. After years of trying quick fixes and gimmicky diets, Cristina decided to try Tiny and Full. She focused on starting her day with a plant-based breakfast like oatmeal and berries. By doing this Cristina set the tone for the rest of day and found herself not cheating and giving into the temptation of high-calorie foods.

After losing 70 pounds, Cristina was able to wear a two-piece for the first time on vacation with her family in Mexico. With this new confidence and willpower there is nothing Cristina can't do. . . including getting her Bachelor's degree in Psychology this year.

"Tiny and Full worked because it allowed me to take the skills and concepts from the book and turn them into a lifestyle. The eating plan was not only delicious, but it helped me get into a healthy routine that I now incorporate into my life every single day. I would have never thought I would be 70 pounds lighter and I couldn't have done it without Tiny and Full."

Real Tips

Find your go-to breakfast. I am very much a creature of habit, so finding a breakfast that I could repeat every day was critical for me. When you start your day with a healthy, filling, plant-based meal you set yourself up for success for the rest of the day. Pick your favorite breakfast and stick to it, because it really helps you start your day with your best foot forward.

Don't miss the scale. When I first read that I should weigh myself every day I was a little intimidated, but I found that it really helped me stay accountable. Every morning, I would weigh myself and I would not only see the progress that I was making, but also I would be reminded of the journey I was on and the choices that I would have to make each day. It's a great way to help re-focus and re-center at the start of each day.

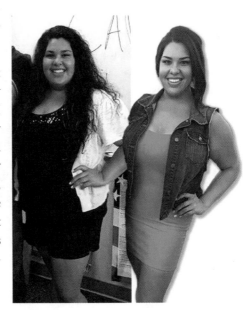

Rick

Lost 55 Pounds

Rick was a former college athlete who turned to food when things were stressful at work. And with his son's wedding around the corner, Rick was determined to lose the weight so that he could not only look great for the wedding, but so he could be around to enjoy his grandsons as they get older.

After years of losing the weight and then gaining it back Rick has finally found the plan that suits him the best. Rick turned to the workout planners instead of food when things got overwhelming at work, and used the meal planners to satisfy and keep him full all throughout the day.

"I would have never thought that at age 53 that I could lose 55 pounds. Tiny and Full has allowed me to turn this diet into a lifestyle. I know I can keep up with my grandkids and turn to the gym whenever I need to blow off some steam. This book has completely changed my life and I now have the tools to stay healthy forever."

Real Tips

Protein power. Every day I would drink a Tiny and Full pea protein shake; it's only 55 calories and it really help turn off my hunger for four hours. Anytime I had a late-night craving or needed something to hold me over between my next meal I would do a shake. It's not only delicious, but it really helps you stay on track and is more filling than whey or soy proteins.

Quench your thirst. Besides protein, I drink a gallon of water every day to stay hydrated and to turn off my hunger. After reading in Tiny and Full that sometimes when we are hungry we are actually just thirsty, I decided to quench my thirst and commit to drinking a gallon a day. This really helped me stay hydrated and control my hunger.

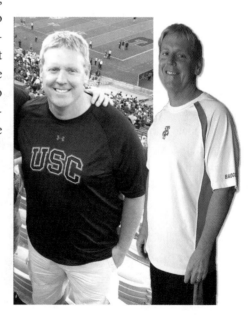

Chloe

Lost 25 Pounds

Before starting Tiny and Full, Chloe was a girl who never really paid too much attention to what she ate or working out. Sure, Chloe tried portion control in the past, but that never really gave her the results she wanted. However, after motivating herself to tone up and look good, she decided to give Tiny and Full a try.

After following the workout planners and meal planners, Chloe's intentions evolved into something more than she could ever imagine. As she pushed herself to be healthy, she was no longer motivated by what she saw in the mirror. By following a Tiny and Full lifestyle, she started sleeping better, thinking better, and working better, but most importantly feeling empowered. Chloe became the strong woman she always was . . . and the results in the mirror just became the cherry on top.

"Tiny and Full isn't just a diet, it's a lifestyle makeover. I lost 25 pounds and have never felt sexier, more confident, and better in my life. No fad diet can even come close to giving you the same results. I have a huge sense of empowerment now and nothing feels better than feeling like you can take over the world."

Real Tips

Snack it up. I am always packing healthy snacks to take with me to the office. Prepping your food and snacks are a real life-saver in the workplace, especially if your co-workers ask you to eat out for lunch. This way you are already fueled for success with healthy snacks and avoid giving into temptation when you see sweets or candy around the office.

Muscle up your mornings. The first thing I do in the morning is a workout. I found that this really helps me manage my time by getting it out of the way first thing in the morning, plus it helps set the tone for the entire day. Not to mention working out helps lower my stress and anxiety so that I don't start my day worrying about all the things I have to do. Instead, I start my day feeling energized and empowered to make healthy choices.

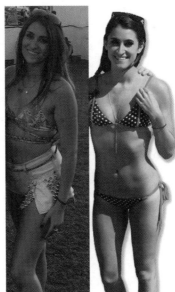

Sam

Lost 20 Pounds

Before Tiny and Full, Sam was a huge workout advocate who was running up to 5 miles a day. Sam was a regular gym rat who used to spend hours at the gym to reveal his six-pack, but always came up short. After trying a variety of fitness programs and going Paleo, Sam was frustrated and lost hope of getting that six-pack he always wanted.

However, by working out less, eating more plant-based foods, and following the meal planners, Sam finally was able to define and tighten his core. Not only did Sam get the six-pack he wanted, he suddenly had clearer skin and more energy.

"For years, I spent countless hours in the gym doing crunches and sit-ups, praying for a six-pack. I would have never thought by just switching up my diet that I would have gotten the abs I've always wanted. Not to mention I now have more energy than ever before and my skin has never been clearer. Tiny and Full has given me a lifestyle that I will continue for the rest of my life."

Real Tips

Don't be a gym rat. I still love working out and gaining muscle, but I realized what Jorge says is true: "You cannot out-train a bad diet." If you like to work out, stick to that routine; but, if you really want to see a difference in the way you look, make sure to watch what you eat. Abs are made in the kitchen, not in the gym.

Spice it up! Growing up, I was always a picky eater when it came to eating veggies. So when I started Tiny and Full I was a bit intimated by all the plant-based foods, but I found that using the right spices like basil, garlic, and cumin really help enhance the flavor and taste of the food. Not to mention most spices are very low in calories, with the majority containing no calories at all. So don't be afraid to use spices with your food. Spices are your friend and really help!

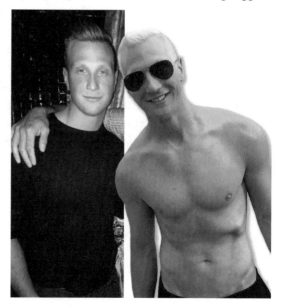

Jorge

Lost 40 Pounds

Growing up in a Mexican family, Jorge was taught that food was love. For years growing up Jorge turned to food because food was his friend that brought him comfort and enjoyment. Over time, Jorge became an emotional eater. Whenever things were tough or stressful, Jorge would turn to food to help him cope.

After gaining 40 pounds, Jorge was determined to make health a priority. He became a fitness trainer and started learning about nutrition. Through his studying and certification Jorge learned that food is medicine.

By focusing on eating more plant-based foods and learning the importance of calorie density, Jorge was able to lose 40 pounds and get the body he's always wanted.

Real Tips

Get support. When starting a new lifestyle you can achieve your goals much faster by creating an environment of support around you. By having a support system or doing the program with a peer you increase you chances of weight loss 3 times more than if you were doing the program on your own. I encourage you to join my support group on my Facebook Live show Tiny Talks. Every day, I bring you guidance, support, and answer your top health and weight loss questions so that you remain focused and stay on track. Join me at facebook.com/jorgecruise.

You can't out-train a poor diet. I've seen so many people try and eat whatever they want and think they can burn it all off in the gym. The truth is that fitness begins in the kitchen. Remember, if you start thinking of food as medicine instead of a comfort you will be able to eat off the pounds.

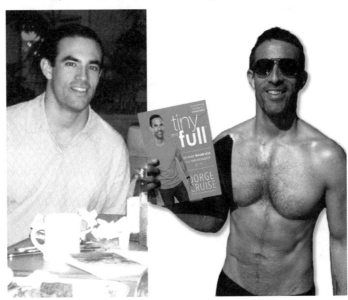

Selected Bibliography

Chapter 1: Ready for Tiny

Alford, Betty, Ann Blankenship, and R. Donald Hagen. "The Effects of Variations in Carbohydrate, Protein, and Fat Content of the Diet Upon Weight Loss, Blood Values, and Nutrient Intake of Adult Obese Women." *Journal of the American Dietetic Association* 90, no. 4 (1990): 534–40.

Astrup, Arne and Søren Toubro. "Randomised Comparison of Diets for Maintaining Obese Subjects' Weight After Major Weight Loss: Ad Lib, Low Fat, High Carbohydrate Diet v Fixed Energy Intake." *British Medical Journal* 314, no. 7073 (1997): 29–34.

Bemis, Thomas, Robert Brychta, Kong Y. Chen, Amber Courville, Emma J. Crayner, Stephanie Goodwin, Juen Guo, Kevin D. Hall, Lilian Howard, Nicolas D. Knuth, Bernard V. Miller III, Carla M. Prado, Mario Siervo, Monica C. Skarulis, Mary Walter, Peter J. Walter, and Laura Yannai. "Calorie for Calorie, Dietary Fat Restriction Results in More Body Fat Loss than Carbohydrate Restriction in People with Obesity." *Cell Metabolism* 22, no. 3 (2015): 427–436.

Braun, Margaret F. and Angela Bryan. "Female Waist-to-Hip And Male Waist-to-Shoulder Ratios As Determinants Of Romantic Partner Desirability." *Journal of Social and Personal Relationships* 23, no. 5 (2006): 805–819.

Dixson, Barnaby J., Gina Grimshaw, Wayne L. Linklater, and Alan Dixson. "Watching the Hourglass." *Human Nature* 21, no. 4 (2010): 355–70.

Dixson, Barnaby J., Alan Dixson, Tim S. Jessop, Bethan J. Morgan, and Devendra Singh. "Cross-cultural Consensus For Waist–Hip Ratio And Women's Attractiveness." *Evolution and Human Behavior* 31 (2010): 176–181.

Faries, Mark D. and John B. Bartholomew. "The Role of Body Fat in Female Attractiveness." *Evolution and Human Behavior* 15, no. 2 (2006): 672–681.

Devil Wears Prada, The. Directed by David Frankel. Performed by Anne Hathaway, Meryl Streep. 20th Century Fox, 2006. Film.

Folsom, Aaron R., Susan A. Kaye, and Thomas A. Sellers. "Body Fat Distribution and 5-Year Risk of Death in Older Women." *The Journal of the American Medical Association* 269 (1993): 483–487.

Goetz-Perry, Catherine. "Diets With Different Targets For Intake of Fat, Protein, and Carbohydrates Achieved Similar Weight Loss in Obese Adults." *Evidence-Based Nursing* 12, no. 4 (2009): 109–109.

Hill, Kyle. "The Twinkie Diet." *Science Based Life,* November 27, 2010. <https://sciencebasedlife.wordpress.com/2010/1½7/the-twinkie-diet/>

Hoover, Adam W., Eric R. Muth, and Jenna L. Scisco. "Examining the Utility of a Bite-Count–Based Measure of Eating Activity in Free-Living Human Beings." *the Academy of Nutrition and Dietetics* 114, no. 3 (2011): 464–469.

Jacobsen, Maryann Tomovich. "The Baby Food Diet Review: Does This Weight Loss Plan Work?" *WebMD,* December 16, 2013. <http://www.webmd.com/diet/baby-food-diet>

Just, David R. and Brian Wansink. "Trayless Cafeterias Lead Diners to Take Less Salad and Relatively More Dessert." *Public Health Nutrition* 18, no. 9 (2015): 1535–1536.

Kalm, Leah M. and Richard D. Semba. "They Starved So That Others Be Better Fed: Remembering Ancel Keys and the Minnesota Experiment." *The Journal of Nutrition* 135 no. 6 (2005): 1347–1352.

Kinsell, Laurance W., Barbara Gunning, George D. Michaels, James Richardson, Stephen E. Cox, and Calvin Lemon. "Calories Do Count." *Metabolism* 13, no. 3 (1964): 195–204.

Neporent, Liz. "Dangerous Diet Trend: The Cotton Ball Diet." *ABC News*, November 21, 2013. <http://abcnews.go.com/Health/dangerous-diet-trend-cotton-balldiet/story?id=20942888>

Nestle, Marion and Malden Nesheim. *Why Calories Count: From Science to Politics.* Oakland: University of California Press, 2013.

Nordqvist, Christian. "Nutrition Professor Loses 27 Pounds on Junk Food Diet in 10 Weeks." *Medical News Today,* November 8, 2010. <http://www.medicalnewstoday.com/articles /207071.php>

North, Jill, James E. Painter, and Brian Wansink. "Bottomless Bowls: Why Visual Cues Of Portion Size May Influence Intake." *Obesity* 13, no. 1 (2005): 93–100.

Oxford Dictionaries. "Oxford Dictionaries.com Quarterly Update: New Words Added Today Include *Hangry, Grexit*, and *Wine O'Clock*." *Oxford Dictionaries Blog,* August 27, 2015. Retrieved September 9, 2015. <http://blog.oxforddictionaries.com/press-releases/ oxforddictionaries-com-quarterly-update-new-words-added-today-include-hangry-grexit -and-wine-oclock/>

Randall, Patrick K. and Devendra Singh. "Beauty is in the Eye of the Plastic Surgeon: Waist–Hip Ratio (WHR) and Women's Attractiveness." *Personality and Individual Differences* 43, no. 2 (2007): 329–340.

Renn, Peter, Adrian Singh, and Devendra Singh. "Did the Perils of Abdominal Obesity Affect Depiction of Feminine Beauty in the Sixteenth to Eighteenth Century British Literature? Exploring the Health and Beauty Link." *Journal of the Royal Society B: Biological Sciences* 274, no. 1611 (2007): 891–894.

Reverby, Susan M. Review of *The Great Starvation Experiment: Ancel Keys and the Men Who Starved for Science* by Todd Tucker. *Journal of the History of Medicine and Allied Sciences* 66 (2011): 134–136.

Salis, Amanda. "The Science Behind Being 'Hangry:' Why Some People Get Grumpy When They're Hungry." *CNN*, July 20, 2015. <http://theconversation.com/health-check-the -science-of-hangry-or-why-some-people-get-grumpy-when-theyre-hungry-37229>

Singh, Devendra. "Adaptive Significance of Female Physical Attractiveness: Role of Waist-to-Hip Ratio." *Journal of Personality and Social Psychology* 65, no. 2 (1993): 293–307.

———. "Female Mate Value at a Glance: Relationship of Waist-to-Hip Ratio to Health, Fecundity and Attractiveness." *Neuroendocrinology Letters* 23, no. 4 (2002): 81–91.

———. " Female Judgment of Male Attractiveness and Desirability for Relationships: Role of Waist-to-Hip Ratio and Financial Status." *Journal of Personality and Social Psychology* 69, no. 6 (1995): 1089–1101.

———. "Mating strategies of young women: Role of physical attractiveness." *Journal of Sex Research* 41, no. 1 (2004): 43–54.

Singh, Devendra and Dorian Singh. "Shape and Significance of Feminine Beauty: An Evolutionary Perspective." *Sex Roles* 64, no. 9 (2011): 723–731.

Singh, Devendra and Suwardi Luis. "Ethnic and Gender Consensus for the Effect of Waist-to-Hip Ratio on Judgment of Women's Attractiveness." *Human Nature* 6, no. 1 (1995): 51–65.

van Ittersum, Koert and Brian Wansink. "Portion Size Me: Plate-Size Induced Consumption Norms and Win-Win Solutions for Reducing Food Intake and Waste." *Journal of Experimental Psychology: Applied* 19, no. 4 (2013): 320–332.

Agnoli, Claudia, Benedetta Bendinelli, Carmela Calonico, Paolo Chiodini, Graziella Frasca, Sara Grioni, Giovanna Masala, Amalia Mattiello, Domenico Palli, Salvatore Panico, Carlotta Sacerdote, Calogero Saieva, Simonetta Salvini, Rosario Tumino, and Paolo Vineis. "Fruit, Vegetables, and Olive Oil and Risk of Coronary Heart Disease in Italian Women: The EPICOR Study." *American Journal of Clinical Nutrition* 93 no. 2 (2011): 275–283.

Alfredo, Martinez, Maira Bes-Rastrollo, Carmen de la Fuente Arrillaga, Miguel Ángel Martinez-González, and Almudena Sánchez-Villegas. "Association of Fiber Intake and Fruit/Vegetable Consumption with Weight Gain in a Mediterranean Population." *Nutrition* 22, no. 5 (2006): 504–511.

Alonso, Alvaro, J. Benuza, Enrique Gómez-Garcia, Miguel Ángel Martinez-González, J. Nuñez-Cordoba, and S. Palma. "Role of Vegetables and Fruits in Mediterranean Diets to Prevent Hypertension." *European Journal of Clinical Nutrition* 63, no. 5 (2008): 605–612.

Amouyel, Philippe, Jean Dallongeville, Luc Dauchet, and Serge Hercberg. "Fruit and Vegetable Consumption and Risk of Coronary Heart Disease: A Meta-Analysis of Cohort Studies." *The Journal of Nutrition* 136, no. 10 (2006): 2588–2593.

S. Arulmozhiselvan, G. Hemalatha, and S. Mathanghi. "Impact of Fruit and Vegetable Intake by Healthy Subjects on the Risk Factors of Cardiovascular Diseases." *The Indian Journal of Nutrition and Dietetics* 52, no. 1 (2015): 80–87.

Appel, Lawrence J., Louise M. Bishop, Hannia Campos, Vincent J. Carey, Jeanne Charleston, Paul R. Conlin, Thomas P. Erlinger, Jeremy D. Furtado, Nancy Laranjo, Phyllis McCarron, Edgar R. Miller, Eva Obarzanek, Bernard A. Rosner, Frank M. Sacks, and Janis F. Swain. "Effects of Protein, Monounsaturated Fat, and Carbohydrate Intake on Blood Pressure and Serum Lipids: Results of the OmniHeart Randomized Trial." *The Journal of the American Medical Association* 294, no. 19 (2005): 2455–2464.

Appel, Lawrence J., George A. Bray, Jeffrey A. Cutler, Marguerite A. Evans, David W. Harsha, Njeri Karanja, Pao-Hwa Lin, Marjorie McCullough, Edgar R. Miller, Thomas J. Moore, Eva Obarzanek, Frank M. Sacks, Denise Simons-Morton, Priscilla Steele, Laura P. Svetkey, Janis Swain, Thomas M. Vogt, William M. Vollmer, and Marlene M. Windhauser. "A Clinical Trial of the Effects of Dietary Patterns on Blood Pressure." *The New England Journal of Medicine* 336, no. 16 (1997): 1117–1124.

Appel, Lawrence J., Jamy D. Ard, Catherine Champagne, Njeri Karanja, Jenny H. Ledikwe, Pao-Hwa Lin, Diane C. Mitchell, Barbara J. Rolls, Helen Smiciklas-Wright, and Victor J Stevens. "Reductions in Dietary Energy Density are Associated with Weight Loss in Overweight and Obese Participants in the PREMIER Trial." *American Journal of Clinical Nutrition* 85, no. 5 (2007): 1212–1221.

Asensio, Laura, Adela Castelló, Manoli Garcia de la Hera, Jesus Vioque, and Tanja Weinbrenner. "Intake of Fruits and Vegetables in Relation to 10-Year Weight Gain Among Spanish Adults." *Obesity* 16, no. 3 (2008): 664–670.

Aucott, Lorna, Alison J. Black, William D. Fraser, Garry Duthie, Susan Duthie, Antonia C. Hardcastle, Susan A. Lanham, Helen M. Macdonald, David M.and Rena Sandison. "Effect of Potassium Citrate Supplementation or Increased Fruit and Vegetable Intake on Bone Metabolism in Healthy Postmenopausal Women: A Randomized Controlled Trial." *Nutrition* 88, no. 2 (2008): 465–474.

Ayres, Ed. "Will We Still Eat Meat: Maybe Not, If We Wake Up to What the Mass Production of Animal Flesh is Doing to Our Health—and the Planet's." *Time*, November 8, 1999.

Barnard, Neal D., Yoshihiro Miyamoto, Kunihiro Nishimura, Tomonori Okamura, Akira Sekikawa, Misa Takegami, Makoto Wantanabe, and Yoko Yokoyama. "Vegetarian Diets and Blood Pressure." *JAMA Internal Medicine* 174, no. 4 (2014): 577–587.

Basu, Samar, Erica M. Holt, Ching Ping Hong, Antoinette Moran, Julie A. Alan R. Sinaiko, Lyn M. Steffen, and Julia Steinberger. "Fruit and Vegetable Consumption and Its Relation to Markers of Inflammation and Oxidative Stress in Adolescents." *Journal of the American Dietetic Association* 109, no. 3 (2009): 414–421.

Bazzano, Lydia A., Frank B. Hu, Kamudi Joshipura, and Tricia Y. Li. "Intake Of Fruit, Vegetables, And Fruit Juices and Risk of Diabetes in Women." *Diabetes Care* 31, no. 7 (2008): 1311–1317.

Beach, Amanda M., Julia A. Ello-Martin, Jenny H. Ledikwe, Liane S. Roe, and Barbara J. Rolls. "Dietary Energy Density in the Treatment of Obesity: A Year-Long Trial Comparing 2 Weight-Loss Diets." *Nutrition* 85, no. 6 (2007): 1465–1477.

Bell, Elizabeth, Liane S. Roe, and Barbara Jean Rolls. "Sensory-Specific Satiety is Affected More By Volume Than by Energy Content of a Liquid Food." *Physiology and Behavior 78*, no. 4 (2003): 593–600.

Bes-Rastrollo, Maira, Frank B. Hu, Tricia Y. Li, Miguel Ángel Martinez-González, Laura L. Sampson, and Rob M. van Dam. "Prospective Study of Dietary Energy Density and Weight Gain in Women." *The American Journal of Clinical Nutrition* 88, no. 3 (2008): 769–777.

Blanck, Heidi M., Laura Kettel Khan, Jenny H. Ledikwe, Barbara J. Rolls, Mary K. Serdula, and Jennifer D. Seymour. "Dietary Energy Density is Associated with Energy Intake and Weight Status in US Adults." *American Journal of Clinical Nutrition* 83, no. 6 (2006): 1362–1368.

Blundell, John, Vicky Drapeau, Eric Doucet, Marion Hetherington, Neil King, and Angelo Tremblay. "Appetite Sensations and Satiety Quotient: Predictors of Energy Intake and Weight Loss." *Appetite* 48, no. 2 (2007): 159–166.

Borenstein, Amy R., Qi Dai, James C. Jackson, Eric B. Larson, and Yougui Wu. "Fruit and Vegetable Juices and Alzheimer's Disease: The Kame Project." *The American Journal of Medicine* 119, no. 9 (2006): 751–759.

Brown, Lisa, Lisa Chasan-Taber, Edward L. Giovannucci, Susan E. Johanna M. Seddon, Donna Spiegelman, and Walter C. Willett. "A Prospective Study of Carotenoid Intake and Risk of Cataract Extraction in US Men." *American Journal of Clinical Nutrition* 70, no. 4 (1999): 517–524.

Buijsse, Brian, Heiner Boeing, Huaidong Du, Edith Feskens, Nita G. Forouhi, Jytte Halkjaer, Marianne U. Jakobsen, Kim Overvad, Domenico Palli, Matthias B. Schulze, Stephen Sharp, Thorkild Sørensen, Anne Tjønneland, Gianluca Tognon, Daphne L. van der A, and Nicholas J. Wareham. "Fruit and Vegetable Intakes and Subsequent Changes in Body Weight in European Populations: Results from The Project on Diet, Obesity, and Genes (DiOGenes)." *Clinical Nutrition* 90, no. 1 (2009): 202–209.

Buring, Julia, William G. Christen, Simin Liu, and Debra A. Schaumberg. "Fruit and Vegetable Intake and the Risk of Cataract in Women." *American Journal of Clinical Nutrition* 81, no. 6 (2005): 1417-1422.

Camilleri, Michael and Anthony Lembo. "Chronic Constipation." *Journal of Medicine* 349 (2003): 1360–1368.

Castellanos, Vanessa, Jason C.G. Halford, Arun Kilara, D. Panyam, C.L. Pelkman, and Barbara J. Rolls. "Volume of Food Consumed Affects Satiety in Men." *Journal of Clinical Nutrition* 67, no. 6 (1998): 1170–1177.

Centers for Disease Control and Prevention. "Low-Energy-Dense Foods and Weight Management: Cutting Calories While Controlling Hunger. http://www.cdc.gov/nccdphp/ dnpa/nutrition/pdf/r2p_energy_density.pdf

Chiang, Yi-Chen, Zhi-Hong Jian, Pei-Chieh Ko, Chia-Chi Lung, and Oswald Ndi Nfor. "Vegetarian Diet and Cholesterol and TAG Levels by Gender." *Health Nutrition* 18, no. 4 (2014): 721–726.

Chylack, Leo T., Susan E. Hankinson, Paul F. Jacques, Marjorie L. McCullough, Suzen M. Moeller, Allen Taylor, Katherine L. Tucker, and Walter C. Willett. "Overall Adherence to the Dietary Guidelines for Americans is Associated with Reduced Prevalence of Early Age-Related Nuclear Lens Opacities in Women." *Journal of Nutrition* 134, no. 7 (2004): 1812–1819.

Cole, Greg, Elizabeth Head, Donald Ingram, and James Joseph. "Nutrition, Brain Aging, and Neurodegeneration." *Journal of Neuroscience* 29, no. 41 (2009): 12795–12801.

Colditz, Graham, Frank B. Hu, Hsin-Chia Hung, Kaumudi J. Joshipura, Tricia Y. Li, Eric B. Rimm, Meir J. Stampfer, and Walter C. Willett. "Intakes of Fruits, Vegetables and Carbohydrate and the Risk of CVD." *Public Health Nutrition* 12, no. 1 (2009): 115–121.

Colditz, Graham A., Frank B. Hu, Hsin-Chia Hung, David Hunter, Rui Jiang, Kaumudi J. Joshipura, Bernard Rosner, Stephanie A. Smith-Warner, Donna Spiegelman, and Walter C. Willett. "Fruit And Vegetable Intake and Risk of Major Chronic Disease." *Journal of the National Cancer Institute* 96, no. 21 (2004): 1577–1584.

De Biase, Simone Grigoletto, João Luiz Garcia Duarte, Sabrina Francine Carrocha Fernandes, and Reinaldo José Gianni. "Vegetarian Diet and Cholesterol and Triglycerides Levels." *Arquivos Brasileiros de Cardiologia* 88, no. 1 (2007): 1678–4170.

Dowling, Emily C., Neal D. Freedman, Stephanie M. George, Albert Hollenbeck, Michael F. Leitzmann, Yikyung Park, Jill Reedy, Arthur Schatzkin, and Amy F. Subar. "Fruit and Vegetable Intake and Risk of Cancer: A Prospective Cohort Study." *American Journal of Clinical Nutrition* 89, no. 1 (2009): 347–353.

Ello-Martin, Julia A., Barbara J. Rolls, and Beth C. Tohill. "What Can Intervention Studies Tell Us about the Relationship between Fruit and Vegetable Consumption and Weight Management?" *Nutrition Reviews* 62, no. 1 (2004): 1–17.

Ellwood, Kathleen C., Claudine J. Kavanaugh, and Paula R. Trumbo. "The U.S. Food And Drug Administration's Evidence-Based Review For Qualified Health Claims: Tomatoes, Lycopene, and Cancer." *Institute* 99, no. 14 (2007): 1074–1085.

Food and Agricultural Organization of the United Nations. "FAO Urges Action to Cope With Increasing Water Scarcity." *FAO Newsroom,* March 22, 2007. <http://www.fao.org/newsroom/en/news/2007/1000520/index.Html>

———. "Livestock a Major Threat to Environment." *FAO Newsroom,* November 29, 2006. <http://www.fao.org/newsroom/en/news/2006/1000448/index.html>

Farmer, Bonnie. "Nutritional Adequacy of Plant-Based Diets for Weight Management: Observations from the NHANES." *Nutrition* 100, no. 1 (2014): 365S–368S.

Giovannucci, Edward, Yan Liu, Elizabeth A. Platz, Meir J. Stampfer, and Walter C. Willett. "Risk Factors for Prostate Cancer Incidence and Progression in the Health Professionals Follow-Up Study." *International Journal of Cancer* 121, no. 7 (2008): 1571–1578.

Grubard, Barry I., Richard B. Hayes, Amy E. Millen, Ulrike Peters, Amy F. Joel L. Weissfeld, Lance A. Yokochi, and Regina G. Ziegler. "Fruit and Vegetable Intake and Prevalence of Colorectal Adenoma in a Cancer Screening Trial." *American Journal of Clinical Nutrition* 86, no. 6 (2007): 1754–1764.

He, Feng J., Lucas, Graham A. MacGregor, and Caryl A. Nowson. "Increased Consumption of Fruit and Vegetables is Related to a Reduced Risk of Coronary Heart Disease: Meta-analysis of Cohort Studies." *Hypertension* 21, no. 9 (2007): 717–728.

He, Feng J., Graham A. MacGregor, and Caryl A. Nowson. "Fruit And Vegetable Consumption and Stroke: Meta-analysis of Cohort Studies." *The Lancet* 28, no. 367 (2006): 320–326.

Kant, Ashima and B.I. Graubard. "Energy Density of Diets Reported by American Adults: Association with Food Group Intake, Nutrient Intake, and Body Weight." *International Journal of Obesity* 29, vol. 8 (2005): 950–956.

Lopes, Carla, A. Oliveira, and F. Rodríguez-Artalejo. "The Association of Fruits, Vegetables, Antioxidant Vitamins, and Fiber Intake with High-Sensitivity C-Reactive Protein: Sex and Body Mass Index Interactions." *Clinical Nutrition* 63, no. 11 (2009): 1345–1352.

Marsh, Kate, Angela Sanders, and Carol Zeuschner. "Health Implications of a Vegetarian Diet: A Review." *American Journal of Lifestyle Medicine* 6, no. 3 (2012): 250–267.

Meengs, Jennifer S., Liane S. Roe, and Barbara J. Rolls. "Salad and Satiety: Energy Density and Portion Size of a First-Course Salad Affect Energy Intake at Lunch." *Journal of the American Dietetic Association* 104, no. 10 (2004): 1570-1576.

Messina, Ginny. "Why Do Some People Fail at Being Vegan?" *The Vegan R.D,* January 6, 2015. <http://www.theveganrd.com/2015/01/why-do-some-people-fail-at-being-vegan.html>

Mohr, Noam. "A New Global Warming Strategy How Environmentalists are Overlooking Vegetarianism as the Most Effective Tool Against Climate Change in Our Lifetimes." *EarthSave International,* August 1, 2005. <http://www.earthsave.org/news/earthsave_global_warming_report.pdf>

Natural Resources Defense Council. "Facts About Pollution from Livestock Farms." February 21, 2013. <http://www.nrdc.org/water/pollution/ffarms.asp>

Penning De Vries, F., Van Keulen, H., and Rabbinge, R. "Natural Resources and Limits of Food Production in 2040." *Systems Approaches for Sustainable Agricultural Development: Eco-Regional Approaches for Sustainable Land Use and Food Production,* edited by J. Bouma, B.A.M. Bourman, A. Kuyvenhoven, J.C. Luyten, and H.G. Zandstra, 65–87. Springer, 1995.

Petrović, Bronislav; Dragana Nikić, and Maja Nikolić. "Fruit and Vegetable Intake and the Risk for Developing Coronary Heart Disease." *Central European Journal of Public Health* 16, no. 1 (2008): 17–20.

Rolls, Barbara J. "The Relationship Between Dietary Energy Density and Energy Intake." *Physiology and Behavior* 97, no. 5 (2009): 609–615.

———. *Ultimate Volumetrics Diet: Smart, Simple, Science-Based Strategies for Losing Weight and Keeping It Off.* New York: William Morrow Cookbooks, 2013.

The United Nations. "Rearing Cattle Produces More Greenhouse Gases than Driving Cars, UN Report Warns." *UN News Centre,* November 29, 2006. <http://www.un.org/apps/news/story.asp?NewsID=20772&Cr=global&Cr1=environment>

Wiseman, Martin. "The Second World Cancer Research Fund/American Institute for Cancer Research Expert Report. Food, Nutrition, Physical Activity, and the Prevention of Cancer: A Global Perspective." *Proceedings of the Nutrition Society* 67, no. 3 (2008): 253–256.

Chapter 3: Ready to Eat

Abou-Samra, Rania, Dino Brienza, Lian Keersmaekers, Katherine Mace, and Rajat Mukherjee. "Effect of Different Protein Sources on Satiation and Short-Term Satiety When Consumed as a Starter." *Nutrition Journal* 10, no. 139 (2011): 139–139.

Baumeister, Roy F. and Matthew T. Gailliot. "The Physiology Of Willpower: Linking Blood Glucose To Self-Control." *Review* 11, no. 4 (2007): 303–327.

Baumeister, Roy F., Matthew Gaillot, C. Nathan DeWall, and Megan Oaten. "Self-Regulation and Personality: How Interventions Increase Regulatory Success, and How Depletion Moderates the Effects of Traits on Behavior." *Personality* 74, no. 6 (2006): 1773–1802.

Baumeister, Roy F. and Andrew Vonasch. "Uses of Self-Regulation to Facilitate and Restrain Addictive Behavior." *Addictive Behaviors* 44 (2015): 3–8.

Baumeister, Roy F. and John Tierney. *"Willpower: Rediscovering the Greatest Human Strength."* New York: Penguin Press, 2011.

Bell, Elizabeth A., Barbara J. Rolls, and Michelle L. Thorwart. "Water Incorporated Into a Food but Not Served with a Food Decreases Energy Intake in Lean Women." *American Journal of Clinical Nutrition* 70, no. 4 (1999): 448–455.

Blundell, John, Eric Doucet, Vicky Drapeau, Marion Hetherington, Neil King, and Angelo Tremblay. "Appetite Sensations and Satiety Quotient: Predictors of Energy Intake and Weight Loss." *Appetite* 48, no. 2 (2007): 159–166.

Butryn, Meghan, Hill, James O., Suzanne Phelan, and Rena R. Wing. "Consistent Self-Monitoring of Weight: A Key Component of Successful Weight Loss Maintenance." *Obesity* 15, no. 12 (2007): 3091–3096.

Centers for Disease Control and Prevention. "Assessing Your Weight." May 15, 2015. <http://www.cdc.gov/healthyweight/assessing/index.html>

Cho, Susan, Ock Kyoung Chun, Chin Eun Chung, Saori Obayashi, and Won O. Song. "Is Consumption of Breakfast Associated with Body Mass Index in US Adults?" *Journal of the American Dietetic Association* 105, no. 9 (2005): 1373–1382.

Cho, Susan, Carol O'Neil, Theresa A. Nicklas, and Michael Zanovec. "Whole Grain and Fiber Consumption are Associated with Lower Body Weight Measures in US Adults: National Health and Nutrition Examination Survey 1999–2004." *Nutrition Research* 30, no. 12 (2010): 815–822.

De Silva, Akila, Waljit S. Dhillo, Paul M. Matthews, and Victoria Salem. "The Use of Functional MRI to Study Appetite Control in the CNS." *Journal of Diabetes Research* (2012).

Diepvens, K., Häiepvens, D., and Westerterp-Plantenga, M. "Different Proteins and Biopeptides Differently Affect Satiety and Anorexigenic/Orexigenic Hormones in Healthy Humans." *International Journal of Obesity* 32, no 3 (2007): 510–518.

Foster, Gary D. and Cathy A. Nonas. "Setting Achievable Goals for Weight Loss." *Journal of the American Dietetic Association* 105, no. 5 (2005): 118–123.

Flood, Julie E. and Barbara J. Rolls. "Soup Preloads in a Variety of Forms Reduce Meal Energy Intake." *Appetite* 49, no. 3 (2007): 626–634.

Flood-Obbagy, Julie and Barbara J. Rolls. "The Effect of Fruit in Different Forms on Energy Intake and Satiety at a Meal." *Appetite* 52, no. 2 (2009): 416–422.

Goldstone, Tony. "Good Breakfast and Good Diet: New Findings Support Common Sense." Lecture presented at Neuroscience 2012, the Annual Meeting of the Society for Neuroscience, New Orleans, October 13–17, 2012.

Hill, James O., Gary K. Grunwald, Mary L. Klem, Cecilia L. Mosca, Rena R. Wing, and Holly R. Wyatt. "Long-Term Weight Loss and Breakfast in Subjects in the National Weight Control Registry." *Obesity* 10, no. 2 (2002): 78–82.

Meengs, Jennifer S., Liane S. Roe, and Barbara J. Rolls. "Salad and Satiety: Energy Density and Portion Size of a First-Course Salad Affect Energy Intake at Lunch." *Journal of the American Dietetic Association* 104, no. 10 (2004), 1570–1576.

Roe, Liane S., Barbara J. Rolls, and Rachel A. Williams. "Assessment of Satiety Depends on the Energy Density and Portion Size of the Test Meal." *Obesity* 22, no. 2 (2013): 318–324.

Chapter 10: Tiny and Full

Alméras, Natalie, Jolanda Boer, Jean-Pierre Després, E.K. Kranenbarg, and A. Tremblay. "Diet Composition and Postexercise Energy Balance." *American Journal of Clinical Nutrition* 59 no. 5 (1994): 975–979.

Alméras, Natalie, Eric Doucet, Pascal Imbeault, and Angelo Tremblay. "Physical Activity and Low-Fat Diet: Is it Enough to Maintain Weight Stability in the Reduced-Obese Individual Following Weight Loss Drug Therapy and Energy Restriction?" *Obesity Reviews* 7 (1999): 323–333.

Alméras, Natalie, Eric Doucet, A. Labrie, Denis Richard, Sylvie St-Pierre, and Mayumi Yoshioko. "Impact of High-Intensity Exercise on Energy Expenditure, Lipid Oxidation, and Body Fatness." *International Journal of Obesity* 25 no. 3 (2001): 332–339.

Bahr, Roald. and Sejersted, Ole. M. "Effect of Intensity of Exercise on Excess Postexercise O2 Consumption." *Metabolism* 40, no. 8 (1991): 836–841.

Bielinski, R., Schutz, Yves, and E. Jéquier. "Energy Metabolism During the Postexercise Recovery in Man." *The American Journal of Clinical Nutrition* 42, no. 1 (1985): 69–82.

Bonen, Arend, Stuart D.R. Galloway, George J.F. Heigenhauser, Lawrence L. Spriet, and Jason L. Talanian. "Two Weeks of High-Intensity Aerobic Interval Training Increases the Capacity for Fat Oxidation During Exercise in Women." *Journal of Applied Physiology* 102, no. 4 (2007): 1439–1447.

Bonen, Arend, George J.F. Heigenhauser, Christopher G.R. Perry, and Lawrence L. Spriet. "High-Intensity Aerobic Interval Training Increases Fat and Carbohydrate Metabolic Capacities in Human Skeletal Muscle. *Applied Physiology, Nutrition, and Metabolism* 33, no. 6 (2008): 1112–1123.

Bouchard, Claude, Jean-Aimé Simoneau, and Angelo Tremblay. "Impact of Exercise Intensity on Body Fatness and Skeletal Muscle Metabolism." *Metabolism* 43, no. 7 (1994): 814–818.

Boutcher, Steve. "High-Intensity Intermittent Exercise and Fat Loss." *Journal of Obesity* (2011).

Boutcher, Steve, D.J. Chisholm, Judith Fruend, and Ethlyn Gail Trapp. "The Effects of High-Intensity Intermittent Exercise Training on Fat Loss and Fasting Insulin Levels of Young Women." *International Journal of Obesity* 32, no. 4 (2008): 684–691.

Cloud, John. "Why Exercise Won't Make You Thin." *Time,* August 9, 2009. <http://content .time.com/time/printout/0,8816,1914974,00.html>

Cohn, V. "Passion to Keep Fit: 100 Million Americans Exercising." *Washington Post,* August 31, 1980.

Craig, C.L., Jean-Pierre Després, Blake Ferris, C. Leblanc, Torrance T. Stephens, and Angelo Tremblay. "Effect of Intensity of Physical Activity on Body Fatness and Fat Distribution." *The American Journal of Clinical Nutrition* 51, no. 2 (1990): 153–157.

Dawes, Jay and Brad Schoenfeld. "General Fitness Training." *Strength and Conditioning Journal* 31, no. 6 (2009): 44–46.

Dionne, Isabell, M. Johnson, Sylvie St-Pierre, Angelo Tremblay, and Matthew White. "Acute Effect of Exercise and Low-Fat Diet on Energy Balance in Heavy Men." *International Journal of Obesity and Related Metabolic Disorders* 21, no. 5 (1997): 413–416.

Ebbeling, Cara B., Henry A. Feldman, Erica Garcia-Lago, David L. Hachey, David S. Ludwig, Janis F. Swain, and William W. Wong. "Dietary Composition on Energy Expenditure During Weight-Loss Maintenance." *Journal of the American Medical Association* 307, no. 24 (2012): 2627–2634.

Fissinger, Jean A., Christopher L. Melby, and Darlene A. Sedlock. "Effect of Exercise Intensity and Duration on Postexercise Energy Expenditure." *Medicine and Science in Sports Exercise* 21, no. 6 (1989): 662–666.

Fogelholm, Mikael and K. Kukkonen-Harjula, K. "000. Physical Activity Prevent Weight Gain: A Systematic Review." *Obesity Reviews* 1, no. 2 (2000): 95–111.

Hamilton, E.J., D. M. Koceja, and W.C. Miller. "A Meta-Analysis of the Past 25 Years of Weight Loss Research Using Diet, Exercise, or Diet Plus Exercise Intervention." *International Journal of Obesity* 21, no. 10 (1997): 941–947.

Hirsch, Jules, Rudolph L. Leibel, and Michael Rosenbaum. "Energy Expenditure Resulting from Altered Body Weight." *New England Journal of Medicine* 332, no. 10 (1995): 621–628.

Jenkins, David G., and Paul Laursen. "The Scientific Basis for High-Intensity Interval Training: Optimising Training Programmes and Maximising Performance in Highly Trained Endurance Athletes." *Sports Medicine* 32, no. 1 (2002): 53–73.

McBride, Jeffery M., Richard P. Mikat, and Mark D. Schuenke. "Effect of an Acute Period of Resistance Exercise on Excess Post-Exercise Oxygen Consumption: Implications for Body Mass Management." *European Journal* of *Applied Physiology* 86, no. 5 (2002): 411–417.

Schoenfeld, Brad. "Does Cardio After an Overnight Fast Maximize Fat Loss?" *Strength and Conditioning Journal* 33, no. 1 (2011): 23–25.

Van Dusen, Allison. "Ten Ways to Get More From Your Workout." *Forbes*, October 20, 2008. <http://www.forbes.com/2008/10/20/exercise-workout-shorter-forbeslife-cx_avd_1020health_slide_5.html?thisSpeed=30000>

Acknowledgments

I owe an incredible gratitude to my client and friend Steve Harvey, thank you for all your support and help in bringing my message to the world. Without your support, Tiny and Full wouldn't be the worldwide phenomenon that it is today.

A big thank you to the amazing BenBella Books team: Adrienne Lang, Sarah Dombrowsky, Leah Wilson, Heather Butterfield, Monica Lowry, Jennifer Canzoneri, Rachel Phares, Alicia Kania—and, most especially, to Glenn Yeffeth, for supporting my vision of this project and helping me share it with the world. Thank you for all of your hard work and support, it means so much. Thank you to the Perseus team as well for helping get this book out: David Steinberger, Elena Chmilowski, Jessie Borkan, Andrea Gochnauer, Sabrina McCarthy, Heidi Sachner, Kim Highland, and Maha Khalil.

A very special thank you to my husband, Sam Cruise. Your support with this project has been incredible. Your insights are invaluable, thank you for all that you did to help me bring this book to life. And to my two sons, Parker and Owen, thank you for being such fun, loving boys. I love watching you grow up and I love being your dad.

I'd also like to thank my friends and supporters: Marjorie Harvey, Gerald Washington, Alex Duda, Meagan Dotson, Thabiti Stephens, Kevin Hurley, Megan Barry, Nelson Carvajal, Jessica Perillo, Terrence Noonan, Jeff Williams, Jay Blahnik, Julz Arney, Richard Galanti, Barrie Galanti, Pennie Clark Ianniciello, Ginnie Roeglin, Tim Talevich, Mary Ellen-Keathing, Edward Ash-Milby, Jon Foro, Sherman Griffin, John Redmann, Leslie Marcus, Lisa Gregorisch-Dempsey, Patty Serato, Carol Brooks, Maggie Jacqua, James Avenell, Christine Byun, Nicolette Gebhardt, Brandon Baiden, Talia Parkinson, Natalie Bubnis, Scott Eason, Lisa Wheeler, Amy Cohn, Marissa McCormick, Maha Tahiri, Patty Neger, Mario Lopez, Tim Sullivan, Dr. Mehmet Oz, Dr. David Katz, Dr. Andrew Weil, Dr. Christiane Northrup, President Bill Clinton, Senator Hillary Clinton, Amanda Molina, Jessica Marlow David Jackson, Jacqui Stafford, Amanda Shaytoya, Marissa Gold, Dory Larrabee-Zayas, Nicole Friday, Lacy Looney, Bob Wietrak, Denise Vivaldo, Jonathan Lizoette, Roger Koehler, Frank Rizzo, Jessica Scosta, Tory Jacob, Nicole Blinn.

About the Author

JORGE CRUISE is internationally recognized as a leading celebrity fitness trainer and is the #1 best-selling author of more than 20 books in 16 languages, with more than 8 million books in print. He is a contributor to *The Steve Harvey Show*, *The Dr. Oz Show*, *Extra TV*, *Good Morning America*, *The Today Show*, *The Rachael Ray Show*, Huffington Post, *First for Women* magazine, and the *Costco Connection*. He hosts his Facebook Live show Tiny Talks with more than 2 million monthly viewers.

Jorge received his bachelor's degree from the University of California, San Diego (UCSD), and his fitness credentials from the Cooper Institute for Aerobics Research, the American College of Sports Medicine (ACSM), and the American Council on Exercise (ACE).

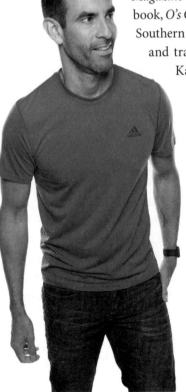

Jorge's career was launched on *The Oprah Winfrey Show* in November of 1998. From there, he was featured in *The Oprah Magazine* in the January 2005 issue and featured again in her book, *O's Guide to Life*. Jorge now trains his celebrity clients in Southern California and New York. He also recently trained and transformed lives on E!'s *Revenge Body* with Khloe Kardashian as one of Hollywood's top trainers.

Celebrities who have since followed Jorge's diet plans include Angelina Jolie, Jennifer Lopez, Lucy Liu, Kyle Richards, Eva Longoria, Countess Luann de Lesseps, and Steve Harvey.

Resource Section
Meet My Health Squad

Anti-Aging & Hormones

Dr. Darren Farnesi
Medical Age Management
(619) 795-6700

When I turned 42, suddenly my hormones changed, I lost all of my energy, and I felt old for the first time in my life. Luckily, I was introduced to Dr. Farnesi and he has helped me diagnose my thyroid condition and re-balance my hormones so that I feel like a kid again.

Dr. Farnesi and his team understand men and women's hormones better than anyone else in the industry. His passion and expertise is the reason he is my own personal doctor as well as the doctor to all of my celebrity clients when it comes to anti-aging medicine, hormones, and thyroid conditions.

If you are struggling with your weight loss goals and feel like your metabolism has slowed down and your hormones are imbalanced (including thyroid), I encourage you to reach out to Dr. Farnesi because he can really help you understand the body's aging process and help you live a better life.

www.manageyourage.com

Dermatology

Dr. Tess Mauricio
M Beauty Clinic
(858) 689-4990

When it comes to skin, no one has you covered quite like America's Favorite Dermatologist Dr. Tess Mauricio. Her passion for healthy beautiful skin has made her one of the world's most trusted dermatologists. Not only is she my dermatologist, she is the dermatologist to many A-listers in Hollywood and thousands of people across California.

Celebrities trust her because she is at the cutting edge in dermatology and has created a variety of services and products that address any skin issue. If you want to look younger, healthier, and more vibrant, Dr. Tess has you covered with her state-of-the-art treatments and care. From her Time Machine procedure to her Venus Legacy treatments, Dr. Tess is at the forefront of medical aesthetics by providing patients with non-invasive solutions to revitalize the skin.

If you are someone who is experiencing skin issues and would like to look your best, I encourage you to consult with Dr. Tess Mauricio because she can really provide you with a comprehensive plan to get your skin looking healthy and beautiful.

www.mbeautyclinic.com

Dentistry

Dr. Robert Schaeffer
Schaeffer Dental Excellence
(858) 481-1148

Achieving quality dental care shouldn't be difficult, that is why I recommend Dr. Schaeffer for making it simple to achieve your healthiest, most beautiful smile. Dr. Schaeffer and his staff are committed to your individual attention and they strive to provide personalized oral health care tailored for your unique dental needs and goals.

Not only is Dr. Schaeffer known for his high levels of accreditation, his commitment to our planet and sustainability makes him California's most respected green dentist. That is why I trust Dr. Schaeffer and his staff for myself and my family's oral health care.

If you are interested in receiving a consultation or investing in your oral health care, I highly recommend you go to Dr. Schaeffer and his staff for your dental needs. Whether it is reconstructive or just a cleaning, Dr. Schaeffer works with your best interest and the earth in mind.

www.schafferdental.com

Optometry

Dr. Michael Gordon
Gordon Schanzlin New Vision Institute
(858) 455-6800

The world is too beautiful a place to not see it clearly. Seven years ago, I met Dr. Gordon and he has changed the way I see the world, literally. He was able to put me at ease, explain things very clearly, and most importantly had a great sense of humor. Dr. Gordon and his staff have been helping myself and my family for several years with our eye health, but what really changed my life was undergoing LASIK surgery, which Dr. Gordon made a wonderful experience for me.

Dr. Gordon and his colleagues at the Gordon Schanzlin New Vision Institute offer an extensive variety of visual correction services for cosmetic and aging eyes. By utilizing the latest in world-class technologies, Dr. Gordon and his staff are capable of fully customizing your treatment plan for optimal results.

If you are someone who is considering vision correction, whether surgical or non-surgical, Dr. Gordon and his team at the Gordon Schanzlin New Vision Institute are truly the leading pioneers in this industry. I highly recommend consulting with Dr. Gordon for any eye health–related issues as he is at the forefront of the latest techniques and technologies in correcting vision.

www.gwsvision.com

Resource Section

Ready to Eat It Off?

Train with me one-on-one **LIVE** in my Tiny and Full club and lose 3x more weight!

- Discover my "Think Fit" affirmations that will ignite your motivation each morning.

- Never let your taste buds get bored using my "Eat Fit" secrets to customize your daily meal plan.

- Feel great with my "Move Fit" Hi-Lo Yoga™ routine that will target your belly fat and help boost your thyroid health.

- Plus: Each week get all-new Tiny and Full meal planners, recipes, and grocery shopping lists.

- Plus: Get access to my personal email for support and to ask any questions.

- Plus: Get access to my "Team Jorge" community where thousands of dedicated members are committed to living a life where fitness begins in the kitchen.

Join today for **FREE** for 7 days!

TinyandFull.com